Interacting with the Dead

Florida A&M University, Tallahassee
Florida Atlantic University, Boca Raton
Florida Gulf Coast University, Ft. Myers
Florida International University, Miami
Florida State University, Tallahassee
New College of Florida, Sarasota
University of Central Florida, Orlando
University of Florida, Gainesville
University of North Florida, Jacksonville
University of South Florida, Tampa
University of West Florida, Pensacola

Interacting with the Dead

Perspectives on Mortuary Archaeology
for the New Millennium

Edited by Gordon F. M. Rakita, Jane E. Buikstra, Lane A. Beck,
and Sloan R. Williams

University Press of Florida
Gainesville/Tallahassee/Tampa/Boca Raton
Pensacola/Orlando/Miami/Jacksonville/Ft. Myers/Sarasota

A record of cataloging-in-publication data is available from the Library of Congress.
ISBN 978-0-8130-2856-9 (cloth)
ISBN 978-0-8130-3317-4 (paper)

Chapter 9, "The Mortuary 'Laying-In' Crypts of the Hopewell Site: Beyond the Funerary
Paradigm," has been adapted from A. M. Byers' The Ohio Hopewell Episode and is printed
here with permission of The University of Akron Press © 2004 The University of Akron. All rights
reserved.

The University Press of Florida is the scholarly publishing agency for the State University System
of Florida, comprising Florida A&M University, Florida Atlantic University, Florida Gulf Coast
University, Florida International University, Florida State University, New College of Florida, Uni-
versity of Central Florida, University of Florida, University of North Florida, University of South
Florida, and University of West Florida.

University Press of Florida
15 Northwest 15th Street
Gainesville, FL 32611-2079
www.upf.com

Contents

Figures

Tables

I

Introduction

Gordon F. M. Rakita and Jane E. Buikstra

Mortuary rites and their materialization in the archaeological record have been of enduring interest to anthropologists since the beginning of the discipline (for example, Kroeber 1927; Bendann 1930; Gluckman 1937; see also Bartel 1982; Humphreys and King 1981; Huntington and Metcalf 1979). Indeed, since mortuary rites involve manipulations of material culture, social relations, cultural ideals, and the human body, they represent a nexus of anthropological interests. Within the closing decades of the twentieth century, mortuary studies became a highly visible focus of anthropological inquiry.

This volume represents the fourth in a series of edited volumes on the archaeology of mortuary behavior, published approximately every ten years since 1971. The first in the series, *Approaches to the Social Dimensions of Mortuary Practices* (Brown 1971a), marked renewed interest in mortuary analysis within archaeology as well as the development of influential new analytical techniques and theoretical frameworks, many of these drawn from general anthropological theory. Subsequent decades have seen the publication of *The Archaeology of Death* (Chapman et al. 1981) and *Regional Approaches to Mortuary Analysis* (Beck 1995), both having expanded the themes, techniques, and scale (both geographically and temporally) of mortuary analysis. Each of these important volumes was based upon papers presented at symposia or conferences. Similarly, this volume is based upon papers presented in two symposia organized by the editors for the Society for American Archaeology (SAA) Annual Meetings held in New Orleans in April of 2001.

Interacting with the Dead: Perspectives on Mortuary Archaeology for the New Millennium continues the tradition of earlier works by exploring the behavioral and social aspects of mortuary behavior in past societies. We expand the interdisciplinary focus of mortuary practices by examining and utilizing a variety of models and theories drawn from ethnohistory, bioarchaeology, and sociocultural anthropology. Subjects that have been of ongoing concern are combined with those that have recently emerged. Because of its wide-ranging scope and interdisciplinary approach, this monograph's relevance extends beyond anthropological archaeology to other social sciences and the humanities.

The first part of this introduction will contextualize this volume within a brief history of anthropological and archaeological works on explaining and understanding mortuary behavior. In doing so, we review the major paradigmatic shifts, key theoretical debates, and methodological advances. We finish with a discussion of the themes developed in this volume. We thus examine the role of the ancestors in the world of the living, the nature and meaning of secondary burials and secondary corpse treatments, and the methodological importance of considering historical, social, cultural, regional, and archaeological contexts in explorations of funerary remains.

Mortuary Studies in Historical Perspective

Modern anthropological approaches to mortuary behavior have emerged in reaction to early-twentieth-century critiques of the assumption that funerary rituals hold social meaning. Kroeber's (1927) classic cross-cultural study of funerary practices is among the earliest and most prominent of such criticism. Kroeber's impetus was his impression that patterns of the disposal of deceased members of native Californian societies seemed uncorrelated to other customs and practices. An examination of mortuary practices from culture areas in South America and Africa appeared to confirm his suspicion. Kroeber (1927:314) concluded, "In their relative isolation or detachment from the remainder of culture, their rather high degree of entry into consciousness, and their tendency to strong emotional toning, social practices of disposing of the dead are of a kind with fashions of dress, luxury, and etiquette. . . . It may be added that in so far as mortuary practices may be accepted as partaking of the nature of fashions, they will tend to discredit certain interpretations based upon them." Although a few anthropologists continued to contribute to the literature on funerary rites (for example, Bendann 1930; Gluckman 1937; Wilson 1939), Kroeber's work was widely cited and appears to have influenced a generation to approach social interpretations of funerary behavior cautiously. As recently as 1969, Ucko echoed this conclusion in his examination of the relevance of ethnographic material on funerary practices in the interpretation of archaeological remains.

However, in 1960, the English translation of Robert Hertz's "Contribution à Une Étude sur la Représentation Collective de la Mort" was published. Focused upon the meaning of extended mortuary rituals and secondary burial, Hertz's influential work was originally published in the *Année Sociologique* in 1907. As it was published in French, it had limited immediate impact upon English-speaking anthropologists, particularly in the Americas. The translation of Hertz's work, along with the simultaneous publication of the English translation of van Gennep's (1960 [1908]) *Les Rites de Passage,* stimulated a florescence of anthropological thought about the role and meaning of mortuary practices in traditional societies.

As part of renewed interest in death rites [or rituals] during the 1960s and

1970s, a number of ethnographic studies explored the nature of funerary practices. These include but are not limited to Forde's (1962) study of Yako mortuary rituals, the study of LoDagaa of West Africa by Goody (1962), Freedman's (1966) examination of Chinese lineages and ancestors, Douglass' (1969) study of Basque funerals, the detailed exploration of Merina mortuary customs by Bloch (1971), and Coffin's 1976 study of American funerary practices. Several of these works (Bloch's and Goody's, for example) explicitly addressed Hertz's earlier assertions concerning secondary burial.

It was within this milieu, though not based explicitly upon Hertz's work, that Arthur Saxe completed his dissertation at the University of Michigan. Saxe's 1970 work is perhaps the most frequently cited unpublished dissertation dealing with mortuary practices. Indeed, Morris (1991:147) noted, "Few doctoral dissertations win a wide readership; fewer still make a lasting mark on archaeological research. Arthur Saxe's *Social Dimensions of Mortuary Practices* (1970) did both." In his dissertation, Saxe attempted to develop a cross-cultural, nomothetic model of how mortuary practices were interrelated with the sociocultural system of the society. Indeed, he suggested that the model should provide a means for "monitor[ing] social complexity" and inferring organizational "type" (Saxe 1970:2). Saxe formulated eight hypotheses that he tested against ethnographic data from three societies (the Kapauku Papuans, the Ashanti, and the Bontoc Igorot). Most of Saxe's hypotheses dealt with ascertaining whether in certain situations the deceased's social persona or the complexity of the sociopolitical organization of the society are represented or symbolically manifest in the mortuary practices of the community. While criticism has been leveled at Saxe's approach (Hodder 1982c; Parker Pearson 1982; see also Brown 1995b:9–12), his dissertation clearly had a profound effect upon archaeological approaches to mortuary studies.

The combination of cross-cultural ethnographic study with formal hypothesis testing encouraged archaeologists to again seek social meaning in mortuary behavior. In addition, Saxe's Hypothesis 8, which linked the presence of formal disposal areas to territoriality, has stimulated further ethnographic and archaeological research by Saxe (Saxe and Gall 1977) and by others (Charles and Buikstra 1983; Goldstein 1980; Morris 1991). We discuss the intellectual extensions of this hypothesis in greater detail below.

In 1971, Memoir 25 of the Society for American Archaeology, edited by James Brown, was published. Brown's introduction acknowledged (1971a:2) the precedence of Saxe's work in regard to themes explored within the chapters of his volume. While Saxe contributed to the 1971 volume, the most widely cited chapters were those by Brown and Lewis Binford. Brown's chapter examined the mortuary practices from the Mississippian-period Spiro site. In analyzing the burial treatments at the site, Brown drew heavily from Saxe's approach. Specifically, he used the same formal analysis technique, a method sometimes referred to as key or paradigmatic diagramming. Brown noted, "A comparison of the burial paradigm [diagram] with the distribution of the most important and precious grave goods shows that there is a correspondence that supports the ranked status inferences drawn from the formal analysis alone" (Brown 1971b:101). While Brown himself did not generalize this inference, his conclusions were used to justify the assumption that the presence of rare or unique items in a burial denoted an individual of high rank or status (Peebles and Kus 1977; Tainter 1978).

Utilizing cross-cultural ethnographic surveys, Binford (1971) identified several behavioral regularities between the subsistence strategy of a society (as a proxy measure for social complexity) and the elaboration of that society's mortuary ritual. He interpreted his results as indicating that as societies move from hunter-gatherer or shifting agricultural strategies to settled agricultural lifeways, burial practices increase in complexity. The interpretative assumption behind this generalization, as with Saxe's work, was that as the number of social roles an individual held during life increased, so too would the number of symbolic representations of those roles. Additionally, it was expected that these symbols would be accurately and unambiguously reflected in mortuary treatments and grave accoutrements.

Binford (1971) also offered an extensive critique of Kroeber's (1927) seminal work on the interpretation of funerary practices. For Binford, this criticism is a crucial preamble to his demonstration that mortuary practices do indeed correlate with other cultural features, such as elevated social status (contra Kroeber). However, Kroeber's point was simply that specific funerary treatment forms (such as burial in trees, pit burials, burial in crypts) are not correlated with "biological or primary social necessities." Binford's argument is slightly different. He asserted that the number of distinctions displayed in funerary practices is correlated with social complexity through his surrogate measure, subsistence strategy. One example is Binford's assertion that "Status was most commonly symbolized by status-specific 'badges' of office and by the quantities of goods contributed to the grave furniture" (Binford 1971:23). Despite his somewhat flawed critique of Kroeber, Binford's observations were widely accepted as firmly establishing that funerary practices do indeed correlate with subsistence practices and by extension with sociopolitical complexity.

The conclusions by Brown and Binford are often summarized to justify the assumption that there is a direct relationship between the social status of the deceased and the relative amount of treatments, grave goods, or energy expended in the burial of the individual (Crown and Fish 1996; Hohmann 1982; Mitchell 1994; Shennan 1975; Tainter 1978; Whittlesey and Reid 2001). Thus, as the complexity of a society increases, so too should the complexity of the burial remains. Frequently, this perspective is simplified even further. Some researchers simply assume that there often is "a direct correlation between higher rank/status of the deceased . . . and the amount of energy invested in grave and body treatment" (Hohmann 2001:99) or that "mortuary practices are a mirror of social organization and the social roles that individuals held in ancient society"

(Whittlesey and Reid 2001). This processual perspective, often referred to as the "Saxe-Binford approach" (Brown 1995b), still represents the dominant interpretive framework for mortuary data throughout much of Americanist archaeology (for example, see chapters in Mitchell and Brunson-Hadley 2001).

The late 1970s and early 1980s witnessed continued visibility for ethnographic studies of mortuary practices, including Huntington and Metcalf's seminal 1979 work. This monograph, reissued as a second edition in 1991, drew inspiration from the fieldwork locations of the authors, Madagascar and Borneo, and the classic theoretical approaches to mortuary practices that had been presented for these locales by van Gennep and Hertz. By emphasizing these world areas and these predecessors, the work naturally focuses upon extended funerary practices and the treatment of the corpse. Humphreys and King 1981, Ariès 1974 and 1981, and Bloch and Parry 1982 are other widely cited monographs from this period. The works by Ariès (1974, 1981) explored the cyclical nature of human social response to the biological fact of death in recent European history. These responses oscillated over time between a metaphorical denial of death and an embracing of death that is tamed. Much like Hertz's secondary mortuary rites model and van Gennep's rites of passage schema, Ariès' approach is intuitively convincing as a descriptive heuristic but deficient in explanatory substance (see also Meskell 2001). Humphreys and King (1981) sought to begin a meaningful conversation between archaeologists, physical anthropologists, and social anthropologists—contrasting the perspectives inherent within each of these subdisciplines as well as cross-cultural comparisons of mortuary rites. Although this book was largely unsuccessful in stimulating subsequent conversations regarding death practices between practitioners from the anthropological subdisciplines, it did demonstrate the utility of cross-cultural, comparative perspectives. The volume assembled by Bloch and Parry (1982) focused upon a perennial anthropological topic—the relationship between death and fertility. Contributors explored facets of revitalization and regeneration among various societies, including those at different levels of sociopolitical complexity. It thus provided a series of new ethnographic case studies for archaeological theorists. Moreover, in their introduction, Bloch and Parry provide a critical overview of key anthropological studies of mortuary practices, including Hertz's seminal work. Such ethnographic or ethnohistoric volumes were complemented by publications within archaeology, particularly studies of prehistoric burial practices in the North American midcontinent (Braun 1977; Brown 1979; Chapman 1977; Tainter 1975a, 1975b) and later from the desert Southwest (Brunson 1989; Hohmann 1982; Ravesloot 1988). Many of these were quantitatively complex and drew inspiration from the Saxe-Binford theoretical perspective.

Two publications in the early 1980s have proved to be enormously influential among students of funerary archaeology. In 1980, Goldstein published a study of two Mississippian-period cemeteries from the lower Illinois River valley. Her study focused upon the spatial dimension of mortuary practices, including a critical reexamination of Saxe's Hypothesis 8. On the basis of her evaluation of globally representative ethnographic data, Goldstein found the relationship between bounded cemeteries to be more nuanced than Saxe had appreciated. She rephrased Hypothesis 8, concluding that "not all corporate groups that control critical resources through lineal descent will maintain formal, exclusive disposal areas for their dead. . . . But if a formal, bounded disposal area exists and if it is used *exclusively* for the dead, [then] the society is very likely to have corporate groups organized by lineal descent" (Goldstein 1980:8). The relationship between bounded cemeteries and resource control was later extended to hunter-foragers (Charles and Buikstra 1983). As we discuss below, more recently Morris (1991) has reaffirmed the ongoing utility of Goldstein's reformulation.

In the sequence leading to this volume, the second influential publication on archaeological approaches to mortuary data was Chapman, Kinnes, and Randsborg 1981. This volume, which included authors from Europe and the United States, focused on "the evolution and critical appraisal of the ideas presented in 1971, as well as the subsequent emergence of new approaches." The influence of the Saxe-Binford approach is apparent in chapters by Goldstein and O'Shea, as well as in the introduction to the volume by Chapman and Randsborg. Chapman's chapter on megalithic tombs in Europe provided new perspective on the meaning of formal disposal areas in prehistoric populations and reinforced the conclusions Goldstein had reached a year earlier. James Brown contributed an important chapter in which he reemphasized the need to consider the full sequence of the rites leading to archaeological residue of funerary practices. That is, the resulting burial is a part, but often only a part, of the full ritual process. Among the newer approaches was Goldstein's chapter on spatial organization. Buikstra and Cook each contributed chapters that illustrated the potential benefits of integrating biological data from the skeletal remains with the material remains of the burial rites.

Critiques of the Saxe-Binford approach were, however, soon to develop. In 1981, for example, Braun developed a nuanced and pointed dissection of the quantitative approaches used by processual researchers, particularly Tainter (1975a, 1975b, 1977a, 1977b). Braun's compelling argument (see also McHugh 1999:8–11) demonstrated that such quantification failed to support Tainter's interpretative model, in part because quantitative ranking of various mortuary treatments was subjective or presented with no explanation for why one treatment ranked higher than another (Braun 1981:407). For example, Braun (1981:402–403) pointed out numerous cases in which classes of objects found in burials were assigned a ranking in terms of energy expenditure relative to other artifact classes that were based upon faulty interpretations of their region of production or origin (local versus imported). A further limitation in such quantification is the difficulty of accounting for nonquantifiable aspects of mortuary behavior, such as variation in the spatial location of burials (McHugh 1999:11).

On the other side of the Atlantic, criticism of the Saxe-Binford approach developed within the symbolic, structuralist, and interpretive theoretical backlash against processual archaeological theory (Hodder 1980, 1982a, 1982b, 1991; McGuire 1988; Miller and Tilley 1984; Parker Pearson 1982; Shanks and Tilley 1982; Tilley 1984). We use the term "postprocessual" here to refer to the multiple theoretical approaches that developed in the wake of processualism. All of these approaches have their own nuanced theoretical arguments. They are united, however, in their indictment of processual thought and their assertion that mortuary rituals are frequently utilized by the living to negotiate, display, mask, or transform actual power or social relations. They further argue that the processual perspective glosses over significant variation that exists in the perception and practice of mortuary rites within a given society. Indeed, they argue that mortuary rites are often an arena in which status and other social distinctions can be negotiated, appropriated, and reappropriated, thus serving as agents of cultural change. Additionally, these scholars asserted that the processual focus upon the identification of vertical social structure obscured or neglected alternative aspects of society (horizontal divisions, for example; see also Whittlesey 1978). Ethnographic (Parker Pearson 1982; Ucko 1969) and archaeological examples (Hodder 1984; McGuire 1992) lent support to these criticisms and led to arguments that cross-cultural generalizations are not appropriate for archaeological contexts; rather, social structure could be inferred only in the context of specific (and historical) cultural traditions. Unfortunately, apt critiques (for example, Parker Pearson 1982; Shanks and Tilley 1982) were seldom linked to convincing archaeological case studies, except in historical contexts.

In an elaboration of ideas first expressed in Parker Pearson's (1982) ethnographic study, Cannon (1989) suggested that while mortuary elaboration is frequently seen as an unbiased indicator of the deceased's social status, a society's mortuary displays are cultural phenomena that are frequently unassociated with social and economic organization. Consequently, the traditional status-based interpretation of mortuary material neglects the historical nature of status symbols and cycles of competitive display. Cannon refined his thesis by suggesting that these cycles often assume a predictable pattern whereby funerary elaboration by elites is followed by adoption (or cooption) of elite symbols by lower-status groups. In response, elites abandon elaborate forms to retain a distinctive funerary symbol set. In his widely cited article, Cannon (1989) provided three examples of this cycle drawn from eighteenth- through twentieth-century England, historic Iroquois groups, and pre-Classic Greece. Cannon also echoes the postprocessual critique's context-specific emphasis (see also Miller 1982).

At the beginning of the last decade of the twentieth century, two scholarly themes regarding mortuary practices developed. The first represented continuing attempts to utilize, support, extend, and respond to criticisms of the Saxe-Binford approach. Examples of attempts to support the Saxe-Binford approach are by Carr (1995) and Kamp (1998), both of whom reassess the cross-cultural evidence lending support to the original nomothetic generalizations of Binford (1971),

Saxe (1970), and others (Peebles and Kus 1977; Tainter 1978). In part, these studies have been successful in underscoring the robusticity of certain generalizations and to a lesser degree in providing a more nuanced interpretation of those generalizations in the same way Goldstein's (1980) work refined Saxe's Hypothesis 8.

Morris (1991) also built upon Goldstein's contributions (1980) and sought to refine Hypothesis 8. Morris focused upon the original anthropological distinction (based on African ethnographies) between funerary rites per se and ancestor cults or rituals relating to continued interactions between the living and the dead. By examining this fundamental distinction, Morris was able to provide a theoretical foundation for Goldstein's reworking of Hypothesis 8.

This late-twentieth-century revision and revitalization of the Saxe-Binford program was capped by the publication of Beck's (1995) edited volume entitled *Regional Approaches to Mortuary Analysis*. The objective of this volume was to extend the geographic scope of studies beyond the examination of intrasite variability in mortuary practices. However, by expanding the geographic focus of such studies, the volume also opened the door to greater emphasis on diachronic variability.

A second theme has emerged from the critical tradition of the postprocessualists. In part, these works have continued to criticize the use of cross-cultural generalizations in mortuary analysis (for example, Parker Pearson 1993). However, these approaches have moved beyond the constraining critiques of the 1980s and have begun to provide relevant and convincing archaeological case studies of their own (for example, Cannon 1995; Curet and Oliver 1998; Hill 1998; McGuire 1992; Parker Pearson 1995; and see Chesson 2001; Silverman and Small 2002). Many of these studies have embraced the idea that the deceased and their death are opportunities for the active manipulation of social, political, ethnic, and material structures. Other researchers have worked to engender studies of the funerary practices of past societies (Crown and Fish 1996; Meskell 2001). Additional productive research venues have included increasingly comprehensive analyses of mortuary ceremonialism in historic archaeological contexts, often using techniques and methods developed within bioarchaeology (Buikstra 2000; Dockall et al. 1996; Grauer 1995; Saunders and Herring 1995; Rainville 1999). Finally, landscape archaeology has moved from a preoccupation with "sacred landscapes," dotted with shrines and monuments to the dead, to a more inclusive and informed broad definition of an imbued landscape that recognizes a deeper meaning to the placement of ancestors (Ashmore and Knapp 1999; Silverman and Small 2002).

An outgrowth of this second theme is a renewed interest, at the end of the past millennium and in these first few years of the new, in the role of the ancestors and the dead in structuring the lives of the living (Buikstra 1995; Curet and Oliver 1998; Helms 1998; Hingley 1996; Parker Pearson 1999; Parker Pearson and Ramilisonina 1998; Rakita 2001). Complementary concerns have, however,

been expressed about the overreliance upon explanations referencing ritual interactions with the ancestors in models of social or cultural change (Bawden 2000;
Potts 2002; Whitley 2002). However, the ancestral-descendant approach remains a robust endeavor, and in many respects this volume draws not only on
these recent works, but also on their theoretical foundations (Morris 1991;
Goldstein 1980; Saxe 1970; Gluckman 1937; Kroeber 1927; van Gennep 1960
[1908]; and Hertz 1960 [1907]). In many ways, these *ancestral* works are structuring the research lives of today's living scholars.

Themes in This Volume

This volume represents a continuation of earlier traditions by exploring the behavioral and social facets of funerary rites in both past and present societies.
These authors expand earlier methodological and theoretical frameworks, drawing inspiration from ethnohistory, ethnography, bioarchaeology, and sociocultural anthropology. In so doing they focus on the overarching themes of variability through time and space, extended and secondary mortuary ceremonialism,
individual agency, and ancestorhood.

The chapters in section one present explorations and extensions of the classi-
cal theoretical developments discussed above. The various authors delve deeply
into the assumptions and expectations of mortuary theories and discuss these in
relation to empirical examples. Charles, for example, reemphasizes the contextualized nature of both mortuary practices and our inferences from the funerary
record. Chapman focuses upon the connection between theory and the empirical
record especially as that connection relates to diachronic analytical approaches.
Cannon is concerned with elucidating how cyclical patterns of funerary "fashion" may be indicative of women's agency. Buikstra and colleagues present their
work with prehistoric Andean mortuary patterns as an example of how an integrated bioarchaeological perspective can enrich an examination of funerary behavior. The final chapter in this section, by Ashmore and Geller, draws on the
comparatively new interest in landscapes and the examination of how the placement of the dead affects the lives of the living.

Section two groups together eight chapters that explore the physical treatment
of the corpse and possible symbolic meaning behind both that treatment and
other postmortem conditions of the body. Rakita and Buikstra, in the first chapter of this section, reexamine Robert Hertz's original formulation and suggest
that an alternative view of mummification and cremation offers a more comprehensive understanding of these treatments. Oakdale presents an ethnographic
perspective on the Hertz–van Gennep sequence, one that should be quite illumi-
nating to those researchers who focus only upon the physical remnants of funerary activities. In his chapter on Ohio Hopewell extended funerary practices,
Byers provides a detailed reminder of James Brown's original warning that recovered funerary features do not necessarily represent the end of the entire mortuary

process. Guillén takes Charles' admonition to heart and provides a rich and contextualized discussion of the Chinchorro mummification practices of Peru and Chile. In a reanalysis of Hohokam cremations, Beck utilizes ethnographic data to infer that some of the recovered cremation features may represent reburning of previously cremated remains. Two chapters, by Weiss-Krejci and Naji, examine historic funerary practices from European contexts. Weiss-Krejci looks at how postmortem treatment of Babenberg and Habsburg dynastic members relate not to ancestor cults but rather to political, economic, or biological constraints. Naji considers diachronic change in interment practices at the abbey of Saint-Jean-des-Vignes near Soissons, France. In the final chapter of this section, Malville describes traditional Tibetan Buddhist practices of exposure or cremation of corpses and how these treatments might appear in the archaeological record.

Section three of the volume contains chapters that expand upon the issues raised in section two, especially as they relate to human sacrifice, cannibalism, violence, and veneration of the dead. The section begins with a chapter in which Duncan, using a theoretical model derived from Maurice Bloch, examines violence against and violation of the corpse as part of Mayan ritual sequences. Stodder describes a possible case of cannibalism from New Guinea, utilizing taphonomic and contextualized depositional information to suggest possible alternative interpretations of the evidence. In two studies from South America, chapters by Verano and Forgey and Williams present discussions of prominent Andean cases of body mutilation in the human sacrifices of the Moche and Nasca trophy heads. Verano combines both archaeological and osteological data to describe how sacrificial displays may have impacted the construction and maintenance of Moche society. Forgey and Williams analyze the formal and contextual variation in Nasca trophy skulls to evaluate current competing theories for the origin and purposes of these ritually charged items. In their chapter on the Cenote at the Mayan site of Chichén Itzá, Beck and Sievert explore the various pathways and processes by which the skeletons of both adults and children were deposited in this specialized location. The final chapter of this section and the volume is by McNeill, who scrutinizes the funerary practices of the Chamorro of Micronesia with special emphasis on the postmortem procurement of human bone for use in manufacturing spear points.

Thus, this volume builds upon earlier theories and methods, refining some and critiquing others. The complexity of interment and other mortuary procedures is emphasized, as is the importance of social, political, and economic contexts in the interpretation of ancient sites. By drawing on interdisciplinary methods and knowledge in ethnohistory, bioarchaeology, and sociocultural anthropology, the various authors in this volume are able to elucidate issues regarding mortuary practices across the globe and through time. Subjects, such as sacrifice and secondary interment, that have been of perennial interest are reexamined, and newly emerging research interests are explored.

As emphasized at the outset, this volume is not the first attempt at addressing the various issues involving human interactions with the dead. Nor is it likely to be the last. It represents, however, an important illustration of a maturing field that has deep roots within anthropological inquiry into the relationship between the living and the dead.

1

Theories, Time, and Space

Gordon F. M. Rakita and Jane E. Buikstra

The chapters in this section deal with several concepts that have been perennial issues in mortuary studies over recent decades: time, space, and the impact of different theoretical and methodological approaches. For example, Charles discusses the relevance of contextual and historical analysis in assessing the meaning of variable mortuary remains in light of contrasting theoretical perspectives. He uses funerary practices from the Archaic and Woodland periods of the lower Illinois valley as illustrative examples of various levels of inference and meaning based upon burial location on landscape, cemetery structure, and specific grave contexts. Charles argues for nuanced contextual analyses of funerary remains and careful scrutiny of the assumptions made in many recent studies of mortuary behavior. Influenced by the postprocessual critique, he also underscores the important point that the place where dead are buried and indeed the information available from the grave itself are not only about mortuary behavior. His study also emphasizes that examinations of mortuary behavior at only one temporal scale can frequently be incomplete or misleading.

Equally self-reflexive in his analysis, Chapman examines the relationship between theory and empirical evidence, paralleling Charles' focus upon time and diachronic analyses. He notes that in many cases both geographic and spatial units seem to be uncritically accepted by researchers. By unpacking the assumptions inherent in these analytical units, Chapman explores the relationship between different theoretical perspectives and how they variously influence methodological practices and units of analysis. Chapman uses examples reflecting 30 years of mortuary analysis in European archaeology: Shennan's study at Branc (Slovakia), Sofaer Derevenski's study of the Copper Age cemetery at Tiszapolgár-Basatanya in Hungary, and early Bronze Age Argaric (Spain) cemeteries. He argues compellingly that focusing on diachronic change across archaeological cultures is potentially an exceedingly productive venue but that this goal requires renewed emphasis on temporal control over empirical data sets.

Cannon extends his earlier (1989) focus upon diachronic change and mortuary "fashions" to cyclical fashion trends and personal agency. He defines agency as "the socioculturally mediated, but individually motivated capacity to act purposefully in such a way as to create archaeologically discernable change in prevailing modes of mortuary practice." Cannon's study examines the role of women, or more appropriately widows, in cycles of ostentation and simplification in funerary practices using data from the seventeenth-century Seneca, fifth- to seventh-century Anglo-Saxon England, Victorian England, and Early Bronze Age Denmark and Central Europe. As with his earlier work, Cannon illustrates the necessity of a fine-grained perspective and rich databases in assessing the forces behind changing mortuary practices.

Buikstra and colleagues present a case study illustrating the significance of an integrated bioarchaeological approach to mortuary site research. They consider information gathered from mortuary analyses and skeletal biology to evaluate the economic and political development of a prehistoric Andean society. Specifically, the authors focus on the Chiribaya polity, formerly thought to be a coastal cultural development following Tiwanaku influence in the south central Andes. New chronometric dates clearly illustrate contemporaneity with this complex Altiplano society and suggest a more complex history for both Chiribaya and Tiwanaku. The authors use artifact distributions, artificial cranial deformation, and isotopic evidence of diet to explore this complexity.

Finally, the chapter by Ashmore and Geller highlights another prominent theme of this volume, namely the spatial dimension of mortuary behavior. Ashmore and Geller argue persuasively that spatial ordering in mortuary remains— the location and placement of burials—can be a valuable tool in the interpretation of prehistoric ideology and cosmology. Using data from a variety of Mayan contexts, the authors examine the location within sites or burial facilities as well as the internal orientation within these facilities. The study demonstrates how spatial patterning of the dead can be used to reconstruct the worldview of the living.

2

The Archaeology of Death as Anthropology

Douglas K. Charles

In general, archaeological mortuary studies, whether seeking processual explanations or contextual understandings, suffer from an assumption that there is a universal link between our chosen analytical procedure—that is, our method and theory—and death: the relative energy expenditure of mortuary ritual is a direct reflection of social organization; formal disposal areas for the dead will reflect the affirmation of corporate group rights over crucial but restricted resources; mortuary ritual is a hegemonic practice that serves to reproduce society and maintain relations of dominance; funerary practices comprise thought and action, forming an inextricable duality that must be understood in terms of people's beliefs and agency rather than simply rationalized in some etic sense. What these assertions share, despite frequent lip service to the contrary, is the assumptive and prescriptive "is." Substitute the possibility of "can," and we approach the archaeology of death in a more realistic and liberating manner.

Lewis Binford trumpeted the birth of the New Archaeology in 1962 with "Archaeology as Anthropology." By 1983, Ian Hodder was arguing for a newer archaeology with, for example, *The Present Past: An Introduction to Anthropology for Archaeologists*. We should take this recurring concern with anthropology very seriously, by confronting and engaging the complexity of human behavior—theirs and ours—in its entirety. Admittedly, many of the contributors to the precursors to this volume (that is, the various authors in Brown 1971a, Chapman et al. 1981, and Beck 1995) would consider theirs an anthropological approach, but overall the theoretical vein encompassed by these collections could be characterized as "processual" and is therefore somewhat limited (compare, for example, Parker Pearson 1999). This polarity represented by the processual and postprocessual approaches to archaeology, and embedded in the above examples as well, also runs through anthropology: emic/etic; ethnography/ethnology; culture/biology; agency/structure; Department of Cultural and Social Anthropology/Department of Anthropological Sciences. A truly anthropological approach embraces this diversity as different approaches to understanding human life, sometimes complementary, sometimes alternative. To the extent that we wish to make these polarities competing approaches, we must acknowledge that this wish is driven by our own personal or political agendas, be they explicit or implicit, acknowledged or disavowed. These differences in anthropological approach reflect at least in part the nature of the behavior that we are trying to understand. Human behavior is varied and inconsistent, it is not necessarily based on universals, and it does not neatly fit within our analytical categories. This chapter will examine one such category, "the archaeology of death."

Mortuary Archaeology as an Approach to Anthropology

There is no inherent reason to believe that the archaeological evidence of mortuary practices is telling us only about the activities surrounding death. As an obvious example, trace element analyses of skeletal material informs us about the diet of the living, which may be completely unrelated to the manner of death of an individual or his or her treatment after death. Likewise, there is no a priori basis on which to assume that all the activities that took place in a particular location are directly related to funerary ritual. Westminster Abbey contains the remains of British monarchs, Isaac Newton, Charles Darwin, and others, but it was not specifically constructed as a monument to the dead. Death is an easy category for archaeology, a conjunction of actual individuals and specific cultural practices, conveniently buried or entombed, thereby increasing the probability of preservation and recovery. But the clues from these assemblages are best "read" by Sherlock Holmes—not through the monolithic and presentist projections of a processualist, a postprocessualist, a selectionist, or a Marxist. The challenge is to see what is (and was) there.

Our attempts to comprehend the past must negotiate myriad intersecting webs of interpretive dimensions. A central dimension is the very disciplinary structure of contemporary academia. At the institution where I teach, the intellectual framework through which we understand our creation myth (that is, the history of *Homo sapiens*) is spread across the campus in an orderly manner. The method and theory through which we model the transition from a quadrupedal hominoid to a bipedal hominid are housed in the Departments of Biology and Earth and Environmental Sciences, which in turn are ensconced in Division III. This division, the natural sciences and mathematics, is physically located at the south end of campus. As we follow along in our creation story, however, the ability of the biological model to illuminate the nature of the plot development decreases. A hunter-gatherer subsistence regime is obviously biological in nature, involving humans interacting with plants and animals, but its effects on human life are economic, social, and political. As the story progresses through the development of domestication and the rise of states and capitalism, the nonbiological factors increase in prominence, and our ability to conceptualize and comprehend them requires the intellectual tools found in the Departments of Economics, Sociology, and Government. Further, the actual study of change per se becomes the domain of history. These disciplines, which fall within Division II, the social and behavioral sciences, are housed in the middle of campus. Beginning with the Upper Paleolithic and the appearance of figurines and cave art, and moving through the inventions of writing, printing, radio, television, and film, additional frameworks become necessary in order to comprehend ourselves. At Wesleyan, the Departments of Art and Art History, English, Romance Languages, Film Studies are grouped as Division I, the arts and humanities, and are clustered on the north end of campus. Finally, the arts and humanities are divided along an east-west axis, with the language-oriented humanities on one side of a north-south street, the nonverbal arts on the other. Thus, at one level, to tell the story of human evolution requires a figurative walk from one end of campus to the other, with a tacking back and forth at the end.

To focus on a particular point in time is not, however, to pause in our perambulation: exploring the Neolithic in Europe, for example, involves running back and forth from one end of the campus to the other, darting in and out of various buildings along the way, as we investigate the physical and chemical properties of ceramics, the coevolutionary process of domestication, the rise of complex polities, and the meaning of Stonehenge. Likewise, the study of a particular phenomenon necessitates engagement with the different disciplines: a thorough investigation of mortuary sites, for instance, can involve the study of soil formation and taphonomic processes, the biology of the skeletons, aspects of social organization and process, and consideration of meaning and symbolism.

Another interpretive dimension is represented, for example, by Braudel's notion that "different historical processes operate at different temporal rhythms or levels" (Smith 1992:25), most famously the tripartite framework of structure, conjuncture, and event, corresponding to the decreasing time frames of the climatic, the economic, and the political (Braudel 1972). As Philip Duke (1991:32; but see also Hodder 1987; Knapp 1992) has noted, the value of Braudel's approach for archaeologists resides in

1. the notion that the historical record is made up of different phenomena, each one of a different time length and with different impacts on human behavior;

2. the development of a model of structure-event as a basis for organizing and understanding the past; and

3. the notion that some of these long-term structures are governed by processes entirely different from those that create the historical and political patterns recognized by culture-history.

Analysis of processes at only one temporal scale can be incomplete. Processes at different levels can interact such that the effects of one are dependent upon the effects of the others. For example, Cobb (1991) relates the successively more elaborate exchange cycles and social organizations associated with the Late Archaic, Hopewell, and Mississippian periods in the American Midwest (at the level of conjuncture in Braudel's terms) to the long-term process of subsistence intensification (at the level of structure [*longue durée*]). Sahlins (1981, 1985) understands, on the one hand, the event of Captain Cook's ill-fated visit to the Hawaiian Islands in terms of the intersection of the conjunctures of two different cultures (that is, traditions, conceptual frameworks, structures of meaning), and on the other, the subsequent transformation of the Hawaiian cultural conjuncture in terms of the event of Captain Cook.

To return to the subject of this volume and the focus of the remainder of this chapter, consider a third interpretive dimension involving the increasingly problematic levels of archaeological inference that must be traversed when approaching mortuary practices:

> Where the dead were ultimately placed, and where at least some of the activities following their deaths occurred, can be addressed in fairly straightforward ways. In the lower Illinois River valley alone, hundreds of Middle and Late Woodland burial mounds have been surveyed and recorded (e.g., Charles 1992). Dozens of mounds have been excavated and reported (e.g., Perino 1968, 1973), and hundreds of skeletons of the dead themselves have been analyzed (e.g., Buikstra 1976). Many bodies were "processed" in centrally located log crypts or other facilities, the partially or fully defleshed remains then moved to peripheral graves (Brown 1979), or even to other sites (Charles et al. 1988).
>
> When a corpse, crypt, or mound was seen or acknowledged, by whom, and under what circumstances are more difficult questions and our interpretations are more provisional. The majority of interments in Middle and Late Archaic cemeteries in the Illinois valley occurred shortly after death, whereas in upland areas away from the main valley the predominance of secondary burials indicates that populations in those regions curated bodies for longer periods of time, and *could have* incorporated them into extended funerary ritual (Charles and Buikstra 1983). From differences in size and form of Ohio Hopewell charnel structures vs. Illinois Hopewell burial crypts we *infer* differences in the numbers of people that could have viewed a corpse at any one time, and in how principles of inclusion and exclusion could have been played out (Brown 1979). In either region the monumentality of the mounds would *presumably* have made them important features of the daily landscape. The orderliness of rows of graves in Mississippian cemeteries *suggests* that individual graves were marked and maintained (Goldstein 1980).
>
> How, when and under what circumstances the dead, individually or collectively, were referenced [that is, the *meaning* of the dead] constitute the

most opaque problems for an archaeology of death. (Charles and Buikstra 2002:13–15)

Aspects of the meaning of the dead for people living during Archaic (ca. 6000–3000 B.P.), Woodland (ca. 3000–1200 B.P.) and Mississippian (ca. 1200–600 B.P.) periods in the American Midwest, in terms of the form and location within the mortuary landscape, have been explored elsewhere (Buikstra and Charles 1999; Charles and Buikstra 2002). A mortuary site is not, however, just a repository for the dead or for information about the dead—it is a window with a much wider view of their world. Furthermore, our understanding of mortuary sites is not solely the recipient of this wider perspective. Looking for the broader view helps create the interpretative context, opening up our anthropological perspective. What follows is an example of the questioning process one might follow in approaching a mortuary site. Decades worth of research in this region has produced contextual information that readily suggests possible answers to some questions but not to others. Questions without answers point toward directions for future research. Indeed, the point is that asking questions of a cemetery can direct us toward avenues of broader anthropological import.

Seeing through Mortuary Practices

Consider, as an example, Mound 7 Burial 9 from the Middle Woodland (c. 1950 B.P.) Elizabeth site in west-central Illinois (Charles et al. 1988:262, Figures 5.22, 5.33, 5.35–5.38). The burial consists of a woman over 50 years of age, plus two infants under a year old. Knowledge relating to aspects of their burial has been systematically collected over the years, but it is only by starting with the burial and working "outward" that the full context and meaning of their interment begins to become apparent, for their contemporaries and for us.

As its designation implies, the cemetery is an earthen mound, one of several located on a ridge on the bluff margin overlooking the Illinois River valley. What does this bluff-top location *mean*? Bluff margins represent one of the two predominant Middle Woodland burial loci in the region, the other being mound sites built on ridges or terraces in the floodplains of the Illinois and Mississippi rivers. This pattern appears to have emerged more than three millennia before, by the end of the Middle Archaic, in a context of fluctuating, but overall decreasing, levels of mobility (Buikstra and Charles 1999; Charles and Buikstra 1983, 2002; Charles 1995). Archaic communities seem to have utilized bluff edge ridges during periods of decreased mobility, presumably to symbolize relationships to specific resource areas. The floodplain sites, conversely, appear to have been periodic multicommunity gathering spots, used during periods of increased mobility, where a number of activities, including burial of the dead, took place. By Middle Woodland times, these locations had become the traditional sites for funerary activity, seemingly within the same symbolic framework. Apparently, the Middle Woodland bluff-top mounds were community cemeteries, while the floodplain mound sites were multicommunity social, ceremonial, and political sites, as they had been during the Archaic. This framework does not, however, accurately describe the context and nature of Mound 7 at the Elizabeth site. The demographic structure of the interments, the diversity of grave goods, and the internal complexity of the mounds at Elizabeth are atypical of bluff-top mound sites. Rather, Elizabeth is probably part of a site complex including the Napoleon Hollow occupation site and the Naples-Russell mound group. Napoleon Hollow is not a base camp, showing instead a number of similarities to floodplain sites like Peisker, considered to be what has been termed a mortuary camp (Struever 1968; Wiant and McGimsey 1986), although this may be an insufficient and even inaccurate characterization. Naples-Russell Mound 8 is a huge loaf-shaped mound of the form otherwise seen at the floodplain mound sites (Charles 1992). This site complex dates to very early in the Middle Woodland sequence in the lower Illinois valley, and it may be that the Archaic spatial distinction between the bluff-top and floodplain sites had not fully reemerged under the new demographic realities, following an Early Woodland hiatus (see below).

The specific form of the cemetery—a log-walled central crypt surrounded by an earthen embankment or ramp—first appeared with the arrival of Middle Woodland populations into the lower Illinois River valley. What does a mound *mean*? The key to understanding this cemetery form may lie in the material used in the construction of the ramp. Recent work at Mound House and other sites has revealed that the characteristic soils, referred to in the literature as "basket-loading," are, in the majority of instances, pieces of sod (Van Nest et al. 2001). The use of sod may relate to the widespread Native American mythology of the Earth Diver, in which dry land was created from a piece of sod or mud brought up by one animal or another from below the water that covered the earth (Hall 1997). The sod may also be relevant to world renewal ceremonies (Hall 1997). It can be further argued (Buikstra et al. 1998; Buikstra and Charles 1999) that the components that comprise the structure of the crypt and ramp complex of a Middle Woodland mound represent a cosmogram of the universe as often represented by Southeastern tribes (Hudson 1976). The clearing of the site for mound construction exposed the damp, dark soils of the Under World, with the Upper World of the sky above. Upon the Under World was spread a circular layer of sand or silt, representing This World. The central crypt was constructed at the center of This World, usually with excavation of the floor of the crypt into the Under World with the log walls of the crypt extending into the Upper World. The crypt was then surrounded by a sod ramp, representing the dry land. Thus, the construction of the mound was potentially a reenactment of the creation of the world. Following death, a corpse would have been carried across the surface of, and placed in the center of, This World. As the body decomposed in the crypt, the "wet" flesh would disappear into the Under World, completing the cycle of life. The remaining "dry" bones would be gathered up and placed in a small pit in the edge of the ramp, that is, buried in the "earth."

Why was this symbolism invoked in this manner only during the Middle Woodland period (if, indeed, the sod and so forth do relate to the Earth Diver and renewal ceremonies)? And why was this behavior so marked in the lower Illinois valley and other places but not in other regions? Ironically, a possible insight into these questions has come in part from aspects of Woodland mortuary behavior of which the participants themselves were not necessarily aware. Because Middle Woodland communities conspicuously interred virtually all of their dead in these mounds (Buikstra 1976) in a region where living sites would come to be buried, plowed, or forested, and thus archaeologically less visible or distinct, we are able to trace changing population distributions through time via mound numbers and locations (Charles 1992). In general, the Middle Woodland period appears to have been one of population aggregation, as increasingly horticulturally oriented communities moved to the major river valleys of the Midwest, where conditions for this form of subsistence would have been optimal (Braun 1987). This movement produced the first wave of the riverine concentration of mounds demonstrably documented by Cyrus Thomas (1894). The material manifestations of what we term the Hopewell Interaction Sphere coalesced at this time. The lower Illinois valley was apparently virtually uninhabited by the end of the Early Woodland period (Charles et al. 1986; Farnsworth and Asch 1986). The earliest Middle Woodland mounds appeared at the north end of the valley, and settlement proceeded southward over the course of the next three centuries (Charles 1992). Thus, the intense ritual activity seemingly invoking symbolism of the cosmos and the creation of the earth appear to correspond to a time of major demographic and social upheaval. Certain areas, such as the lower Illinois valley, where population went from nil to very dense over a matter of a few centuries, constitute extreme examples of this process. Subsequent Late Woodland mounds, ubiquitous throughout the valley and reflecting geographical stability of populations, lack the ramp and crypt structure and are more accurately described as accretional (Kerber 1986).

Among the artifacts buried with the adult female in Burial 9 were a platform pipe, two clusters of bird bone pins, and five mussel shells with serrations cut along part of their margin. What do these artifacts *mean*? Pipes in burials are rare in this region, but they occur equally with males and females (table 2.1)—all older adults in those cases where age at death could be determined. Pipes have been suggested to be important in mourning and greeting (calumet) ceremonies (Hall 1997) or to be associated specifically with shamanistic practices (James Brown, personal communication 2000). In either case, their equal association with males and females is intriguing. The bird bone pin clusters are even more enigmatic, but one possibility, also related to shamanism, would be that they were used in divination. The serrated edge of one of the mussel shells appears to match the dentate design on several vessels interred with an infant in a subcrypt

Table 2.1. Distribution by Sex of Grave Goods at Selected Illinois Valley Mortuary Sites

Form	F	M	I	F/I	M/I	F/M	?
Vessel	6	1	8	5	3	0	1
Bladelet	9	0	3	1	0	1[a]	2
Biface	0	1	1	0	0	1	3
Pipe	3	3	0	0	0	0	4
Hopewell[b]							
Copper	0	2	3	1	0	2	2
Marine shell	0	1	4	1	1	0	5
Mica	0	1	0	0	1	0	3

Source: For Bedford, Elizabeth, Gibson, Klunk sites, data compiled from Leigh 1988:Tables 10.3–10.9.

Notes: Cell counts = presence of an artifact form in a grave containing only indicated sex(es): that is, vessels occurred in six interments (on a surface or in a grave or crypt) containing only females (one or more), one interment containing only males, and so forth. Abbreviations: F = female, M = male, I = indeterminate (the majority are subadults), ? = unknown age and sex, / = both categories present.

[a] Found with F/M/I interment.

[b] Indicates items from outside general region: for example, bladelets and pipes may be made from materials available elsewhere in Illinois.

chamber that was created prior to the actual construction of the mound (Charles et al. 1988:71).

The apparent importance of this woman in Burial 9 belies the gendered nature of Illinois Hopewellian society. In terms of grave goods, nonlocal items such as copper, marine shell, and mica are found only with males and/or subadults, while ceramic vessels and stone bladelets are associated almost exclusively with women and/or subadults (table 2.1). At these same sites, males are found twice as frequently in crypts as either females or subadults (10 versus 6 versus 5, respectively [Charles et al. 1988; Perino 1968; Farnsworth and Wiant 2005]). In general, the exchange and mortuary activities characterizing Hopewell appear to have been conducted or controlled by men, whereas women increasingly dominated the horticulturally based economy (Charles 1998a, 1998b, 2000). Exchange and funerary activities as male concerns probably also emerged at least by the Archaic. The presumed increasing control over the subsistence economy by women was a more recent development (but again with roots in the Archaic), based on the importance of starchy seeds in the Middle Woodland diet. Advances in ceramic technology may have been crucial to this new diet (Braun 1987).

Mortuary ostentation, of the sort that might relate to the status of the group or individual responsible for the funeral rather than to the status of the deceased, appears to have been focused on crypts. Items in individual graves were more likely to have belonged to the person(s) with whom they were buried. In that case, apparently both men and women used pipes, possibly suggesting important social and/or ritual roles for both genders. By the same logic, exchange and/or manufacture of nonlocal Hopewell items and materials would seem to be associated with men, while ceramic and bladelet use and/or manufacture were apparently the province of women. The association of nonlocal items with men and ceramics with women is not unusual from a cross-cultural perspective. The fact that all bladelets as grave goods have been found with women or subadults, a pattern also recognized at the Gibson/Klunk mound group by Buikstra (1976:35, Table 16; see also Morrow 1988, 1998), suggests that we need to review the use of bladelets in other contexts. The role of bladelets in Hopewell societies has long puzzled archaeologists. Recent studies in Illinois by McGimsey (1995), Morrow (1987, 1988), and Odell (1985, 1994) found no functional or locational difference between bladelets and other comparable tool categories (for example, flakes or bifaces)—in other words, they could offer no explanation for the correlation of bladelet technology and Hopewell, a correlation so close that bladelets are considered a Hopewell diagnostic. The only suggestion was that bladelets were important socially, rather than functionally (Morrow 1987, 1988; Odell 1994). What none of these studies specifically investigated was the possibility that the use, and even manufacture, of bladelets was associated with a particular gender. The mortuary evidence suggests that bladelets were women's tools, perhaps something like the *ulu* among Arctic populations. If this is the case, a question asked about a cemetery now invites a reconsideration of occupation site data. For example, what other items are found, or not found, associated with bladelets in different depositional contexts? Such patterns might shed light on the gendered structure of activities at living sites.

Conclusion

The study of mortuary sites should be a means to an end, not an end in itself. A traditional Binford (1971)/Saxe (1970) approach to a cemetery would focus on the variability in burial treatments, not on the nature of the elements comprising the cemetery (for example, Tainter 1977a). While such an exercise would tell us something about Middle Woodland funerary behavior in the region surrounding the lower Illinois River valley, it would not have directed us to ask about the bluff-top versus floodplain mound locations, the chronological distribution of mounds, the nature of the soils constituting them, or the significance of specific artifact forms. The settings chosen for mounds would seem rather arbitrary, viewed only in a synchronic context of the Middle Woodland Midwest. Within a longer historical context, we see that by Middle Woodland times ridges on the margins of the bluffs or floodplain terraces were *traditional* locations. The origin of these loci can be traced several millennia earlier and relate to long-term trends toward sedentism (J. Brown 1985).

A postprocessual approach might well have led to the last question, concerning the construction materials, but would likely have shied away from the type of distributional study cited (Charles 1992), because it is derived from Saxe's Hypothesis 8 (Parker Pearson 1999:132–141). However, the diachronic, rather than synchronic, framework of the mound study offers an empirical foundation (Kuznar 1997:88–89) generally missing from recent phenomenological approaches (for example, Tilley 1994). As Parker Pearson (1999:141) notes, Tilley's "arguments often lack a range of corroborative evidence which would help to give validity to a single observation." Thus, the creation of a cemetery whose symbolic form and content locate it at the center of one's universe—that is, the everyday world—begins to make sense when we can suggest a context in which the redistribution of communities across the landscape make the space of everyday life contested space. But to reiterate, our understanding of the demographic transformation of the lower Illinois valley region is derived from the mortuary site distributions. Occupation site and more general ceramic distributions (Farnsworth and Asch 1986; McGregor 1958) had only hinted at the pattern. Furthermore, the mound distributions, originally based on external shape and certain locational criteria, have recently been "tested" and supported by ^{14}C dates (Kut and Buikstra 1998).

In a similar vein, it is one thing to suggest that Hopewellian exchange and mortuary ritual were male operations increasingly emphasized as women came to dominate the subsistence economy (Charles 1998a, 1998b, 2000); it is something more to begin to corroborate the hypothesis from the differential distribution by sex of particular artifact forms. Perhaps even more significant, the mortuary patterning of bladelets may direct us toward an understanding of their use and distribution in occupation sites, which is to date one of the enigmas of Hopewell. Rather than seeing occupation sites as simply generated from a subsistence system, as is too often the case in Eastern Woodland archaeology, perhaps we can begin to tease out a more realistic political economy of Hopewell life, one that is not gender neutral (Charles 2000). Perhaps we can pursue the archaeology of death as anthropology.

3

Mortuary Analysis

A Matter of Time?

Robert William Chapman

During the past four decades archaeology has become obsessed with theory and theories drawn from the social and natural sciences. It would be difficult to find an "-ism" in the sciences and the philosophy of science that has not featured in archaeological debate. In some cases it can be argued that the works of the gurus responsible for these theories have achieved greater notoriety in Anglo-American archaeology than in their own disciplines or countries (for example, Coudart 1999:162). Their theories are adopted and/or discarded by different "schools" of archaeology, archaeologists are classified according to which theoretical position they hold or "school" to which they belong, and archaeological theory is now recognized as a subarea of our discipline.

The history of this theoretical debate reveals two interesting observations. First, there would appear to be a major difference of opinion between those who regard these theories and "schools" as being mutually exclusive articles of faith and areas of practice and those who recognize permeable boundaries between them. Second, I see comparatively little explicit reflection in the Anglo-American world on the relationship between these theories and archaeological practice by analysis of published work. Do different theories determine, as logic would dictate, different sets of practice, different analytical concepts, different units and scales of analysis, and different methods? The answers to these questions may only be determined by careful scrutiny of case studies drawn from our disciplinary practice, thus contributing to the development of a philosophy of archaeology.

In this chapter I wish to consider one aspect of the relationship between theory and practice in mortuary analysis. From the seminal works of Lewis Binford (1971) and Arthur Saxe (1970), as well as the SAA Memoir edited by James Brown (1971a), it has been clear that mortuary analysis depended upon prior conceptions of society and social change. If the aim was to reconstruct past societies, then we had to be clear about what society was, how it was structured, and how it changed. Although permeable boundaries may be recognized, and bridges built, three major theories of society have been used in mortuary analysis: neo-evolutionism, Marxism, and practice theory. Advocates of these theories are found in a variety of case studies, but we need to reflect on whether and how these theories have changed the way in which we *do* mortuary analysis.

My interest here is in issues of scale and the chronological units of analysis we use in studying the dead. A concern with time is nothing new in mortuary analysis. The relative chronology of burials, whether determined by grave good typologies and associations or determined by the horizontal stratigraphy of cemeteries, played a key part in the nineteenth-century periodization of the prehistoric past. The increase in chronological resolution that was introduced by radiocarbon dating and dendrochronology in the twentieth century depended very much on the preservation of suitable dating materials and the perception of a need for the independent measurement of absolute time. The units of time used in mortuary analysis since the early 1970s have varied widely. For example, the volume I co-edited, *The Archaeology of Death* (Chapman et al. 1981), included studies of samples dated to within one (O'Shea 1981) and two (Goldstein 1981) generations, as well as Buikstra's (1981) analysis of 28 individuals spread over 3,000 years of occupation of the Modoc Rock Shelter. Elsewhere cemeteries were dated to cultural periods, and some "classic" analyses provided reinterpretations of mortuary data for which there was poor control over context and chronology (for example, Peebles 1971; Larson 1971). In my own reanalysis of the Copper Age cemetery of Los Millares in southeast Spain, I had to sift carefully through the uneven excavation and publication records of tombs and grave goods that could have been built and deposited over 700–900 years (Chapman 1981, 1990:178–195). Elsewhere quantitative methods were used to define significant associations, clusters, and patterns in mortuary data that provided the basis of inferences on social differentiation. In some cases quantitative methods, including seriation and cluster analyses, were evaluated on data from cemeteries (for example, Kendall 1971).

My impression of mortuary analyses during the 1970s and 1980s is that the spatial scale was given greater emphasis than the temporal scale. The use of cultural phases provided coarse chronologies that relegated change to breaks between them and also failed to fully disentangle chronological as opposed to social causes of variation in mortuary practices. One of the few practitioners to address the issue of scale during this time has been John O'Shea. In his major analysis of mortuary variability, he focused attention on change in mortuary rituals through time and what he called the archaeological "dilemma": "a short use-life minimizes the potential for diachronic change, but may provide an insufficient sample for meaningful analysis, whereas the large cemetery, ideal for social analysis, often has the greatest potential for diachronic distortion" (O'Shea 1984:14). Running the risk of such distortion is clearly the preferred strategy in using large-scale samples of burials for analysis. In a later paper, O'Shea

(1995:126) criticizes the analysis of individual mortuary sites such as cemeteries in isolation from their regional contexts. Such an emphasis on the individual site may focus attention on a limited range of mortuary rituals, both in space and time, and may provide too small a sample for social reconstruction. O'Shea advocates a "top down" approach, with the region as the unit of analysis.

While there is logic to O'Shea's argument, we are still left with the problem of time. What are the chronological units of analysis, and how easily can we distinguish change in mortuary rituals that is the consequence of social change as opposed to changing representations of existing social relations? Clearly what is needed is independent dating, as O'Shea acknowledges elsewhere (1996:16), and on a larger scale than has mostly been applied in mortuary analysis. Here there is an argument for aspiring to a regional scale of analysis, but working from the "bottom up," building finer-scale chronologies in relation to individual sites first.

In what follows I will begin with a critical examination of two case studies of mortuary analysis, one from the 1970s and the other from the 1990s. While their aims and theoretical approaches differ, both studies use "coarse" rather than "fine" chronologies and leave open the effects of time on intracemetery patterning. Then I will present some of the results of an attempt to build a "fine" chronology, working from the local to the regional scale, from the Bronze Age site of Gatas in southeast Spain.

A Tale of Two Cemeteries

The two case studies I have selected are both analyses of later prehistoric cemeteries in central Europe, derived from doctoral dissertations and published in the journal *Antiquity.* In 1975 Susan Shennan published an analysis of social organization at the Early Bronze Age cemetery of Branc in Slovakia (Shennan 1975). She took the cemetery as her unit of analysis, aiming to trace the development of social hierarchy and stratification through the recognition of patterning in artifact associations and distributions, and the correlation of cultural and biological data. Analysis of the individual cemetery was a "building-block" in the reconstruction of Early Bronze Age society on a more regional scale. Given that the 308 inhumation graves were spread out over a period of 200–400 years, and there were no radiocarbon dates for the cemetery, Shennan used diagnostic artifacts to argue for a linear expansion of graves from south to north through this time period. Quantitative analysis was then carried out to determine correlations between age and sex, on the one hand, and the types of grave goods, the orientation of the body, and the side on which it was interred. Assumptions were made that grave goods reflected status at death and that the costumes in which the dead were buried marked out that status. Here Shennan (1975:283) drew upon the theoretical arguments of Binford and Saxe. She concluded that the evidence for ascribed wealth at birth indicated the existence of social stratification.

If Shennan's analysis was of its time, then so is Joanna Sofaer Derevenski's

(1997) study of the Copper Age cemetery at Tiszapolgár-Basatanya in Hungary. Here the theoretical arguments are concerned with the cultural construction of gender and with changes in "gender perception" through the life cycle of individuals. Rather than assuming that mortuary practices reflect social identity, Sofaer Derevenski argues that the rituals surrounding the disposal of the dead reflect the "social perceptions" of the deceased by the living (1997:875). But once again the cemetery, this time of 156 graves, is the unit of analysis. Quantitative analyses and tests of significance are used to identify patterning in the relationship of sex to the side of burial and the deposition of grave goods, and to the changing relationship between age and grave goods of different types and materials. The conclusion is reached that there are age-related gender statuses, which may have been based upon different social and economic activities at different stages in the life cycle.

These two case studies start from different theoretical positions, although both take the cemetery as the unit of analysis and both use quantitative methods to identify normative patterns and deviations from those patterns. Although Shennan was concerned with "Society" with a capital "S," she accepted the need to work from the local to the regional scale (1975:279). Departures from the norm of biological sex-based burial differences were less important to her than they would be today in a study of gender construction. Neither study discusses the extent to which the buried individuals were representative of the living population, and neither situates the treatment of the dead in the context of social production among the living.

A further similarity concerns the temporal scale of analysis. Although Shennan traced a relative chronology of graves, the analysis was still carried out over the entire Branc cemetery, with its chronology of up to 400 years, or at least 12 generations. The use of the Tiszapolgár-Basatanya cemetery spanned the period c.4500–3600 cal B.C., which is at least 27 generations, or one grave for just under every six years. For the purposes of analysis, Sofaer Derevenski divides the graves into two periods, Early and Middle Copper Age, but does not give the span of each in centuries. Radiocarbon dating does not yet enable a clear distinction to be made between these two periods, especially c.4000–3600 cal B.C. (Forenbaher 1993:Figure 3).

This use of "coarse" chronologies in cemetery analyses is also seen in two recent studies of gender relations in the Central European Early Bronze Age. Rega (1997) has studied 268 skeletons from the cemetery at Mokrin but argues that the available radiocarbon dates do not support any internal phasing in the date range of 2100–1500 cal B.C, treating the cemetery as one unit of analysis over 600 years. Similarly Weglian (2001) treats the cemetery of Singen am Hohentwiel as "belonging to one mortuary archaeological phase," c.2300–1700 cal B.C. But if, as is argued in much recent literature, archaeologists should now be focusing greater attention on the small scale and the short term—on class factions and gender, or on social practices—then surely we need to look more closely at the scale of the temporal units we use in our analyses of mortuary practices, let alone other aspects of past societies. Indeed, whatever our focus, time remains a critical dimension in the definition of our units of analysis. To illustrate this point, I now turn to a further Bronze Age case study, this time in southeast Spain.

Building a Finer Chronology: The Gatas Cemetery

For over a century it has been known that the disposal of the dead in the Early Bronze Age of southeast Spain took the form of intramural burial, mainly for individuals, in artificial caves, pits, stone cists, or pottery urns (Siret and Siret 1887). These are found underneath floors and embedded in the walls of domestic structures on artificial terraces in naturally defended hilltop settlements. Speculation on the nature of this Bronze Age society centered on a small number of particularly rich assemblages of grave goods. But the identification of such socially important individuals took second place to that of this Argaric "culture" as a distinctive ethnic group (see, for example, Siret 1913). Blance (1964, 1971) proposed an influential division of this Argaric material into two periods, A and B, based on the typologies and associations of artifacts from 366 graves published by Siret and Siret (1887) for the type-site of El Argar. Absolute dating was by cross-dating to Central Europe and the eastern Mediterranean. Exceptional burials that did not fit into either of these periods, such as Grave 9 at Fuente Alamo (which was a cist burial of Argar A but included grave goods such as a sword, segmented faience beads, and a silver diadem characteristic of Argar B), were attributed to local chieftains. Occupation phases within newly excavated Argaric settlements in southeast Spain were then attributed to these two periods.

Criticisms of Blance's periodization included the observation that the numbers of artifact types exclusively associated with containers such as cists or urns were in the minority and the fact that there were no tests of significance for any of the claimed associations (Lull 1982, 1983). When the first radiocarbon dates were published, it was noted that some of the dates for Argar B were as early as those for Argar A (Chapman 1990:92). In spite of these contradictions, the division of the Argaric into these two periods (and their subdivisions) continued to be used (for the most recent examples, see Brandherm 2000; Schubart et al. 2000).

The construction of a finer, independent, absolute chronology for the Bronze Age was one of the aims of the Gatas project, which began in 1985. The site is located on a foothill of the Sierra Cabrera, on the southern edge of the Vera Basin, in Almería Province, southeast Spain (figures 3.1–3.3). Evidence for Bronze Age structures and burials was found in 1886 (Siret and Siret 1887:165–177) and, as with other Argaric sites in this region, provided the basis for inferences of social stratification and models as to how this stratification emerged (see Chapman 1990 and 2003). The selection of samples for ^{14}C dating from closed domestic and burial contexts was one part of the critical evaluation of these models (for the

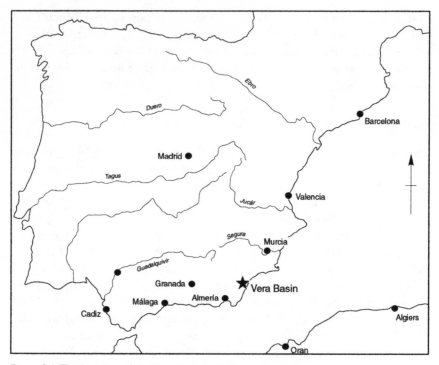

Figure 3.1. The location of the Vera Basin in Spain.

project as a whole, see Castro et al. 1999a, 1999b, 2000). Conventional ^{14}C dating was used for domestic contexts, unless short-lived samples such as carbonized seeds were available, while AMS dating was used on human bone from burial contexts. After the initial excavation of small sondages (S1–S4), attention has focused on the well-preserved stratigraphic occupation sequences of domestic structures and burials in Zones B and C on the lower slopes of the north-facing hill (figure 3.4). In addition to the 18 tombs studied in 1886 (Siret and Siret 1887; Chapman et al. 1987:112–115), which are known to have come from the top of the hill, a further 25 tombs were excavated before 2002. AMS dates have been obtained (through the collaboration of the NERC facility at Oxford University) on 14 tombs from the new excavations and 4 tombs from the 1886 excavations (through the collaboration of the museums in Almería, Madrid, and Brussels). Double burials (figure 3.5) were found and dated in 2 tombs. In all, some 56 percent of the newly excavated tombs and 42 percent of all the tombs at Gatas now have independent, absolute dates, and all tombs from the new excavations are tied into stratified domestic contexts. Indeed, it is the stratified record (or its absence in cases where burials are located on different terraces from each other and postdepositional processes have removed the deposits that originally linked them) that has been the main determinant of the selection of tombs for AMS dating.

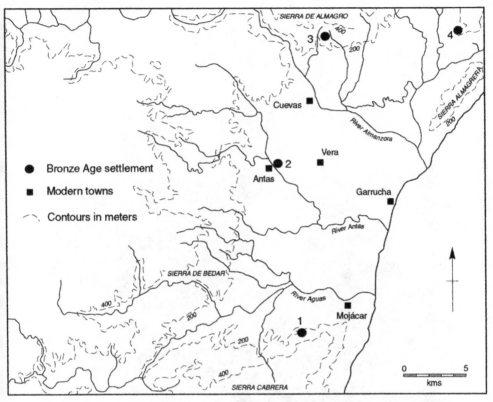

Figure 3.2. The Vera Basin, showing the location of Gatas and the other main Bronze Age settlements mentioned in the text: (1) Gatas, (2) El Argar, (3) Fuente Alamo, (4) El Oficio.

AMS radiocarbon dating was also extended to Argaric burials from other settlements in southeast Spain, again in collaboration with the NERC facility at Oxford University and using samples taken from museum collections in Almería and Brussels. These samples include burials from excavations in the 1880s at El Argar and El Oficio (both in the Vera Basin), Ifre and Zapata (in southern Murcia) and modern excavations at Fuente Alamo (in the north of the Vera Basin), El Picacho, and Lorca. This gave an additional 18 dates, including three further examples of double burials (for details, see Castro et al. 1993–1994; Lull 2000). There are two main aims of this dating program: to see how far regional horizons can be detected in the deposition of particular grave goods and to provide dates for double burials (see below and Lull 2000). In the case of burials excavated in the 1880s, there is no stratigraphic information, although in some cases plans exist that show their location in particular houses (for example, at Gatas). The opportunity was also taken (by Jane Buikstra and Cristina Rihuete) to restudy the human remains in these tombs.

Of the 117 ^{14}C dates for the Argaric assembled by Castro and colleagues

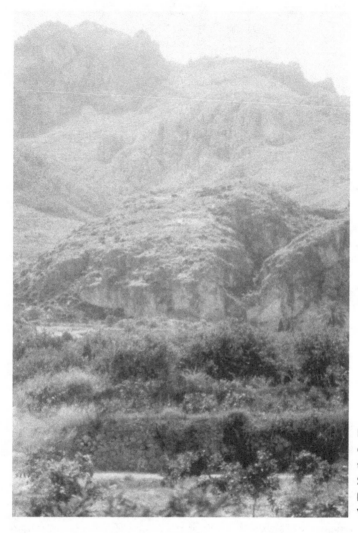

Figure 3.3. The hill
of Gatas seen from
the north, with the
Sierra Cabrera be-
hind. Photograph by
Vincente Lull.

(1993–1994), 36 percent came from Gatas. The Argaric is now known to have
lasted for just over 700 years, c.2250–1500 cal B.C., with at least three main
periods within that time span at Gatas (2250–1950 cal B.C., 1950–1700 cal B.C.,
and 1700–1500 cal B.C.). This is a much longer time span than that included in
the Argar A-B periodization. According to that scheme, artificial caves and stone
cist burials preceded the deposition of the dead in pottery urns. While ^{14}C dating
confirms the very early dating of some artificial cave burials and the late dating
of some urn burials (Castro et al. 1993–1994:85), it also shows that the dead
were deposited in such containers, as well as pits and stone cists, throughout the
period c.2100/2000–1700/1600 cal B.C. Cists and urns (figure 3.6) occurred in

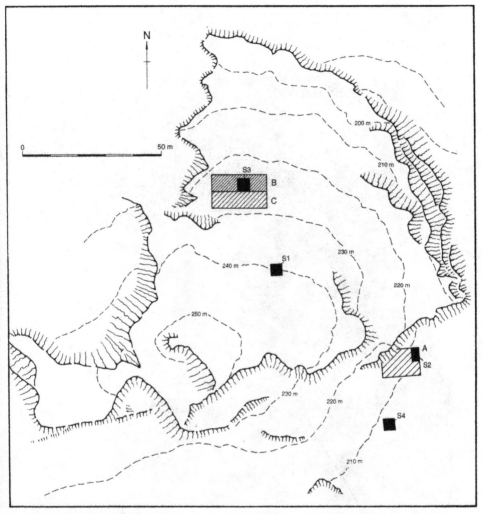

Figure 3.4. Map of Gatas, showing the location of excavated sondages (S1–S4) and open area excavations (A–C).

the greatest frequencies overall. Recent excavations also suggest that cist burials continued until the end of the Argaric.

Although we cannot yet measure the relative frequencies of burial containers used at particular times, it is clear that all were available for social selection during most of the Argaric. The exception to this relates to regional differences between the coastal and interior areas of the Argaric: in the latter, urn burials are much less frequent, while pit burials are more numerous (Lull and Estévez 1986). The earliest dated Argaric urns were used for the interment of infants, and only later were adults included in this type of container. The absence of dated urns and infant burials before c.2000 cal B.C. needs to be tested by further AMS dates but

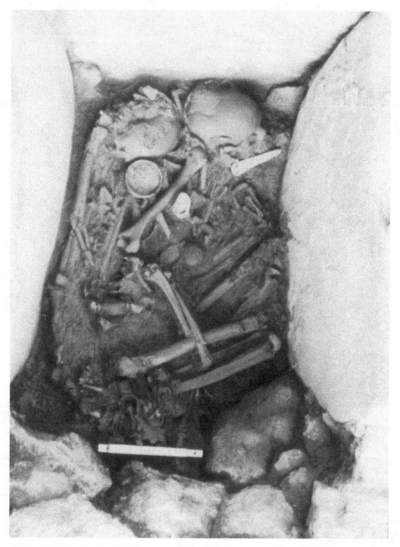

Figure 3.5. Double burial in a cist (Tomb 33) from Gatas. Photograph by Vincente Lull.

suggests the hypothesis that infants and children were not given social recognition through intramural burial in the first two centuries of the Argaric Bronze Age.

The AMS dating of double burials in four cists (Gatas T33, T37; Fuente Alamo T75; Madres Mercedarias T11, Lorca) and one pit (Calle de Los Tintes T2, Lorca) has also demonstrated that such interments did not represent individuals of the same generation but were separated by up to three generations (Castro et al. 1993–1994:88–89; Lull 2000:587–588). In the cists the adult fe-

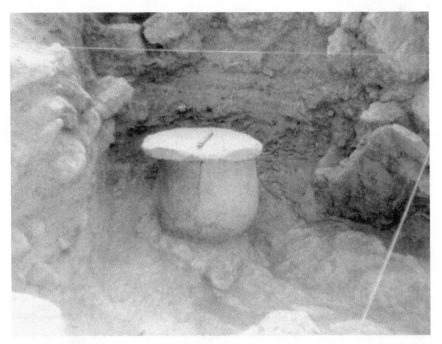

Figure 3.6. Urn burial (Tomb 22) from Gatas.

male was interred before the adult male, and this pattern appears to be repeated in other nondated double burials in southeast Spain. Once again the use of AMS dating has contributed to a change in our understanding of the mortuary rituals. Rather than being married couples, as was previously inferred, the double burials may represent the marking out of intergenerational ties of kinship, perhaps through the female line.

Not only was there no exclusive division of burial containers by period in the Argaric, but ^{14}C dating is now beginning to show which grave goods were deposited during which periods of time. For example, objects of silver (mainly ornaments) are found almost exclusively in funerary rather than domestic contexts but throughout the period c.2100/2000–1600 cal B.C. (Castro et al. 1993–1994:100) and not just at the end of the Argaric, as was previously argued on the basis of typological and association arguments (for example, Blance 1964). In contrast, the chalice or cup (pottery type 7) has a late dating supported by initial ^{14}C dates, and copper halberds appear to have been deposited in graves c.2000–1800 cal B.C., or in the early half of the Argaric, as proposed by Blance (1964). In the case of copper daggers and knives, which have been ^{14}C dated in 15 tombs, there is little support for simple typologies based on increasing complexity of artifact form through time (Lull 2000:Figure 3).

Observations on Argaric grave goods across southeast Spain suggest some sharp divisions between male and female associations. Metal weapons such as halberds, swords, and axes are associated overwhelmingly with older adult males of higher social position, while the dagger-awl association is exclusively associated with females of the third level in Argaric society (Lull and Estévez 1986). The dagger by itself also occurs in male burials. The application of AMS ^{14}C dating has cast new light on these male and female associations. The dated male burials with halberds all fit tightly within a period of some 200 years, c.2000–1800 cal B.C., or six to seven generations, while axes were deposited after c.1800 cal B.C. Elsewhere it has been proposed that the use of the halberd to mark out adult males of the most important position in Argaric society gave way to the use of the long sword (Castro et al. 1993–1994:91–97). The date of c.1800 cal B.C. also seems to mark a change in the use of the dagger in adult male and female graves, with the dagger being added to the graves of subadults as well. However, the use of the dagger-awl association to mark out females of the third level in Argaric society continues throughout the Argaric period.

What this all means is that the extensive ^{14}C dating program on burials is beginning to enable us to separate out chronological from social variation, to test arguments based on artifact form and association, and to establish a finer scale of chronological resolution. This is enhanced by the fact that the burials are stratified within the deposits of successive occupations of Early Bronze Age sites such as Gatas. For example, within Zones B and C, in an area of approximately 225 square meters, 25 urn and cist burials (12 of them dated by ^{14}C) were deposited within a period of about 400 years in domestic spaces on two adjacent terraces.

The observed distribution of the dead so far at Gatas shows a peak of individuals under 5 years of age, a small number of subadults, and a further, though smaller, peak between 50 and 60 years of age. Young adults (20–30 years) and those aged in their late 30s and 40s were absent (see Buikstra et al. 1995:Figure 7). This is a higher infant mortality than is seen at the contemporary sites of El Argar and El Oficio, where the age at death decreased continuously from 20 to 60 years. These differences could be explained in a number of ways, including a higher infant mortality at Gatas, that is, real demographic (a growing population?) and health differences between individual Argaric settlements. But this explanation assumes that the excavated burials from these sites are a representative sample of the population that lived and died in them. This assumption has been questioned on the basis of calculations of the predicted number of burials per century from nine Argaric sites, where we know the number of excavated burials and can estimate the occupation duration in calendar years, the percentage of the site that has been excavated, and thus the total number of burials that would originally have been made on each site as a whole (Chapman 1990:200–201). A further assumption that burials were evenly deposited across these settlements underpins these calculations, but it seems justified given the argument that the nuclear family was the basic burial unit (Lull 2000:585). When the predicted burials per century are compared against the estimated populations, it seems reasonable to infer that not all the dead were disposed of within the settlement; for example, the predicted burials per century for Ifre (10) and Zapata (54) seem low compared with an occupation of some 300 people. We know that a small number of Argaric burials in both the coastal and the interior areas of southeast Spain were deposited in megalithic tombs (Chapman 1990:196).

If such calculations are regarded as dubious, given the assumptions they invoke, then the figures for the number of tombs and burial by age in the successive occupation phases in Zones B and C at Gatas show marked variations. For the first Argaric phase, c.2250–1950 cal B.C., there is one possible cist (T42) late in the sequence, containing an adult female. For the second phase, c.1950–1700 cal B.C., there are two double cists (T33, T37), each with an adult male and a female aged around 50 years, two cists with individual burials, one aged 40 years (T26) and the other older (T41), and four urns containing infants (T24, T28, T32, T36). For the third phase, c.1700–1500 cal B.C., there is only one cist (T35), containing a double adult burial, and some 13 urns containing mainly infant burials. Only one infant and two child burials were excavated in the 1880s, so the peak in observed infant mortality at Gatas is mainly the result of the last phase of Argaric occupation. The burial figures also raise the question as to whether the houses excavated so far are representative of other areas within the settlement, in terms of health and mortality and in terms of the extent to which all the dead were accorded burial within the domestic unit. Future excavations might expect to determine whether any differences in access to production were related to differences in health and mortality.

In a wider context, it is worth noting that the available ^{14}C dates for Argaric burials in southeast Spain as a whole strengthen this pattern of predominantly adult burials before c.1900 cal B.C. and mainly infant, child, and juvenile burials c.1700–1500 cal B.C. (Castro et al. 1993–1994:90). As was mentioned above, the absence of infants and children before c.2000 cal B.C. may indicate the absence of their social recognition in intramural mortuary treatment at that time. For the first six or seven generations of the Argaric, infants and children received mortuary rituals that left no material trace. A rather different situation is suggested for adult males between 20 and 30 years of age, which are notable for their scarcity throughout the occupations of Gatas and Fuente Alamo (on the southern and northern edges of the Vera Basin), as opposed to El Argar. The central location of this site (approximately 10 kilometers from both sites), coupled with its evidence for metallurgy and wealth deposition with over 1,000 burials, has led to the inference that it acted as the major political center of this region. Did this have some effect on the location for burial of adult males, no matter where they resided in life? Study of phenotypic variation within the Argaric population (Buikstra and Hoshower 1994) has suggested that males were five times more heterogeneous than females, leading to the inference that males changed residence on marriage. This inference now needs further testing by such methods as isotopic analysis, using samples taken from across the full chronological range of the

Argaric. Taken together, the skeletal data and demographic profiles suggest that there is good reason for inferring mobility in life and death related to Argaric social practices.

Conclusions

I began this chapter by wondering generally about the relationship between theory and practice in mortuary analysis. Do we do it differently now, in our supposedly enlightened "post" years, compared with that rather naïve, primitive, "new" era of 30 years ago? When we look at the units of time that are used to structure our mortuary data, there is some evidence to suggest that little has changed. My purpose in the main body of the chapter has been to use the example of the Gatas project to show how finer chronologies can be constructed and what they can tell us. By making the measurement of time independent of the dating of the material objects placed with the dead, we can avoid such problems as the "heirloom effect," by which longer circulation times on a local or regional scale, or relating to some artifacts and not others, can be hidden from view in supposedly homogenous typological units. Short-term differences in demography and in the social representation of the dead may now emerge from what had been thought to be longer-term homogenous units. Changes may emerge in the representation of what are continuous social differences. This applies as much to what are now regarded by some as the more "traditional" inferences of social rank and status as it does to current gender analyses.

The Gatas example shows how such finer chronologies can be built, selecting short-lived samples (the dead themselves) in relation to existing knowledge of local chronologies of graves and artifacts, as well as the evidence for their stratigraphic relations. In the case of Gatas, we are fortunate in having intramural mortuary rituals that can be related to specific domestic contexts. One of the future aims of research will be to situate the disposal and representation of the dead within these domestic units to have access to, and control over, the production, distribution, and consumption of the basic necessities of life, which are the foundations of social stratification. Like the Gatas burials, this involves a "bottom up" approach, starting with the individual tombs within the domestic unit and moving up to the groups of such contemporary domestic units within the settlement and then to the contemporary occupations of settlements within the region. The finer chronology is then linked to a sliding series of spatial scales.

It may seem self-evident that smaller-scale approaches to past societies require smaller-scale analyses in time and space and that we need to divorce chronological and social causes of variability in mortuary practices, but how often are these requirements recognized or put into practice as fully as they deserve? With the large cemeteries and samples of burials that offer the best potential for studying the biological characteristics and social practices of past populations come the problems of "diachronic distortion" noted by O'Shea (1984:14). The scale of ^{14}C dating used in the Gatas project seems to be a rarity in mortuary analysis (compare Savage 2001:124–125 on a comparable project to establish an absolute chronology for Predynastic Egyptian cemeteries). It depends heavily on the active collaboration of radiocarbon-dating facilities. Without such collaboration it is difficult to imagine the financial resources being more routinely available for large-scale AMS dating of burials in cemeteries.

Given that we cannot expect to date every burial in a cemetery, it is clear that careful thought has to be given to the selection of samples for dating. This sampling has to occur within the contexts of the size of the burial population, resource availability, and the specific problems under study, as well as in relation to other studies of human bone (for example, isotopic analyses). This is all part of the initial research design. We might expect this to be a different sampling process with intramural disposal, where vertical stratigraphy gives us our relative chronology, than in more extensive, open-air cemeteries, where instances of horizontal stratigraphy (for example, intercutting of burial pits) may occur only in small numbers. But in both cases it can be argued that absolute dating programs are required to test hypotheses based on the fundamental archaeological evidence of stratigraphy, spatial patterning, artifact typology, and association. On a regional basis, one strategy might be to make an initial, intense, investment in AMS dating of burials from a well-controlled cemetery excavation and then use such dating more selectively for other cemeteries in the region to evaluate the extent to which time-specific disposal patterns extended more widely.

It might be suggested that I am chiding archaeologists about the importance of time in mortuary analysis, while not suggesting something that can be done about this problem as part of regular fieldwork and analysis. I hope that I have addressed this issue and that the case study presented in this chapter will stimulate others to consider more carefully the relationship between scale and the kinds of problems we seek to study through mortuary analysis. At the very least we should look critically at research that claims to study finer-scale problems with rather coarse data. This is no more than the basic recognition that the scale of the archaeological record is one measure of the strength of what are claimed to be sound inferences of past societies.

Acknowledgments

I would like to thank the editors for the invitation to attend the symposium on which this book is based and the British Academy for a grant from its Overseas Conference Fund that allowed me to attend the meetings of the Society for American Archaeology in New Orleans in April 2001. Revision of this chapter has not taken into account the small number of new burials excavated in the most recent fieldwork at Gatas in the fall of 2002. As always I acknowledge the following friends for their energetic and stimulating collaboration on the Gatas project: Pedro Castro, Trini Escoriza, Sylvia Gili, Vicente Lull, Rafa Micó, Cristina Rihuete, Roberto Risch, and Ma. E. Sanahuja. The research of Jane Buikstra has dramatically changed our knowledge of human skeletal remains at Gatas and other Argaric sites in southeast Spain, and I am, as always, in her debt. I would also like to thank the staff of the Almería and Brussels museums, as well as excavation directors, especially Hermanfrid Schubart, for providing the samples of human bone for dating and the Radiocarbon Unit of the University of Oxford for carrying out successive programs of dating. John O'Shea kindly read a draft of this chapter and offered constructive comments toward its revision.

4

Gender and Agency in Mortuary Fashion

Aubrey Cannon

Fashion is a powerful process focused on emerging styles and individual expression. Understanding fashion's role in shaping burial trends in a variety of archaeological and historical contexts helps to explain the role of individual agents in creating and transforming patterns of mortuary treatment. Identifying women as initiators of change in some cases further refines the concept of agency to highlight the personally motivated choices of specific people influenced on one level by fashion trends but equally important in setting those trends in motion.

Archaeological interpretation of mortuary patterning is more likely to be based on structural correlates of large-scale variation than on an understanding of the influences and motivations that affect individual choice. Burial treatments are known to vary among individuals and to change over time, of course, but these sources of variability are more often controlled in the process of interpretation than viewed as both the source of structural variation and a focus of interpretation in their own right. Long-term trends in mortuary patterns have been explained in relation to broader contexts of social and political development (Buikstra and Charles 1999; Parker Pearson 1993) or inherent limits of elaboration and comparison (Cannon 1989, 1995), but relatively little attention has been given to individual agents or motivations responsible for change. With the notable exception of Chapman's (2000) study of Late Neolithic burials from Hungary, considerations of agency in mortuary analysis have also tended to focus only on elite expressions of status and power (Arnold 2001; Cannon 2002; Gillespie 2001). Mortuary trends, however, are clearly the product of more than just media constraints and opportunities and are motivated by more than simply the need or desire to express social status and power relations (Tarlow 1997: 109). Influence over long-term trends in treatment and commemoration of the dead is also not restricted to the elite and powerful but is equally evident in the actions of individuals within broader social categories, such as those based on gender, and discernible in the burial patterns for which they are responsible.

Agency is defined here as the socioculturally mediated but individually motivated capacity to act purposefully in such a way as to create archaeologically discernible change in prevailing modes of mortuary practice (compare Ahearn 2001:112). Agency, of course, can also refer to actions that maintain prevailing practice (Cowgill 2000:57) or to actions that bring about unintended consequences (Dobres and Robb 2000:10), but the focus here is on deliberate creation of variation perceived as beneficial to the responsible agent. The agency of women, in particular, is suggested in the differential mortuary treatments of men and women in a variety of archaeological contexts, in which interpretation might more commonly focus on differences as the passive reflection of relative gender status. It is especially evident in the differential rates by which new modes of burial and commemoration are adopted and come into general usage. A focus on the agency of women in these cases does not derive from an overt effort to redress their neglect in this respect. Instead, it derives from observations of temporal trends in historic and prehistoric contexts that are consistent with the agency of women in the initiation and direction of mortuary fashion.

Whether fashion is the appropriate way to view variability and change in mortuary practice has long been debated (for example, Binford 1971; Kroeber 1927), but fashion-based interpretations have been applied to mortuary patterns in contexts ranging from Early Bronze Age Central Europe (Shennan 1982) to Victorian England (Cannon 1989). The appropriateness of fashion to explain trends in these contexts is plain from its contemporary definition as a process of change in material or clothing style characterized by sequential phases. These include invention and introduction, leadership in adoption among the most fashion conscious, increasing social visibility, conformity within and across social groups, social saturation, and decline and obsolescence (Sproles 1985:56). To the extent that fashion adoption, emulation, saturation, and obsolescence also drive the process of change in mortuary expression, fashion-conscious individuals can be identified as the responsible agents. The extent and rate of conformity they inspire through emulation is also a measure of their social prominence and influence.

Rapid fashion change may be more characteristic of recent times than of most archaeological contexts (Cannon 1998), but the basic features of the process are clearly evident archaeologically. Although he did not use the term, fashion comparison and change was highlighted in archaeology by Miller (1982), who drew inspiration for his discussion of socially based material differentiation and emulation in part from the work of sociolinguist William Labov. Among his findings, Labov (1972:290) showed that linguistic forms initially adopted by higher-status social groups often are subsequently adopted by less prestigious groups. Labov also noted that some individuals, and those within some groups in particular, appear to be more aware of the prestige value of innovative speech variants. These could be described as more fashion conscious individuals, to use Sproles' (1985:56) characterization of leaders in the fashion process, though Miller (1982:91) notes that emulation among social groups can occur without individuals actually being aware of the process or of the changes taking place. In keeping with the definition of agency as purposeful action, however, all choices could be described as consciously mediated by the desire either to conform with or to depart from prevailing practice, while some departures are also consciously motivated by the desire to emulate prestige variants.

Miller illustrated the material culture implications of the process of differentiation and emulation in the introduction and adoption of pot types in India. He also (1982:96) noted the potential applicability of this process to the explanation of any pattern of change in material culture, such as those that are the basis for seriation in archaeology, where material forms show gradual increase and later decrease in popularity over time. The same process of fashion change should be and is evident in historical and archaeological examples of changes in burial mode, but the identities of the agents responsible for this change are less evident in gross temporal patterns. To move beyond identification of socially based fashion as a disembodied process underlying burial trends to identify those individuals responsible for the process requires an examination of differential practice and, more important, differential rates of change in practice among identifiable groups, such as those based on gender or social class.

Although recent studies have highlighted the ambiguity of gender categories (Lucy 1997:154–155; Stoodley 1999:5; Weglian 2001), divisions defined with respect to biologically determined sex are consistently available in the majority of burial contexts. Differences in mortuary treatment, often used to define "status" differences between men and women, may provide better insight into their differential agency in the creation and transformation of mortuary practice. The examples below highlight gender-based agency and illustrate the problems and ambiguities that arise in its investigation in a variety of archaeological contexts.

Victorian England

Trends in Victorian grave monument design exhibit all the characteristics of the typical fashion process (Cannon 1989, 1996; Parker Pearson 1982). In villages in rural south Cambridgeshire, England, for example, stone grave monuments from the early to the mid nineteenth century primarily commemorate members of socially prominent families. They only gradually came to be associated as often with members of more middle- or laboring-class families. This emulation encouraged differentiation in monument design among leading members of rural society, but eventually, as the medium of monumental expression became accessible to all social classes, it reached a level of social saturation, and ostentatious styles became obsolete. Subsequently, the prevailing mode of monumental commemoration was and has remained one of relatively small and homogenous headstones.

Specific patterns of differentiation and emulation of monument style are difficult to trace among the great diversity of styles that developed and proliferated over the course of the nineteenth century, but a group of designs based on the Gothic Revival movement in architecture (Clark 1962) provides a notable excep-

Table 4.1. Number and Relative Popularity of Gothic-Style Monuments among 3,553 Nineteenth-Century Gravestones Recorded in 50 Villages in Rural Southern Cambridgeshire

Decade	Headstone		Coped stone		All Gothic styles	
	n	%	*n*	%	*n*	%
1891–1900	56	9.8	14	2.5	72	12.6
1881–1890	64	11.1	32	5.6	98	17.1
1871–1880	58	11.4	31	6.1	97	19.0
1861–1870	49	10.2	28	5.8	90	18.7
1851–1860	21	7.0	15	5.0	42	14.0
1841–1850	7	2.8	8	3.2	19	7.6
1831–1840	5	1.8	2	0.7	10	3.6
1821–1830	2	0.9	0	0.0	5	2.3
1811–1820	2	1.0	0	0.0	2	1.0
1801–1810	0	0.0	1	0.6	1	0.6

Note: Percentage figures are based on all monuments recorded for each decade; the total number of Gothic styles includes combinations of headstones and other forms of grave marker.

tion. This group exhibits a smooth trend in overall popularity and in its rate of adoption within and between social divisions. These Gothic styles, which consist of the coped stone (figure 4.1) and various forms of headstone featuring elaborated and often encircled cross motifs (figure 4.2), were prescribed by ecclesiastical reformers as proper Christian memorials (Burgess 1963:31–36). As such, they were promoted in design catalogues that subsequently became the basis for

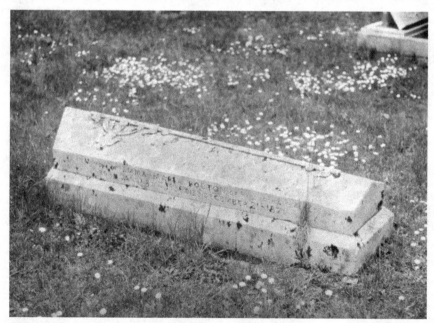

Figure 4.1. The coped stone style of Gothic grave marker.

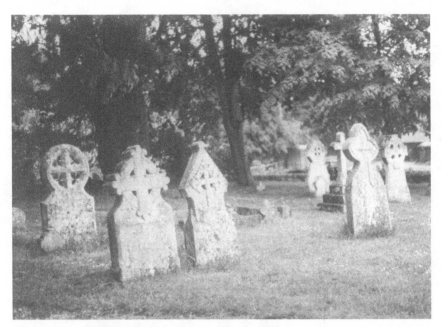

Figure 4.2. Cruciform Gothic headstones.

masons' pattern books. The popularity of these designs follows a classic growth curve over the course of the nineteenth century (figure 4.3, table 4.1), and their varying popularity among different social classes provides a perfect illustration of socially based differentiation and emulation.

Over the last half of the nineteenth century, for which census data showing occupation categories are available, it is clear that Gothic forms occur initially most often in association with higher-status members of rural communities, represented by farming families and members of the clergy (figure 4.4, table 4.2). They were subsequently increasingly popular among middle-class families, represented by tradespeople and craftspeople, and only later became associated in greater proportion with the graves of agricultural laborers. Of course by this time Gothic styles were starting to become increasingly unfashionable among the general population.

When viewed in relation to social class, the process of differentiation and emulation is clearly evident. Individuals from higher status groups were the fashion-conscious leaders who adopted Gothic monument styles nearer to the time when they were initially introduced. Members of lower status groups lagged behind in their emulation of those same styles. While this social pattern is consistent with observations of the fashion process in other contexts, the representation of men and women on Gothic-style grave monuments shows essentially the same pattern. Men led in their association with Gothic styles, while women lagged behind (figure 4.5, table 4.3). Women were represented by an equal proportion of

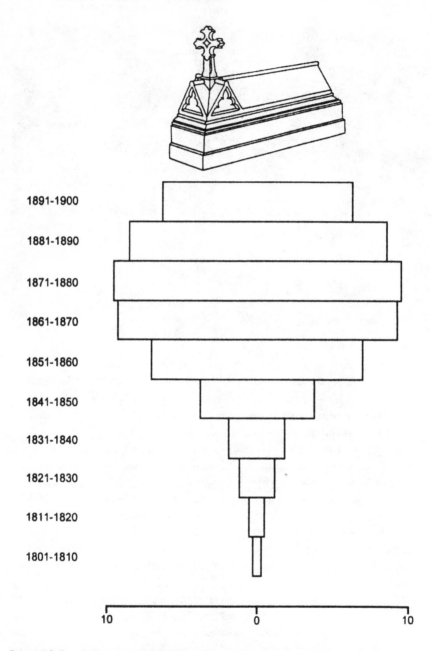

1891-1900

1881-1890

1871-1880

1861-1870

1851-1860

1841-1850

1831-1840

1821-1830

1811-1820

1801-1810

10   0   10

Figure 4.3. Popularity curves of Gothic-style monuments among 3,553 nineteenth-century gravestones recorded in 50 villages in rural southern Cambridgeshire (bar widths indicate the relative popularity of Gothic forms among the total number of monuments recorded for each decade).

Table 4.2. Association of Gothic-Style Grave Monuments with Occupation Classes by Decade

	Clergy/large-scale farmers		Trades/craftspeople		Agricultural laborers	
Decade	*n*	%	*n*	%	*n*	%
1891–1900	6	40.0	4	26.7	5	33.3
1881–1890	10	38.5	9	34.6	7	26.9
1871–1880	10	41.7	10	41.7	4	16.7
1861–1870	15	45.5	15	45.5	3	9.1
1851–1860	13	76.5	3	17.6	1	5.9

Note: Percentage figures are of Gothic-style monuments per decade distributed among the three occupation categories.

Gothic monuments only at the end of the century, when these styles were becoming generally less fashionable.

At face value, this pattern of gender representation could suggest that women were of lesser status. Their lagging association with new prestige monument designs could be considered an appropriate reflection of their lesser status, whether the choice to differentially commemorate men and women was conscious or not. The alternative, in keeping with the active, socially based fashion process evident in Gothic style selection, would require that individuals in different social groups be differentially aware of shifting fashions or differentially inclined or motivated to adopt more fashionable styles. The clear problem in applying this argument to gender-based style associations is that the dead are unlikely to be the primary agents responsible for their own mode of burial. Following the often-cited maxim that the dead do not bury themselves (Parker Pearson 1993:203), the dead also would not normally be fashion leaders or followers with respect to their own commemoration. An explanation for differen-

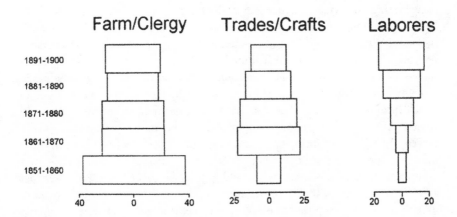

Figure 4.4. Popularity of Gothic-style monuments among social classes.

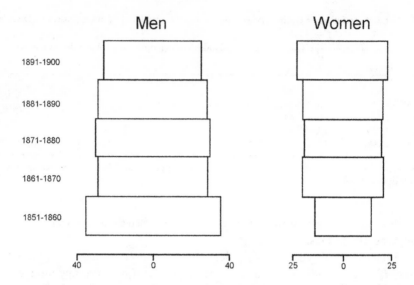

Figure 4.5. Popularity of Gothic-style monuments by gender of burial.

tial rates in the adoption of Gothic styles is more likely to be found in the choices of survivors, which would generally be family members of the deceased.

Only a relatively few monument inscriptions identify who was responsible for the erection of the stone. Of the 3,553 monuments recorded in rural south Cambridgeshire, only 50 identify the individual or individuals who commissioned the stone. These include a diverse array of relationships with the deceased, including sons, daughters, children more generally, a granddaughter, a nephew, sisters, brothers, employers (particularly in the case of servants), a mother, parishioners, and friends. A surviving wife is identified as responsible for monuments in only four cases; a surviving husband is not identified in any. There is a very slight tendency for daughters more often to erect monuments for their fathers, but this is evident in only a very few cases. Generally the gender identities of the persons selecting the stone are evenly distributed with respect to the gender identities of the persons for whom the stone is erected. If there is a differential gender bias in monument selection, it can come only from a majority of the unnoted cases in which monuments were selected by either a wife or husband for a departed spouse. Although inscriptions normally identify the marital relations of the deceased, the possessive form, as in "my husband" or "my wife," does not come into common usage until the twentieth century. Nonetheless, the selection of a monument for a man or a woman would in some large proportion of cases specifically be the responsibility of the surviving spouse. Although surviving children, other family members, or even the deceased could have chosen monument styles in a large number or even the majority of cases, the death of a married man

Table 4.3. Association of Gothic-Style Grave Monuments with Men and Women by Decade

Decade	Men		Women	
	n	%	n	%
1891–1900	24	52.2	22	47.8
1881–1890	42	58.3	30	41.7
1871–1880	48	60.0	32	40.0
1861–1870	43	58.1	31	41.9
1851–1860	29	70.7	12	29.3

Note: Percentages are of Gothic-style monuments identified as commemorating men or women.

or woman at least increases the likelihood that the choice would be made by the surviving spouse.

The question this raises is why widows or other family members more often chose a more fashionable mode of commemoration for men, while widowers or other surviving family members were less inclined to make the same choice for women. One possibility is that women were more often concerned about the perception of their relative status in the absence of a husband, while men did not perceive the same need or opportunity for status expression on the occasion of their wife's death. Certainly, a woman's social position and financial security were in greater jeopardy on the death of a husband than a man's position was on the death of a wife (Jalland 1996:230–254). These differential concerns, however, do not explain why a surviving husband or other family member would choose to commemorate a woman with an increasingly unfashionable style of monument. This is particularly difficult to explain at the end of the century when Gothic forms were becoming predominantly associated with lower social classes.

The preferential choice of more fashionable commemoration earlier in the century for men may have been in keeping with perceptions of men's greater social prominence. Commemoration of women with those same styles at the time when they were becoming less fashionable, however, is unlikely to have been a deliberate attempt to mark a lower social status for women. Why would surviving widowers or other family members knowingly choose unfashionable styles to commemorate deceased women? The answer to this question need not assume either that the burial of men was a more prominent social event or the even less realistic possibility that unfashionable styles were knowingly selected for women. An alternative is suggested by another result of Labov's sociolinguistic studies.

Labov and other linguists have consistently found that women show a greater propensity to use prestige variants of language. Studies have also shown time and again that women tend to lead men in the adoption of new language variants, sometimes by as much as a generation (Labov 1972:301–302; Wolfram and Schilling-Estes 1998:187). The reasons for these widespread observations are still poorly understood and are widely debated, but linguistic studies in a variety of contexts suggest that women are more likely than men to favor incoming prestige language variants. Labov maintained that women were more prestige conscious and therefore more aware of prestige forms and more likely to lead in their adoption, though he acknowledged that other factors also played a role. Other linguists have also attempted to explain why women might be more prestige conscious than men are. Women's apparently greater awareness of prestige forms has been attributed, for example, to a desire to further the social prospects of their children. Alternatively, linguists cite the historically insecure social position of women, which may lead them to place more emphasis on signaling social status, or a greater propensity for women to be "rated" more on the basis of appearances (Trudgill 1983:167–168). All these explanations in turn derive from sociological generalizations to the effect that status consciousness is generally more pronounced among women than among men (Martin 1954:58).

Recent extensive review of linguistic research concludes that it is an oversimplification to suggest that women generally use more prestige forms than men and confirms that there is no simple link between the female sex and a heightened focus on social prestige (James 1996). Nevertheless, the specific and significant role of women in effecting linguistic change remains firmly established (Labov 1972:303). The reasons why women lead in the adoption of new language variants probably vary in different contexts, but the generalization that women in some circumstances at least are more concerned with social prestige still holds as an explanation for their differential adoption of prestige variants (Wolfram and Schilling-Estes 1998:192).

The same pattern also appears to be evident in the selection of monument styles in rural Victorian England. Gothic styles, which were actively promoted by leading members of the Anglican clergy, clearly originated "from above" in relation to the social spectrum. Their differential adoption among members of different social classes also follows from above to below. Women initially were either more aware of or more inclined to adopt these new prestige-associated styles and to select them for the commemoration of men, which is why they are found in greater numbers earlier in association with the graves of men. Men's preferential choice of the same monument styles to commemorate women only became as common once the style had already become established. In later periods men may simply have been unaware that the style preferences they thought were established were no longer fashionable.

Beyond simply following fashion's lead in the commemoration of their husbands, sons, and fathers, women could also be seen as having created the fashion trend toward and later away from Gothic-style monuments. Women, in other words, were the agents of style change in this instance. The lag in the style of women's monuments represents selection of an established mode of commemoration. If we assume that men made this choice, they were not expressing women's lower status in their selection but instead were simply choosing what was, to the best of their knowledge, current fashion. In effect women made a greater contribution toward the creation of a stylistic pattern or norm, which ironically became the basis for their own representation even as other women continued to act toward the establishment of newer modes.

Gender associations with mortuary patterns over time and the process of style change this represents therefore give us insight, in this case, into women's roles as agents of change, and provide us with a direct link between individual action and longer-term trends. Gender and agency are not just revealed in this instance; they are intrinsic to trends observed over time. These trends and archaeologists' ability to use them to document the agency of women in mortuary change are not restricted to the well-controlled contexts of dated monuments and documented individuals. Nor are they confined to recent historic contexts, in which the communication of style trends was conveyed in part by the printed page. Similar patterns suggestive of women's active role in directing mortuary trends are evident in a variety of archaeologically documented contexts.

Sixteenth- and Seventeenth-Century Seneca of New York State

The ideal archaeological contexts in which to seek evidence of the active agency of women in mortuary fashion would be burials that are well dated and consistently sexed on the basis of biological indicators and that exhibit clear evidence of differential mortuary treatment for women and men. Identification of differential rates in the adoption of common mortuary treatments also requires very fine chronological control, which is often lacking outside of historically documented contexts. Not surprisingly, archaeological examples that exhibit this type of gender-based pattern together with control over chronology and biological sex determination are more readily available closer in time to the present.

Additional evidence regarding the specific individuals responsible for mortuary treatments is often ambiguous in even the most well documented of historic contexts, as it is in Victorian England. In the absence of clear documentation, the inferred likelihood that a spouse would have some responsibility for the choice of burial treatment can be based only on the probability that he or she would be included among the survivors ultimately responsible for the burial. An example from the post-European-contact Iroquois meets these rather stringent criteria for dating and biological sexing and provides a modicum of documentary evidence for the active role of men and women in burial practice. Although the role of men and women in the provision of goods can be only loosely inferred from the available documentary sources, this example illustrates the likelihood of a more general role for women in the development and transformation of mortuary practices, beyond the limits of Victorian England.

In a series of well-dated sixteenth- to seventeenth-century Seneca cemeteries from New York State, Sempowski (1986) documented persistent inequality in the grave-good associations of male and female burials. In all time periods repre-

Table 4.4. Percentages of Male and Female Graves in Seneca Sites Containing Weapons, Tools, and Ornamental Objects

	Tools and weapons		Ornamental objects	
Year	Male	Female	Male	Female
1570	65	27	29	36
1590	28	26	28	26
1610	83	31	32	31
1630	—	—	—	—
1650	70	27	80	51
1670	73	49	68	60
1680	85	58	58	65

Source: After Sempowski 1986:42.
Note: Dates are the approximate midpoints of site occupations. Dash indicates absence of data.

sented in the sequence, fewer female than male graves contained goods of various kinds, including weapons, tools, and adornments (table 4.4). Sempowski interpreted this consistent pattern as an indication that Iroquois women may have enjoyed lesser status than men, contrary to common assertions concerning the relatively high social status of Iroquois women. The provision of goods is assumed to reflect more or less accurately a status derived from one or more factors including individual wealth, community perceptions of prestige, and social position.

Since a sizeable proportion of graves of both men and women lack any goods, it is unlikely that the provision of goods was a standard reflection of gender status. The alternatives are supported by ethnohistoric accounts describing the solicitude with which the Seneca placed grave goods beside bodies (Wallace 1970:94). Chiefs were described as being buried with their best clothes, guns, traps, and knives, and it was noted that even the poorest people would scrimp and save to buy a respectable robe for their departed friends. Provisioning for the dead could therefore readily be viewed as a function of both individual wealth and community esteem. Eighteenth-century accounts indicate that women's funeral rites were as important as those of men, and one account describes a woman's burial in new clothes decorated with a copious amount and variety of silver and shell ornaments (Beauchamp 1900:90). Interpretation of differential provisioning of the graves of men and women as a reflection of relative status is therefore reasonable insofar as it is based on the role of individual wealth and community participation in burial rites. Its weakness is its lack of consideration for the specific role of women and men in the provision of grave goods, and its failure to account for variable temporal trends, especially the opposing trends in burials with ornamental objects.

Ethnohistoric accounts of the Seneca and related Iroquoian groups indicate a prominent role for women in funeral rites, including digging and preparation of the grave, preparation and burial of the body, and subsequent mourning (Beauchamp 1900:88; Thwaites 1896–1901:39:29–31; Wallace 1970:98). Among the Huron, the death of a wife or a husband required the spouse to remain in mourning and not remarry for a full year (Thwaites 1896–1901:10:273). Iroquois women and men also participated equally in the giving of gifts as condolences at funeral feasts; the equal liberality of women in gift giving was specifically noted by a Jesuit missionary in attendance at one funeral (Thwaites 1896–1901:43: 269). The provisioning of grave goods was widely shared among friends and relatives, but the Franciscan missionary Sagard noted one particular example of a Huron man who remained impoverished because he had given so much to his dead wife (Wrong 1939:213). The scarce data and mix of ethnohistoric sources are insufficient to document who would have had primary responsibility for provisioning the burials of Seneca men and women, but either surviving spouse likely would have had equal opportunity and motivation for contributing to adequate and respectful treatment of the dead.

If Seneca women and men enjoyed variable wealth, and if the burial of either was likely to invoke generous provisioning of grave goods from friends, relatives, and spouses, then why, as Sempowski documents, were fewer women's graves provisioned with durable goods? Initial consideration might suggest either that more men had more goods or that more men were held in esteem among the wider community that provided goods. Alternatively, in keeping with the selection of Victorian Gothic-style monuments, this pattern might show that the provision of grave goods for the dead was a greater concern earlier among women than among men. The latter suggestion is also supported by specific trends in the provisioning of grave goods.

The Seneca burial data for the late sixteenth to mid seventeenth centuries show a roughly equal propensity to inter ornamental objects in the graves of males and females. They show an uneven mix of patterns with respect to the provision of tools and weapons, though the overall percentage of male graves with these items is much larger. In the series of three sites from the latter half of the seventeenth century the trends are much clearer. The percentage of male graves with tools and weapons is much larger but increases relatively little over time. The percentage of female graves provisioned with the same goods more than doubles over a period of approximately 30 years. This pattern may reflect a "trickling down" of utilitarian European trade goods from men to women over time, but it is also consistent with women and men differentially including these items in the burials of their respective spouses. Women's fashion lead would be expressed in the earlier inclusion of tools and weapons in a greater percentage of male graves, while men's lagging adoption of the same practice would be expressed in the increasing percentages of women's graves similarly provisioned. The evidence for this pattern and its interpretation in the same terms as the

Victorian example would be weak if based on these trends alone, but it is strengthened by the observation of opposite trends in the provisioning of men's and women's graves with ornamental objects.

If the provisioning of graves is an expression of wealth, status, or prestige, then the greater percentage of male graves with ornamental objects around 1650 is easily interpreted as an expression of greater relative status. The decrease in male graves and increase in female graves with ornaments over the course of the following 30 years cannot be interpreted in those same terms unless the wealth and status of females was rising just as it was falling for men. Men were either leading a fashion trend away from wearing ornaments, while women lagged behind, or women were leading mortuary fashions away from the inclusion of these items with the dead, while men were still actively adopting the fashion for provisioning female graves in this manner. Either alternative is equally likely, but since the provision of grave goods depended on more than just inclusion of the deceased's personal possessions, the latter alternative may be slightly more likely.

The mode of female burial lags behind that of men in both the common trends toward increasing inclusion of tools and weapons and in the opposite trends for inclusion of ornamental objects. Consistent lag in mortuary fashion can be explained as an expression of either women's lesser wealth and status or their more active role in the creation and transformation of burial fashion. The former explanation requires that survivors passively inter the dead with goods appropriate to their individual wealth and status, while the latter allows for a more active role on the part of survivors in the creation and manipulation of burial modes. This latter perspective is more consistent with recent theoretical trends in mortuary archaeology but also seems more consistent with the limited ethnographic information available, which shows an active role for survivors in the provisioning of graves.

The implication in this case goes well beyond the role of women in establishing and actively transforming modes of burial and commemoration. If the disposition of goods, including European trade goods, was, to some extent at least, in the hands of women, then Iroquoian women's role in the development of the fur trade may have been much greater than has been recognized (see Conkey and Spector 1984:11). Based on trends over time rather than static associations at any one point in time, the patterns Sempowski documented could be used to argue that women's status, as measured by their role in driving economic and cultural developments, was greater than that of men. There is certainly no reason to think that women's roles were any less active and effective in relation to internal social representation or external trade, whatever their ultimate status may have been.

The Seneca example is sufficient to extend the idea of women's agency in the creation and adoption of mortuary fashion into an archaeological context more typical than that of the Victorian cemetery. The precise timing of mortuary practices and the relative roles of men and women in burial treatment, however, are much less likely to be readily discernible and are much more likely to be ambiguous and open to dispute in archaeological contexts where the quality of data is necessarily lacking. The Seneca example also highlights a problem not encountered in the study of specialized mortuary treatments such as Victorian gravestones or other constructions created by the living solely on behalf of the dead. When burial distinctions are marked by the tools, weapons, and adornments used in life, it can be impossible to attribute their provision unambiguously either to the agency of the deceased in amassing the items in life or to the agency of the survivors in contributing them after death. The Seneca burial trends minimally indicate that women and men actively engaged in the fashion process either in providing for themselves in life or in contributing to the dead. In the latter case, the further implication is that women were prominently among the leaders in mortuary fashion, as expressed in the male-biased trends in grave-good associations.

The variable and generally lesser quality of data available in most archaeological contexts makes precise dating almost impossible. Variable preservation can also make it difficult to sex burials accurately and consistently. Normally there is also a complete lack of information regarding who should be considered responsible for the treatment of the dead. Added to these circumstances is the ambiguity that must accompany attribution of grave goods either to ownership by the deceased or to contributions from the living. All of these conditions together mean that a different approach than that applied in the Victorian and Seneca examples is needed to recognize gender-based agency in more remote and much less well documented archaeological contexts. The type of agency revealed in these contexts may also differ in many respects from that which can be shown or inferred in historically documented circumstances. Nonetheless, differential burial treatments of men and women and broader changes in burial mode over time can still provide equally suggestive evidence for the active agency of women in effecting changes in mortuary fashion.

Late Fifth- to Early Seventh-Century Anglo-Saxon England

English Anglo-Saxon burial analysis has a long history, but the past two decades have seen a number of broader scale, synthetic analyses designed to elucidate the social implications of patterns and trends in grave-good associations and grave construction (Arnold 1980; Härke 1990; Lucy 1998). Increasingly, attention has focused on this rich though somewhat uneven body of data to interpret gender roles and status (Lucy 1997, 1998:32–50; Pader 1982; Stoodley 1999). The study of gender in Anglo-Saxon burial contexts has developed over a short period of time. Relatively simple comparisons of wealth based on the number and variety of associated grave goods (Arnold 1980) have quickly given way to contextual analyses of gender- and age-based differences in the type and meaning of goods

(Pader 1982). Recently, broader synthetic overviews have sought to understand in detail the meaning of the forms, variability, and trends in grave goods (Härke 1990, 1992; Stoodley 1999).

Pader's (1982) study clearly showed the difficulties involved in making individual status or social structural interpretations based on simple counts or diversity of grave goods. She particularly noted the difficulties involved in gauging the relative status of men and women on the basis of what are for the most part very different types of goods. Härke's (1990, 1992) elegant multidimensional analysis of Anglo-Saxon weapon burials and their interpretation as warriors' graves showed that it is a mistake to assume that goods interred with an individual were necessarily used by them. He makes a convincing argument that weapons in graves do not indicate real warrior status but instead display the status of the individual's family and symbolically express an ethnically, socially, or ideologically based warrior status to which the family considered itself and the deceased entitled. Stoodley (1999) has extended this same approach to the analysis of engendered burials of men and women to examine questions of when, why, and how grave goods engender burials.

All recent studies agree that there is little if any basis for direct comparison between the grave goods of men and women. Grave-good assemblages that Stoodley (1999:75) has characterized as masculine and feminine exhibit minimal overlap in specific artifact types or symbolic meanings. Therefore, despite the large sample of detailed grave-good descriptions for male and female graves in Anglo-Saxon England, there is seemingly very little basis for the investigation of women's agency in the creation or transformation of grave-good fashions. Anglo-Saxon archaeology has heeded the postprocessual critique (Hodder 1980) and has moved away from interpretations of goods as passive reflections of social status. Instead, stress is placed on the symbolic role of grave goods as signals of gender and other aspects of identity. The individual life and status of the deceased is less the subject of interpretation than is the community of survivors that grant material mortuary expressions to the deceased (see, for example, Stoodley 1999).

Typically, masculine grave-good assemblages are more constrained and standardized to include a limited range of items (Hirst 1985:96; Stoodley 1999:78–79, 136), principally weapons, leaving little room for the agency of women in their variability. Furnished male graves also exhibit little change over time. They show only a sharp increase in numbers from the first half of the fifth century to a peak about the middle of the sixth century, followed by gradual decline and disappearance by the end of the seventh or early eighth century (Härke 1990:30). Female-associated items, consisting largely of dress fittings and jewelry, in contrast, show much greater variability at all times but indicate little evidence of the systematic fashion process based on emulation of prestige-conscious leaders. Nor is it clear who would be the agents of systematic change, since interpretations now attribute the engendering of burials to the family or descent group (Härke

1992:155) or to an undifferentiated burying "community" (Lucy 1997:162; Stoodley 1999:76).

Despite these problems that seemingly preclude application of the same model for mortuary fashion change developed to account for the Victorian and Seneca examples, there are indications of a superficially similar process in limited examples of Anglo-Saxon cemeteries. But rather than serving to extend the same model, analysis of these examples serves instead to highlight the difficulties that might more generally be faced in trying to apply the same understanding of women's agency to more remote, much less well documented, and less chronologically controlled archaeological contexts. It also shows the complications that arise when goods or other mortuary treatments have gender-specific meanings that extend beyond their role as prestige stylistic variants. Comparison of trends in grave-good associations in Anglo-Saxon burials suggests a very different type of agency, though women are still likely to have been active agents. Women's agency in the creation and adoption of mortuary fashions, which is expressed in the Victorian and possibly the Seneca examples in treatments of male burials, is replaced in this case by their active creation of their own material representation in life as much as in death.

Data from three cemeteries—Holywell Row and Westgarth Gardens in Suffolk (Pader 1982) and Sewerby in Yorkshire (Hirst 1985)—show limited patterns of differential adoption of mortuary fashion that, superficially at least, seem similar to those described for Seneca grave goods and Victorian Gothic grave monuments. Although engendered grave assemblages are generally different, two common items, the knife and the buckle, show widespread distribution in the graves of both men and women (Stoodley 1999:30, 34). The available data from Holywell Row, Westgarth Gardens, and Sewerby show a consistent lag in the association of these items with the graves of females.

Studies of these cemeteries have been criticized for their reliance on grave goods for sexing burials and for their basis in partial excavations of cemeteries of unknown overall size (Lucy 1997:152–156; Stoodley 1999:6). Criticism of the use of goods to sex burials has been particularly vociferous (for example, Lucy 1998:34), though controlled comparisons of biological sexing and grave goods have shown that only a tiny number of burials are likely to be mistakenly sexed on the basis of grave goods (Hirst 1985:96; Stoodley 1999:29, 74). In any case, misidentification of the sex of individual burials is unlikely to create false temporal trends. The partial nature of the excavated assemblages introduces an unknown distortion to the data and their analysis, but again this is unlikely to create significant directional trends. Once these cautions are taken into account, the temporal comparison of sex associations of knives and buckles shows some interesting results (table 4.5).

At all three cemeteries, among the burials with grave goods that can be roughly categorized into chronological periods, males lead in their associations

Table 4.5. Male and Female Burials Associated with Knives and Buckles over Time in the Anglo-Saxon Cemeteries of Holywell Row, Westgarth Gardens, and Sewerby

Cemetery	Burials with knives	Burials without knives	Burials with buckles	Burials without buckles
Early period				
Male				
Holywell	9*, 38*	68	9*, 68	38*
Westgarth	10, 11*, 18*, 41 49, 50, 51, 62	25	10, 11*, 41, 50, 51	18*, 25, 49, 62
Sewerby	45, 55	—	55	45
Female				
Holywell	37, 39, 48, 52, 99	10, 13, 46, 47, 69, 82, 89, 92	37, 89	10, 13, 39, 46 ,47, 48, 52, 69, 82, 92, 99
Westgarth	52, 55, 61	7*, 9, 13*, 16*, 26*, 31*, 36, 48	61	7*, 9, 13*, 16*, 26*, 31*, 36, 48, 52, 55
Sewerby	8*, 12*, 15, 35*	57	15, 35*, 57	8*, 12*
Late period				
Male				
Holywell	4, 15*, 29*, 56, 60, 91, 93	30*	4, 30*, 56, 91, 93	15*, 29*, 60
Westgarth	8*, 66*	—	8*, 66*	—
Sewerby	—	—	—	—
Female				
Holywell	1, 11, 14, 16, 21*, 70, 79*, 98	31, 43, 83	11, 21*, 31, 43, 79*	1, 14, 16, 70, 83, 98
Westgarth	27	—	27	—
Sewerby	23*, 49	19, 24	19, 23*	24, 49

Source: For burial numbers shown, see Pader 1982 and Hirst 1985.

Notes: Early period burials include those dated as late fifth to early sixth centuries, early sixth century, mid sixth century, or sixth century generally. Late period burials include those dated as late sixth century, late sixth to early seventh centuries, or seventh century.

* Burials sexed on basis of skeletal elements (all other burials sexed on basis of grave good associations).

with knives and buckles, and females lag behind. Female burials show roughly equal associations with these items only by the late sixth to the early seventh century. Restricting analysis to only those burials sexed on the basis of skeletal indicators (marked with an asterisk in table 4.5) greatly reduces the overall numbers, but the trends remain the same. Over time the association of female burials with knives and buckles becomes comparable to the association of male burials with these items.

The chronological periods are necessarily crude and overlap to some extent, but these problems should serve to obscure rather than to create temporal patterning. The temporal pattern is significant in these three cemeteries and is superficially the same as the temporal trends in Victorian Gothic monuments and in Seneca grave goods, which were used to argue for women's agency in the transformation of modes of burial treatment. The differences between those examples and the use of buckles and knives as burial equipment in Anglo-Saxon England, however, are extensive and inform a wide range of considerations that must be taken into account in seeking to define agency in archaeological contexts.

The difficulty in sexing poorly preserved skeletal remains and the potential circularity of using grave goods to sex graves is amply attested to in this example, though the trends in this case hold for even the small number of biologically sexed burials. The need to use partial and potentially biased samples of cemeteries is also an acknowledged problem. The chronological control needed to follow the social focus and agency of fashion trends is also lacking in this case, though it is still far more refined than is likely to be available in more remote archaeological contexts. All of these issues limit the size of samples available for comparison, which hinders any effort to trace and compare mortuary fashion trends between gender groups.

Combining cemeteries from different regions can increase sample size but is likely to obscure local trends if regional variability in their timing and direction is pronounced. Pader (1982:183), for example, noted the Droxford cemetery in Hampshire as a regional exception for its early association of female burials with knives and buckles. Its inclusion in the sample listed in table 4.5 would have completely obscured any temporal pattern. Regional differences in Anglo-Saxon burial treatments, which are increasingly evident, have led some researchers to advocate more localized studies (Lucy 1998:21). Others continue to support broader regional comparisons, though on a less refined scale of analysis and with due attention to regional differences (Stoodley 1999:11).

Similar problems with sample size and representativeness, chronological control, and regional variability are likely to be common in most archaeological contexts, and in most will be even more pronounced than in the Anglo-Saxon example. All of these problems will obscure and may render hopelessly ambiguous any systematic trends in gender-based differentiation and emulation. Variation in the nature of goods and in the meaning of their association with the dead is an additional problem. The difficulty in attributing grave goods to the agency of particular individuals or groups, alluded to in the Seneca example, is even more pronounced for the Anglo-Saxon period and for almost all prehistoric contexts, in which independent documentary evidence of who was responsible for burial treatment is completely lacking. If burial involves grave goods owned and used by the deceased in life, then who is the agent responsible for their association with the dead? Certainly someone among the living was responsible for the placement of the objects in the grave, but was that someone making a choice from among a range of possible options or merely following prescribed practice in burying with the dead those objects with which an individual was rightfully associated in life? In the latter case, agency to transform burial fashion is within the power of the deceased as much as that of the survivors, if not more. Ironically, the agency of the deceased in creating their own mortuary representation has been all but ignored in some recent Anglo-Saxon studies as a result of efforts to stress the active and dynamic role of the living in creating representations of the dead (for example, Lucy 1998:104, 107).

Härke (1990, 1992) has demonstrated conclusively that weapons often found in male graves are symbolic representations of the status and identity of those with whom they are interred. His results indicate that weapons represent much more than the items used by an individual warrior in life. Their restricted variety also makes it clear that weapons were not a free expression of mere wealth or status aspirations. Competitive differentiation and emulation may be evident in the multiple numbers of some individual weapon types or in the increase in weapon graves up to the mid sixth century, but the limited number and diversity of goods in most weapon burials indicate that they were not elements of unconstrained fashion. Male graves show little change over time. Later decline in the number of weapon graves could be a sign of a practice that had reached social saturation, but the earlier increase in weapon graves could as easily indicate population growth within the segment of society entitled to this display rather than wider dissemination of the practice. Härke (1990:38–39, 1992:154) has shown a consistent stature difference between male burials with and without weapons, which he attributes to ethnic distinctions. The breakdown of the stature differential might indicate that broader emulation of this style of mortuary treatment occurred only in the seventh to eighth century, just as the weapon burial rite was coming to an end.

All indications, then, are that male-associated weapon burials represent the display in death of items with which the same individuals likely would have been associated in life, though not necessarily as the functional weapons of active warriors. Burial may not be a passive reflection of status in life in this case, but it is likely much closer to that reality than it is to one involving the active creation of mortuary representations by the living. The choice for the living seems restricted to whether to inter weapons or not; their choice does not seem to have been open to the creation of new and distinctive modes of burial for men.

Female Anglo-Saxon burials show much more variability in the numbers and diversity of grave goods, and there is greater evidence for competitive emulation and differentiation in the adoption of material display. Although weapons are found with a small number of women's burials, there clearly was little widespread emulation of male burial treatments for women. The increasing association of knives and buckles as part of women's burial costume, in contrast, may represent an active effort among women within at least some communities to adopt particular items previously associated more with men as additions and enhancements to an existing assemblage of dress accessories and jewelry. There is further limited support for this interpretation in the fact that burials associated with amber beads in the Sewerby cemetery are also much more likely to be associated with buckles and knives than are burials associated with blue glass beads (Hirst 1985:76). The timing of the relative popularity of these bead types is not completely clear, but the weight of opinion is that amber beads became more popular (in comparison to the more common glass beads) later in at least in some regions (Hirst 1985:75). The implication, then, is that fashion consciousness expressed in the display of knives and buckles was also expressed in the selection of amber beads. Fashion leadership is also evident in the fact that two of the amber bead burials with knives and buckles (burials 15 and 35) date to the early sixth century, well before these items became more widely associated with women's burials.

The question is whose agency is expressed in the burial of Anglo-Saxon women. The nature of the objects and their age associations suggest that the burial mode for women was a product of their own agency in the acquisition of items and in the adoption of new styles of dress and adornment. Stoodley's (1999:108–110) analysis shows that burials of females between the ages of 20 and 40 exhibit the most jewelry and other items, while young girls and older women have considerably fewer grave goods. This pattern is consistent with a process of inheritance in which mothers passed on to daughters some proportion of their jewelry and other items of display at around the age of puberty. Women between 20 and 40 years of age would still possess and thus would be more likely to be buried with their own goods; any daughters they might have would be less likely to have reached the age of inheritance. Stoodley (1999:132) makes this point with respect to a pair of burials in a single cemetery and cites a similar argument by Halsall (1996:19–20) for Merovingian burials. The implication is that female burials *are* a reflection of their own individual status, wealth, and identity as displayed in life. Certainly this is true on the group scale. Burials associated with engendered items typically also show better health and less evidence of hard labor than female burials that lack these items (Stoodley 1999:124, 138). The same also appears to be true on the scale of individual identity; a woman who died at an age when her display of material wealth in life was most pronounced was also appropriately arrayed in those same items in death.

Stylistic changes in female grave goods therefore indicate women's agency in adding new items to those they might have inherited from either their own or their husbands' families. Whether women or men were also agents with respect to the choice of goods to inter with individuals other than themselves is not known or accessible in this case. The likelihood remains that women were responsible for the choice of goods found in association with female burials, whether it was their own burial or the burial of others for whom they were responsible. The Anglo-Saxon burial example is sufficient to show an active role for women as agents of fashion change. Their motivation to express social status and their ability and desire to direct resources toward the acquisition and ultimate disposition of material symbols of wealth and status is evident in what they may have worn in life or offered to commemorate the dead.

The complexities of the Anglo-Saxon example raise questions about whether fashion concepts based on differentiation and emulation evident on the scale of individual graves within the fine temporal resolution possible in more recent historic contexts, such as Victorian England or the seventeenth-century Seneca, are more widely applicable. The appropriateness of analogies drawn from well-documented and well-dated historic contexts for the interpretation of burials in more remote prehistoric contexts has been questioned before (Bartel 1989). The Anglo-Saxon example is actually a perfect illustration of the problem, since it rests on the cusp between historic contexts from which analogies are drawn and the much cruder scale of temporal resolution and contextual information available in situations in which they are typically applied. The solution is not to apply analogies directly to data of inappropriate quality or resolution, nor to admonish archaeologists that they must somehow seek to improve the quality of their data in order to make such applications possible. Instead, the solution is to seek means of applying the more fundamental principles derived from analogical contexts.

In this case, the analogous principle is the agency of women in consciously creating and adopting prestigious material fashions and in transforming burial practice through either their own choices of adornment or their selection of items or memorials in honor of the dead. The further indication is of women's active role in the transformation of cultural patterns and their role in driving economies predicated on the acquisition and display of prestige goods. Other examples of this broader form of agency are available from more remote prehistoric contexts.

Early Bronze Age Central Europe and Denmark

Gender-based differences and transitions in the relative wealth of European Bronze Age graves have been a common focus of interpretation. Susan Shennan's (1975, 1982) study of successive Early Bronze Age cemeteries in Slovakia, for example, shows a trend toward increasing richness of women's burials over the course of 200–300 years at the very beginning of the Early Bronze Age at around 2000 B.C. The relative number of graves described as rich was approximately equally distributed between men and women at the beginning of this period, but women's graves had increasingly greater numbers of goods in succeeding periods, though men and women were generally associated with different types of artifacts (Shennan 1975:285). Shennan (1982:30–31) explicitly cited the role of emulation and competitive display in the transformation and elaboration of mortuary expression, noting that certain artifact types that came into general currency in the later period were restricted to rich graves in earlier cemeteries. She also noted that a larger proportion of female graves were poor in the earlier than in the later phase, though the average wealth of the richer female graves was the same in both periods. She attributed this pattern to the increasing availability of metal in the later phase and thus to the possibility that metal lost some of its value as a result and therefore became more generally accessible.

The patterns in Early Bronze Age Slovakia exhibit all the hallmarks of the fashion process, with acknowledged fashion leaders, widespread emulation, and relatively rapid change. As in Anglo-Saxon England, the majority of items contributing to burial richness are those associated with a standard female costume worn at burial. The prestige aspirations of women and their role in driving the process of competitive material display are expressed through their own burial with the ornaments they could have worn in life. Although Shennan (1982:30) tentatively attributed the grave-good associations in female graves to the achievement of their status, possibly on marriage, the temporal pattern strongly suggests that women played an instrumental role in the development of this particular prestige economy. The gender-based distinctions in artifact types placed in burials also suggest that trends in men's and women's burials cannot be compared directly, except in relation to an abstract concept of relative richness. The patterns observed might be less an indication of changes in the style of burial than a suggestion of the amount of metal goods owned and worn in life and only incidentally deposited in the grave at death. Nevertheless, this example supports the wider case for women as fashion leaders and as agents of change in mortuary expression. The structure of gender-based status distinctions, if any ever existed, will always be ambiguous when based solely on personal adornment (Cannon 1991), but the importance and the context of women's roles in prestige economies and social competition are more directly open to investigation.

This is the direction that has been taken recently in studies of the early Danish Bronze Age. There a similar albeit less dramatic pattern of increase in the relative richness of women's graves has long been noted and widely interpreted (Gibbs 1987; Gilman 1981:1; Levy 1995, 1999; Randsborg 1973, 1975, 1984). The measures used in the comparison of grave goods vary from weights of bronze and gold to the diversity of items, but the general consensus is that though women were generally buried with a lesser amount and variety of goods the relative richness of their graves increased over time. This pattern is particularly evident between Early Bronze Age Periods II and III, a span of 300–500 years around 1600–1100 B.C., though Gibbs (1987:84) shows a longer trend in the increasing diversity of women's grave goods dating from the Late Neolithic in northeastern Zealand.

The mortuary data from Early Bronze Age Denmark generally have been interpreted in relation to potential changes in the status and role of women in society over time. Levy (1999:66), however, has recently viewed the trends in grave goods and later hoards of bronze objects as an indication that both women and men wore, displayed, and manipulated valuable ritual objects made of exotic raw materials and that metal wealth was controlled by both men and women. The role of women could also be as evident in the decision to inter metal goods in the graves of men as it is in the trend toward increasing display of metal adornments worn by women. The shift toward cremation and the eventual lack of gender distinctions in grave goods in the later Bronze Age could further be seen as the long-term culmination of a cycle of display led as much by women as by men, if not more. By then the display of material wealth was expressed in the deposit of ritual hoards rather than in burials, but female-associated artifacts are dominant in the ritual hoards, especially in the Late Bronze Age (Levy 1999:68).

Summary and Conclusion

All these examples of gender-based differential forms or rates of change in burial treatment illustrate a fashion process involving deliberate differentiation and emulation. The process in these cases develops over relatively short periods of time, from less than 50 to no more than 400 years. They all show evidence for fashion leaders who initiate what later become more widespread standards of mortuary expression. The examples also show some evidence that the agency of change in mortuary expression is attributable to women, regardless of whether trends are expressed in the burials of men, for which women may have been responsible, or their own burial with the adornments they wore in life. The evidence also suggests that women were more active in material display and fashion trends by virtue of their greater awareness of prestige forms.

These examples highlight the agency of women, but they do not support any broader generalization that women are inherently more prestige or fashion conscious. This generalization has proven untenable in linguistic studies (James 1996), despite ample empirical evidence for women's lead in the adoption of prestige language variants in a variety of cultural contexts. The examples of gender-based differential mortuary practice described here were selected to make the case for women's agency; other examples might equally illustrate the agency of men or agency shared between gender divisions. As in linguistic studies, the challenge is to use these empirical results as a basis for determining the particular contexts that might favor women's enhanced awareness of prestige fashion and encourage their agency in effecting change in mortuary or other forms of material expression. Investigations to document the mobility of women or patterns of marriage or kinship, for example, might provide evidence that enhanced prestige consciousness was a product of interaction within a wider social sphere. The argument that women's fashion awareness is in some cases a product of social vulnerability in circumstances of change, especially on the death of a husband, could also be the subject of investigation.

Certainly the role of women in the development and operation of prestige economies should not be underestimated. Despite assertions to the contrary (for example, Clark and Blake 1994:30), some women in various circumstances aspire and act to acquire prestige and whatever power may derive from its possession. The differential adoption among women of prestige variants of burial display also indicates that agency is not homogenous with respect to gender any more than it is with respect to social class or people in general. Differences in timing among women and between women and men in the adoption of new forms of mortuary expression indicate some propensity among women to use styles of adornment and mortuary expression to achieve and maintain prestige recognition. Whether this implies "a resort to subtler contrivances" to express status (Kehoe 1999) is still open to interpretation and debate, but the effect in creating and transforming prevailing modes of material and mortuary expression in particular is undeniable.

Investigation of the reasons for women's particular fashion consciousness or agency in effecting change in mortuary practices is an enormous undertaking in itself. All that has been illustrated in the examples presented here is that it is possible to identify agency in a variety of ways in the patterns of mortuary representation that are archaeologically available. These examples also serve as additional caution, if any is still needed, against the simple equation of status with differences in mortuary treatment. The focus instead is on change and on the role of individual choice in effecting change (see Conkey and Spector 1984:22–23). The further emphasis is on locating this particular type of agency differentially within gender or other social groups. Mortuary analysis focused explicitly on change is less concerned with the establishment of individual or group identity than with the evolving process of identity negotiation (for example, Sofaer Derevinski 2000). The examples described here illustrate the active negotiation and representation of identity among women, among families on the part of women, and between women and men. This process is partially expressed in burial treatments but in different ways, using different media, and principally directed by different agents at different times. Explicit focus on the role of women in effecting change highlights the type of agency and individual motivation that must ultimately be invoked in any effort to explain change in mortuary practice. This focus stands in contrast to more common and much simpler approaches that have sought only to assess relative gender status on the basis of variation in burial treatment.

The patterns illustrated here may represent only a small fraction of the total range of temporal trends in burial treatment, and the active role of women that they suggest may be only one factor among several responsible for change in even these contexts. The complexities of burial data increasingly are seen to preclude simple interpretations in mortuary archaeology (Whittle 2001:45), but it is precisely this complexity that makes the study of agency, agents, and the contexts for differential agency both possible and necessary. While opportunities for simple classificatory interpretation of the past are thereby diminished, the prospects for understanding everyday lives and perceptions and their role in the creation of culture patterns are immeasurably enhanced.

5

Chiribaya Political Economy

A Bioarchaeological Perspective

Jane E. Buikstra, Paula D. Tomczak, Maria Cecilia Lozada Cerna,
and Gordon F. M. Rakita

Over the past 30 years, mortuary site studies have become increasingly integrated into the fabric of Americanist archaeology. During this period, data derived from both ancient and modern cemeteries have been used to address issues ranging from health to cosmology. In this study, based on excavations of millennium-old sites from the west coast of South America, we will discuss the emergence of social, political, and economic complexity through the investigation of ancient cemeteries and the materials recovered therein. At the outset, it must be emphasized that this is a thoroughly collaborative venture, with key contributions made by each of the coauthors.

Chiribaya

The ancient Andean Chiribaya culture is commonly described as a late Middle Horizon/Late Intermediate coastal phenomenon, influenced by preexisting altiplano and coastal traditions alike (Dauelsberg 1972–1973a, 1972–1973b; Lumbreras 1972, 1972–1973; Nuñez Atencio 1972–1973; Owen 1993; Rice 1989; Stanish 1992). Diagnostic Chiribaya materials, primarily ceramic technical attributes and decorative motifs (Belan Franco 1981a, 1981b; Ghersi Barrera 1956; Jessup 1990a, 1991; Owen 1993; Santos Ramirez 1983), have been found from the coastal Tambo valley on the north to the Azapa valley within northern Chile. While the distribution of Chiribaya ceramics extends into the sierra (Stanish 1992), the most complex sequence is centered within the coastal Osmore drainage of southern Peru (figure 5.1). Many Chiribaya sites appear to have been positioned to maximize the extractive potential of various resource zones, for example, San Gerónimo on the coast, Chiribaya Baja, Loreto Viejo, and Algodonal within the inland agricultural valley of the Osmore River (Jessup 1987, 1990a, 1990b, 1991; Owen 1993; Stanish 1992). Evidence of complexity is well documented at the site of Chiribaya Alta, where over 15 hectares bear evidence of agricultural terraces, more than nine cemeteries, residential and public spaces, a "defensive" wall, and both elaborate and simple tombs (Buikstra 1988, 1995; Jessup 1991).

The chronological development of the Chiribaya tradition, based primarily upon information derived from cemetery contexts, is interpreted variously. Within the Azapa valley, radiocarbon dates as early as the ninth century A.D. have encouraged archaeologists to emphasize local continuity from Middle Horizon times, while recognizing cultural influences from the altiplano (Dauelsberg 1972–1973a, 1972–1973b; Foccaci Aste 1981, 1983; Muñoz 1983; Tartaglia 1980). Archaeologists working within the Osmore drainage, however, have argued that Chiribaya is exclusively a post-Tiwanaku late Middle Horizon phenomenon that emerged in the wake of a "collapse" of Tiwanaku administrative control emanating from the middle Osmore valley (Bawden 1989; García Márquez 1988; Owen 1993; Stanish 1989, 1992; Stanish and Rice 1989; Sutter 1997). Tiwanaku colonies were well established within the middle Osmore valley, with maximum density during Tiwanaku V times, A.D. 725–950 (Goldstein 1989a, 1989b, 1993). In a recent paper, Goldstein and Owen (2000) suggest that this Tiwanaku or Chen Chen phase may have developed slightly later, approximately A.D. 800–1050.

Although initial radiocarbon dates from the Osmore drainage supported a Late Intermediate timing for Chiribaya peoples, recent investigations have placed initial Chiribaya development well within Tiwanaku (Middle Horizon) times (Buikstra et al. 2001). This revision suggests that the relationship between Chiribaya and Tiwanaku peoples may have been more complex than is presumed by the standard culture-evolutionary paradigm. Here we consider this complexity from the perspective of cemetery excavations at the Chiribaya sites of San Gerónimo, Chiribaya Alta, and El Yaral (see figure 5.1). Lines of evidence include artifact distributions, artificial cranial deformation, and isotopic evidence of diet. Variation in these attributes is explored, followed by the implications of these data for the interpretation of local political economies.

The Sites

The site of San Gerónimo is located approximately 200 meters from the ocean, at the mouth of the Osmore River. The site was first reported as "Boca del Rio" by Ghersi Barrera (1956) and continues to suffer the ongoing impact of an active barrio of the municipality of Ilo. Although the total area of ancient occupation is much more extensive, estimated by Jessup as covering a natural terrace of 200 x 500 meters, the materials discussed here were recovered during a 1988 rescue excavation within a 21 x 21 meter block (Jessup 1990b; Jessup and Torres Pino 1990). While diagnostic Early Ceramic, Tiwanaku, Estuquiña, and Historic materials were encountered during the 1988 excavation, the major site compo-

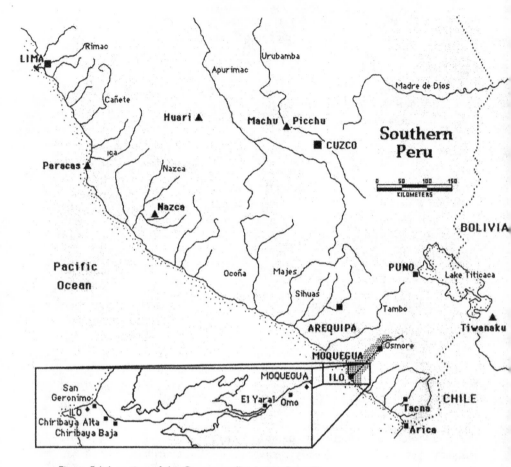

Figure 5.1. Location of the Osmore valley in southern Peru.

nent was clearly Chiribaya, including ceramics described by Jessup (1990a, 1990b, 1991) as belonging to Chiribaya's Middle (Yaral) and Late (San Gerónimo) phases. None of Jessup's Early Chiribaya wares (Algarrobal) were discovered. Rectangular tombs and ostentatious grave wealth characterize San Gerónimo, as do artifacts emphasizing marine resource extraction.

During 1989 and 1990, excavations were conducted at Chiribaya Alta, which is both the largest and the most complex Osmore valley Chiribaya site discovered to date (Buikstra 1995; Jessup 1991; Owen 1993). The site is located approximately 5 kilometers from the coast, on an escarpment overlooking the Osmore valley. As illustrated in figure 5.2, nine distinct cemeteries across the approximately 600 x 600 meter site were sampled, yielding a total of 307 tombs (Buikstra 1995). Diagnostic ceramics from each of Jessup's phases were recovered. Radiocarbon dates indicate that the earliest Chiribaya interments within the Osmore drainage were located at Chiribaya Alta. These were encountered within Cemetery 7, which extends under the "defensive" earthwork that encircles a portion of the site. Other cemeteries document the full temporal extent of the Chiribaya occupation within the Osmore valley (Buikstra et al. 2001).

The site of El Yaral (1000 meters above sea level) is located at the base of the middle Osmore valley, adjacent to the point at which the river becomes subterranean prior to its emergence within the lower valley (García Márquez 1988; Rice 1989, 1993). Two distinct cemeteries were sampled (Buikstra 1995; Lozada Cerna and Torres Pino 1991), yielding a total of 99 individuals. From Cemetery 1, 47 tombs were excavated; these included a few remains associated with very late Tiwanaku (Tumilaca) diagnostic artifacts. Cemetery 2 yielded the remains of

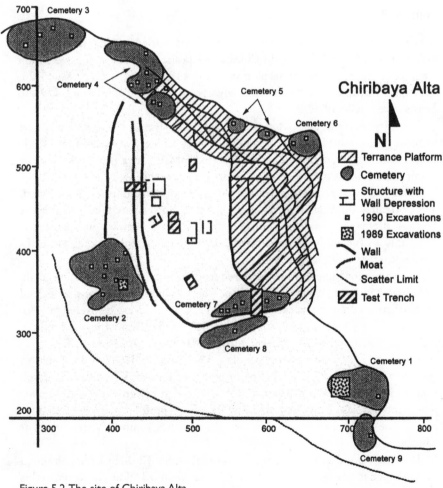

Figure 5.2. The site of Chiribaya Alta.

52 individuals. Ceramics recovered in both cemeteries could be identified as Algarrobal and Yaral types. No San Gerónimo vessels were recovered at this site.

Grave-good assemblages at El Yaral are clearly less rich overall than those from sites such as Chiribaya Alta and San Gerónimo. One or two baskets, one or two ceramic vessels, and one or two gourd containers typically accompanied the deceased. This distinctive funerary pattern, which lacks the ostentation of the lower Osmore valley sites, may reflect a long-standing tradition that extends across millennia (Buikstra 1995). This does not mean, however, that the ritual life of those living at El Yaral was impoverished. On the contrary, nine camelid sacrifices were associated with a large public structure, and an adult male wrapped in camelid skins was buried at the door of another building (Buikstra 1995; García Márquez 1988; Rice 1993).

Tomb 419

While the tombs within and between the cemeteries varied considerably, the most elaborate was Tomb 419 from the Chiribaya Alta site (figure 5.3). Located within Cemetery 4, near the edge of the plateau, Tomb 419 was excavated on March 23, 1990. To provide a context for other analyses of tomb complexity, Tomb 419 will be described in detail here.

Funerary offerings associated with the capping layer of the tomb included 4 camelid skulls, camelid feet, a broken pitcher, and 3 large wooden litters. While only 4 other occurrences of litters are reported for Chiribaya Alta, they are more common at San Gerónimo, where 17 were encountered.

Tomb 419 was rectangular, with the long axis oriented northeast–southwest. The horizontal dimensions of the tomb, 3.5 x 0.6 meters, are unique within the Osmore drainage. The depth, however, of less than a meter is unremarkable. Long axis walls exhibited stone construction with mud chinking; the short walls were not lined.

Three mummy bundles were recovered from within the tomb, all facing north. Offerings had been clustered around each corpse. Preservation of textiles and other organic remains was excellent. Most grave goods were recovered in association with a 40–50-year-old male (Specimen #3704) located in the southern aspect of the tomb base. Adjacent to the male was a 40–50-year-old female (Specimen #3758), with a slightly younger (35–45 years old) female positioned to the north (Specimen #3610). Having three sets of remains within a single tomb was itself unusual, as was the nature of the associated 137 grave goods. The male interment was associated with as many objects as both females considered together. The quantity of metal items also distinguishes Tomb 419 from others at Chiribaya Alta.

This grave-good assemblage is thus unusual within Chiribaya Alta, although similarly rich tombs were encountered at San Gerónimo. Unique, however, to this site is the presence of three interments that appear to have been entombed at the

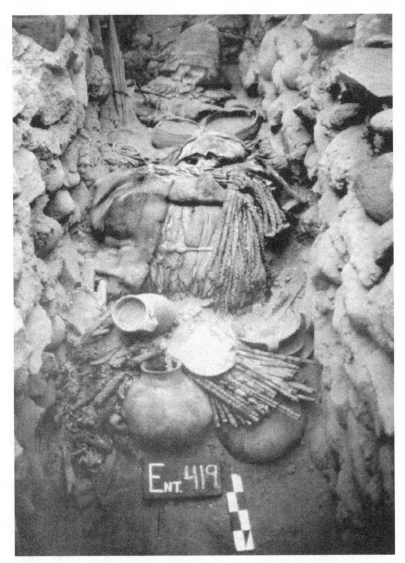

Figure 5.3. Tomb 419 at Chiribaya Alta. Photograph by the Chiribaya
Project, Programa Contisuyo.

same time. Each was positioned in precisely the same manner, seated with the legs
flexed toward the chest and arms slightly flexed and encircling the knees. The
composition of the enclosing wool cordage as well as both the internal and the
external knots used in mummy bundle construction were virtually identical
across all three interments. According to Juana Lazo (personal communication),
who has unwrapped more than 100 Chiribaya mummy bundles preparatory to

textile analysis, such knots are unique among the Chiribaya Alta, El Yaral, and Algodonal samples.

All three bodies were dressed in four garments. The male's shirt was short and trapezoidal in outline, with a *taparrabo* or loincloth being the other interior garment. The internal clothing for both females comprised a long dress; the external for each was an unusually large shawl, similar to a cape. While the internal textiles for all three individuals exhibited evidence of wear, the additional shirts and dresses were new, of unusual proportions, and not finished in the manner typical of items worn on a daily basis. It appears, therefore, that the innermost clothing constituted personal items while the remaining layers were prepared specifically for the funerary context. Numerous *panuelos* (bags containing coca) were recovered within each of the mummy bundles.

Given the richness of this tomb, located within the largest and most complex of the Chiribaya sites, it is important to establish the chronological placement of Tomb 419 within Chiribaya Alta and in relationship to other Chiribaya sites.

Time

The Chiribaya culture was first defined ceramically as a coastal entity that developed during the Late Intermediate period (A.D. 1000–1476). It has been characterized as postdating direct Tiwanaku influences and predating the expansion of the Inca Empire (Bawden 1989; García Márquez 1988; Owen 1993; Stanish 1989, 1992; Stanish and Rice 1989; Sutter 1997). Until recently, most of the temporal associations for Chiribaya were based upon stratigraphic relationships and ceramic seriation. Ceramic-based chronologies have been used to argue that late Tiwanaku (or Tumilaca) peoples predate and were perhaps ancestral to several temporally sequential, ceramically distinct, coastal Chiribaya groups.

The earliest of the Chiribaya sequence is characterized by Algarrobal ceramics, linked to Tumilaca by stylistic tradition (figure 5.4). Following the Algarrobal series is the Yaral assemblage, defined in terms of standardized design elements and uniform forms. The San Gerónimo tradition succeeds Yaral and is characterized by a virtual explosion of forms, simplified designs, and a paste similar to that for the Yaral materials. This typology, laboriously developed through considerations of site stratigraphy and ceramic stylistic and technical analyses, has guided most studies of Late Intermediate sites from the south central Andes (Bawden 1989; Jessup 1991; Lozada Cerna et al. 1996). In the course of our current work, we decided to develop a series of collagen ^{14}C dates from human remains recovered with the distinctive ceramic styles (Buikstra et al. 2001).

Thirty-four dates were dendrochronologically calibrated and 41 years subtracted to balance the differences in atmospheric ^{14}C between the northern and southern hemispheres. As illustrated in figure 5.5, even when corrected for the "old carbon problem," the earliest dates clearly identify a Chiribaya presence by

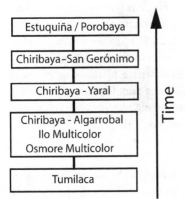

Figure 5.4. Development of
Chiribaya pottery design styles.

A.D. 900, which is approximately two centuries earlier than most published start-dates for the Late Intermediate period on the southern coast of Peru. Interestingly, when dates associated with specific ceramic types are compared to typological dating, most types, with the exception of Tumilaca materials, are shifted to earlier times (Buikstra et al. 2001). Thus, it appears that Chiribaya peoples were living on the coast while Tiwanaku colonies were flourishing within the middle valley at sites such as Omo M10, where a temple complex replicates the

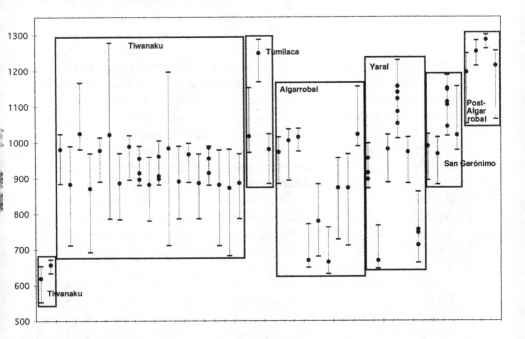

Figure 5.5. Method A intercept dates from Tiwanaku, Tumilaca, and Chiribaya contexts, grouped by ceramic association.

Akapana, located at the site of Tiwanaku itself. There is strong archaeological evidence that the mid-valley colonists followed altiplano traditions and provided surplus agricultural products to the Tiwanaku state (Goldstein 1989a, 1989b, 1990a, 1990b). The apparent boundary or frontier between the middle and lower Osmore valleys may reflect distinctive, contrastive histories of political alliance formation. Active conflict between Chiribaya and Tiwanaku peoples is not documented archaeologically, however, suggesting the presence of a per-ceived but not defended frontier. Distinctive genetic differences between the lower-valley Chiribaya and mid-valley Tiwanaku peoples (Lozada Cerna 1998) reinforces this construct.

The newly generated radiocarbon dates also permit the development of a chronology for the cemeteries excavated at Chiribaya Alta (figure 5.6). Cemetery 4, which contains Tomb 419, dates to the middle period of occupation, when several other cemeteries were also active. The three earlier mortuary areas, cem-eteries 7, 3, and 9, may reflect sequential use. There are two cemeteries (6 and 8) with more recent dates.

Diet

The next data set to be considered characterizes resource consumption, which is assumed to be related to economic factors, especially food production. Appropri-ate techniques for such paleodietary reconstruction are stable carbon and nitro-gen isotope analyses, which clearly separate groups who consumed primarily marine foods from those who consumed more terrestrial resources (Ambrose 1993; Ambrose et al. 1997; Chisholm et al. 1982; Hutchinson et al. 1998; Norr 1995; Schoeninger et al. 1983; Walker and DeNiro 1986). Bone collagen has been the most commonly analyzed tissue fraction; however, recent studies dem-onstrate that carbon atoms of collagen come primarily from dietary protein, rather than from protein, carbohydrates, and lipids (Ambrose and Norr 1993; Tieszen and Fagre 1993). Thus, when individuals consume protein and nonpro-tein resources, collagen isotopic values may not accurately reflect the whole diet (Ambrose et al. 1997). The difference between collagen values and diet is known as the diet-to-collagen fractionation factor and is dependent on the isotopic com-position of dietary protein relative to the whole diet (Ambrose and Norr 1993). As a result, collagen isotopes do not have a consistent fractionation factor. By contrast, bone apatite carbonate ratios reflect the whole diet (Ambrose and Norr 1993; Tieszen and Fagre 1993).

In this chapter we present carbon isotope results from bone collagen analysis. These results are consistent with recently developed results for bone carbonate (Tomczak 2001). Results will be compared to a model local food web, which is corrected for depletion of historic carbon (figure 5.7). We present data for 58 samples from Chiribaya Alta, along with 18 from San Gerónimo and 28 from El

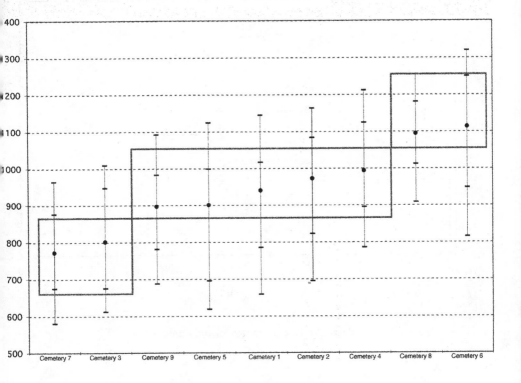

Figure 5.6. Distribution of ¹⁴C dates for Chiribaya Alta. Cemeteries are grouped into early, middle, and late periods of occupation.

Yaral (Tomczak 1995). Tiwanaku data reported by Sandness (1992) from the mid-valley Omo skeletal series are also considered.

Looking first at an evaluation for the three spatially distinct Chiribaya sites, along with the comparative Tiwanaku sample (figure 5.8), we find that the isotope distributions clearly reflect proximity to the coast. San Gerónimo and Chiribaya Alta present strong evidence for marine resource consumption, which is less evident at El Yaral. Even so, El Yaral shows some marine dependence, which contrasts with patterns developed for mid-valley Tiwanaku sites such as Omo, where terrestrial resources such as maize dominate.

Turning to the nine cemeteries at Chiribaya Alta (figure 5.9), we can clearly see that the earlier cemeteries (3, 5, and 7, all of which predate A.D. 1000) show strong marine signals. By approximately A.D. 1000, however, marked intercemetery dietary differences develop, with Cemetery 4 (including Tomb 419) presenting the most extreme evidence for marine resource consumption of any Chiribaya

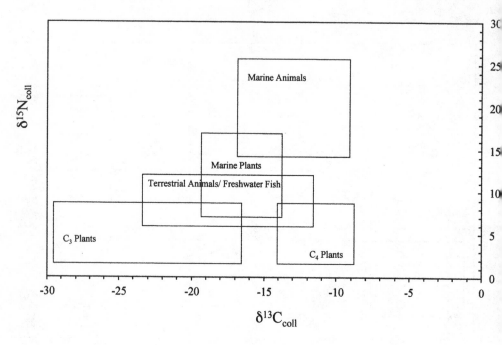

Figure 5.7. Carbon and nitrogen isotopic ranges for the Osmore valley.

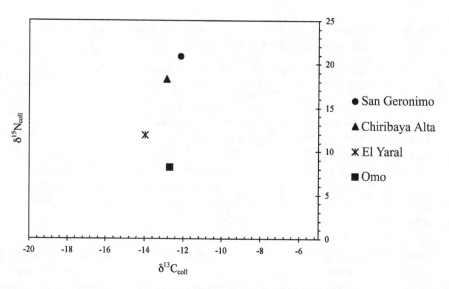

Figure 5.8. Carbon and nitrogen isotopic values within the Osmore valley.

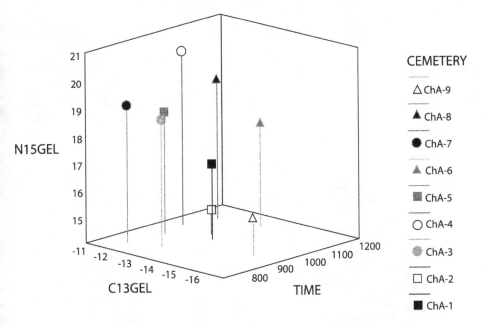

Figure 5.9. Carbon and nitrogen isotopic values within the Chiribaya Alta cemeteries.

Alta cemetery. Other contemporaneous cemeteries, however (such as 1, 2, and 9), denote significantly different dietary profiles. Thus, at Chiribaya Alta, marine resource dependence dominates during earlier periods, while diversity characterizes the post–A.D. 1000 time frame. Within this post–A.D. 1000 diversity, tombs associated with massive grave wealth maintain evidence of marine resource consumption.

Cranial Deformation

Recently, Lozada Cerna and colleagues (1996; also Lozada Cerna 1998) conducted an analysis of cranial deformation found within the three sites used in this analysis. They discovered that 40 percent of the skulls were normal and 60 percent were deformed. A significant portion of the skulls from Chiribaya Alta Cemeteries 4 and 7 as well as at San Gerónimo were deformed (Lozada Cerna et al. 1996). Conversely, very few skulls from El Yaral were deformed (Lozada Cerna et al. 1996). Of the deformed skulls, Lozada and colleagues (1996) identified four distinct types of deformation: annular (turban type), fronto-occipital flat, fronto-occipital round, and fronto-occipital slight (figure 5.10).

While there was no clear patterning according to gender, there were significant correlations between ceramic associations and type of deformation (Lozada Cerna et al. 1996). The association of Algarrobal ceramics with individuals with

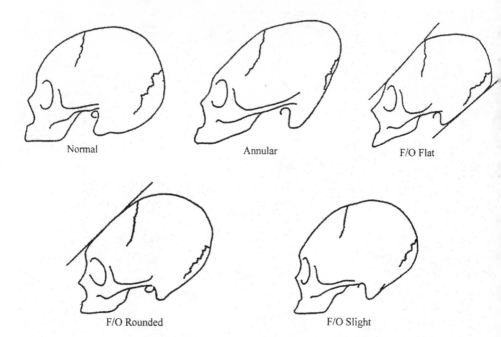

Normal

Annular

F/O Flat

F/O Rounded

F/O Slight

Figure 5.10. Cranial deformation types (F/O indicates fronto-occipital).

fronto-occipital slight deformation indicates that this type is common in the earliest Chiribaya phase (Lozada Cerna et al. 1996). In contrast, annular deformation seems to have been a late Chiribaya phenomenon, since individuals exhibiting it were buried almost exclusively with San Gerónimo ceramics (Lozada Cerna et al. 1996).

The correlations between ceramic type and cranial deformation also translate into patterns of deformation by site and cemetery. Individuals at the San Gerónimo site and Cemetery 4 at Chiribaya Alta most frequently exhibit annular deformation, while those at Chiribaya Alta Cemetery 7 exhibit the fronto-occipital flat deformation (Lozada Cerna et al. 1996). The fronto-occipital slight type is present only in individuals buried at Chiribaya Alta Cemeteries 1 and 2, El Yaral, and the Tumilaca site of Algodonal (Lozada Cerna 1998; Lozada Cerna et al. 1996). Most individuals buried at Chiribaya Alta Cemetery 4 exhibit the same deformation type as those at San Gerónimo; this is a type of deformation different from that common to individuals buried in the contemporaneous Cemeteries 1 and 2. Similarly, individuals interred at Chiribaya Alta Cemetery 7 exhibit a type of deformation distinct from that which characterizes individuals from the contemporaneous Cemeteries 3 and 5 (Lozada Cerna 1998; Lozada Cerna et al.

1996). These patterns suggest social links that mirror those indicated by dietary and artifact analyses.

The females within Tomb 419 display the annular type of cranial deformation typical of San Gerónimo and associated by Lozada Cerna (1998) with occupationally specialized *pescadores*. The male from Tomb 419, while he displays the isotopic signature associated with marine resources, presents the fronto-occipital deformation typical of the agricultural *laboradores*. His grave-good assemblage also contains the occupational signatures of the laboradores, along with musical instruments, quantities of llama remains, and *keros* (ceremonial vessels). Lozada Cerna (1998), adapting an ethnohistoric model developed by Rostworowski (1977, 1981, 1989, 1991), interprets the male as a paramount lord of the Chiribaya *señorío*. Lozada Cerna's (1998) study of inherited skeletal attributes suggests, however, that unlike Rostworowski's example, the Chiribaya señorío was not genetically differentiated. Occupational specialization did not correlate with marriage patterns.

The Big, Speculative Picture

In sum, our suite of radiocarbon dates indicates that there were Chiribaya peoples on the Osmore coast at the same time Tiwanaku peoples were cultivating maize within the middle valley. Marine resource consumption is signaled within the earliest cemeteries at Chiribaya Alta and maintains a high profile among the elite when evidence of sociopolitical inequalities develops around A.D. 1000.

To further explore the meaning behind these patterns, the latter portion of the central-valley Tiwanaku occupation must be elaborated. As indicated in figure 5.8, the Tiwanaku V peoples from the Omo site were not consuming marine resources. They were, most probably, growing and eating significant amounts of maize while contributing surpluses to the altiplano Tiwanaku state. With waning influence from the Lake Titicaca region, evidence of hostility emerges within the middle Osmore valley. The temple complex at Omo M10 suffered depredation, while defensive earthworks emerge as boundaries for the later Tumilaca sites such as M11 (Buikstra 1995; Goldstein 1989a, 1989b). It is obvious that the so-called Pax Tiwanaku was over and that alliances with altiplano *ayllus* (a type of social group unique to the Andean region) were no longer sufficient to buffer local political stresses. In this circumstance, it would appear that new partnerships were being sought by late Tiwanaku peoples, notably with coastal lineages associated with productive marine food webs. It is at this juncture, circa A.D. 1000, that evidence of social inequalities emerges on the coast, and it is at this time that marine resources become evident in mid-valley diets in sites such as El Yaral. Elaborate coastal tombs, such as 419, include several keros and multiple camelid remains. We consider this evidence of *chicha* (maize beer) consumption and feasting symbolically linked to distant altiplano rituals.

The boundary or frontier between Chiribaya and Tiwanaku peoples had thus become permeable by A.D. 1000. Late Tiwanaku (Tumilaca) peoples actively sought alliances with coastal groups to establish new power relationships in the absence of Tiwanaku state control. From coastal sites flowed goods and labor for food production, resources previously distributed and monitored under altiplano influence. In complementary fashion, such relationships enhanced the significance of foreign goods and exotic rituals for the Chiribaya people, leading to social inequalities based upon economic production and trade and reinforced by ideology.

However speculative this interpretation may be, it does provide a point of departure for further problem-oriented studies. It also serves to illustrate the importance of bioarchaeological data derived from mortuary sites in addressing political and economic issues.

Acknowledgments

This work has benefited from the support of the National Science Foundation (BNS89-20769), the Bioanthropology Foundation, Centro Mallqui, Fundación Contisuyu, the University of New Mexico, and the University of Chicago.

6

Social Dimensions of Mortuary Space

Wendy Ashmore and Pamela L. Geller

Spatial dimensions are well established as informing archaeologists' mortuary analyses. Earlier compendia on the archaeology of death highlight contributions from processualist archaeology, especially systems models, and from early critiques (for example, Brown 1971a; Chapman et al. 1981). In these and related works, analysts frequently draw attention to space and examine burial locations and distributions as indices of social role and rank of the deceased (for example, Peebles and Kus 1977). The much-discussed Saxe/Goldstein hypothesis also deals centrally with space, in linking existence of discrete burial grounds to the importance of competition among corporate groups for critical localized resources (for example, Charles and Buikstra 1983; Goldstein 1976, 1981; Saxe 1970). Such analyses, involving individual and community social scales, continue to provide extremely fruitful inferences (for example, Brown 1995b; Buikstra and Charles 1999; Morris 1991). With Beck's (1995) volume, *Regional Approaches to Mortuary Analysis,* emphasis on space took explicit center stage, its contributors arguing both that treatment of the dead could be an elongated process rather than a discrete event and, of equal importance, that understanding mortuary processes requires a regional scale of analysis. As Larsen (1995:261) comments in closing the Beck volume: "Previous work in mortuary archaeology—although certainly not all—focused on single burials within the confines of individual archaeological sites. However, time and again, the contributors to the volume demonstrate that representation is potentially compromised by study of only part of a mortuary landscape."

Inferences drawn from spatial dimensions have thus grown in overall range of pertinent scales. They have also expanded in concert with changes in theoretical perspectives, in both spatial and mortuary studies (for example, Silverman and Small 2002). While acknowledging that social information in mortuary space has been explored unevenly across traditions of archaeological inquiry, we focus here on mortuary spaces of one cultural tradition and consider how studies of the ancient Maya and their neighbors illustrate interpretive potentials of particular kinds of spatialized mortuary studies.

Mayanist Patricia McAnany and her colleagues characterized concisely the ways in which mortuary analyses, generally, changed in the last third of the twentieth century. In their words: "The archaeological study of mortuary ritual has expanded theoretically from a reconstruction of status grades based upon burial accoutrements and interment facility . . . or of territoriality maintained through descent lines . . . to include a semiotic study of the messages and symbolic language encoded in mortuary customs by and for the living" (McAnany et al. 1999:129). The same authors acknowledge other important changes. These include heightened recognition of cross-cultural diversity in beliefs about the partibility of the human body at death; in some societies and cultures, crania, femora, or other isolated skeletal elements are often subject to differential postmortem treatment, thereby providing clues to worldview and beliefs about the individual (for example, Bradley 1995; Joyce 1998). Other analytic avenues include attention to the sensual aspects of death, including sensory involvement with corpses as well as emotional expression of mourning and loss (for example, Kus 1992; Meskell 2000; Parker Pearson 1999; Tarlow 1999). Several analysts urge more fully nuanced examination of the social fabric enfolding the living and the dead, attending much more closely to dimensions of gender, class, faction, age, sexuality, and individuality (Geller 2000; Haviland 1997; Joyce 1999; Meskell 1999, 2000; Reeder 2000). Even as we explore new potentials for more sophisticated social understandings from mortuary analysis, we continue to recognize that the social implications of mortuary remains are often intricately subtle and ambiguous (for example, compare Duncan, this volume).

Social information about individuals, groups, and worldview is often materialized in spatial arrays. In this chapter, we consider *mortuary space* as an analytical domain embracing scales ranging from within individual interments and other forms of disposition, to distributions of burial sites across the landscape. At any scale, key attributes of spatial structure are location, orientation, and arrangement. Mindful of the compelling need for a regional scale when analyzing mortuary—and other—practices (for example, Billman and Feinman 1999), we point here to select extant examples of analyses set specifically at smaller scales within the Maya region. In so doing, we also call for regional reassessment of the expanding information set of which these instances are a part (for example, Bradley 1995; Welsh 1988).

The very deliberateness that characterizes much mortuary behavior facilitates archaeological study, protecting any spatial order intended by those who placed the deceased at rest. At the same time, apparent preservation of spatial structure impels us to proceed cautiously. Mortuary remains have lost their signaling innocence, and we risk overinferring symbolic messaging where none may have been intended. Observed patterns in location, orientation, and arrangement may materialize nonreflective aspects of style and custom rather than reflective and iconic expressions of social standing or worldview. Conversely, apparent *lack* of spatial patterning may be quite socially informative, indicating more fluid social

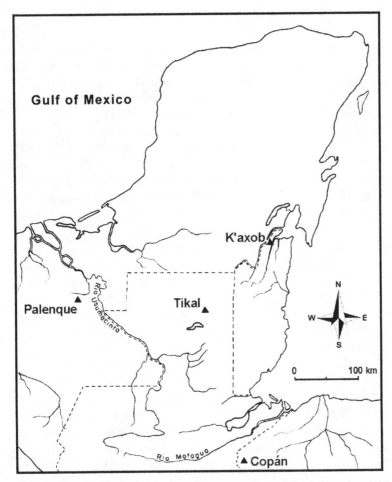

Figure 6.1. The Maya region of Mesoamerica, showing places mentioned in the text.

identities for the dead and for their relations to the world of the living (for example, Geller 2000). Drawing from regional analytic contexts may clarify patterns (or their absence) by removing obscuring effects of more limited samples (for example, Beck 1995; Buikstra 1981). The key to social inference on any sample, of course, is critical invocation of analogy and social theory (for example, Geller 2000, 2004; Joyce 1998, 1999; Meskell 1999).

In this chapter, we illustrate concretely only a few of the social dimensions of mortuary space, with select recent examples from the ancient Maya and their neighbors, the societies and cultures we know best (figure 6.1). The examples we cite are drawn from periods known conventionally as the Formative or Preclassic (ca. 1000 B.C.–A.D. 250), Early Classic (ca. A.D. 250–700), and Late Classic (ca. A.D. 700–1000).

Maya Space: Location of Interments

We begin with location of mortuary sites and arrangement or distribution of sets of burials. We focus on two classes of inference: location relative to landscape and construction and location relative to other decedents. Each of these is instructive in relating individuals to society, and both to worldview.

With regard to landscape and construction, Maya burials are now customarily described as being placed in caves within earth mountains (for example, Brady and Ashmore 1999). Although the chambers involved were sometimes "actual" geological caves, diverse metaphorical caves are identified in graves, formal tombs, and such other artificial hollows as *chultuns* (figure 6.2). Human remains are also found in the absence of a discernible chamber, especially within construction matrix. Like burial sites elsewhere, all of these Maya forms are liminal spaces, breaching boundaries of time at the edge of human life, as well as boundaries of space between earthly and supernatural realms. Specifically, burial chambers situate the deceased in the underworld, whether literally or by metaphor. They also allude to womblike places of birth and emergence (for example, Brady 1988; Gillespie 2000:158, 2002; Heyden 1981:22). As in other societies, transcendence of such boundaries of human life and worldly existence makes Maya burial sites appropriate places for transforming the deceased and commemorating ancestral continuities.

Cross-culturally, of course, burials imply proprietary links to land, and as claims, sequential burials within the same chamber parallel sequential creation of new superimposed or closely juxtaposed spaces of equivalent form (for example, Bloch and Parry 1982; Buikstra and Charles 1999; Charles and Buikstra 2002; Parker Pearson 1999; Saxe 1970). McAnany and her colleagues have interpreted both kinds of interments at Formative and Early Classic Maya K'axob to mark the "gathering together" of particular families' ancestors and ancestral authority, the practice intensifying with institutionalization of sociopolitical hierarchy (McAnany et al. 1999). Although correlating with the emergence of state-level polities, this form of "gathering together" is far from universal across the Maya region, its most prominent exemplars concentrated along the length of Belize (for example, Chase and Chase 1996; Hammond et al. 1975; McAnany 1995, 1998).

Most broadly, location emphasizes the critical role of burials in social reproduction, in charting continuity of kin and community. In 1956, Michael Coe (1956, 1975) argued that the frequent identification of Maya tombs as dedicatory to funerary temples actually inverted the anciently intended message and that the architecture was commemorative of human interment (also Chase and Chase 1998:302). Drawing on a more inclusive social cross-section at K'axob, Patricia McAnany and her colleagues (1999:141) likewise suggest that burials were important in "'completing' or 'ensouling' a structure that may have been dedicated to the deceased, rather than the opposite case." Just as pyramid mountains were settings for funerary caves, so too did domestic house platforms and

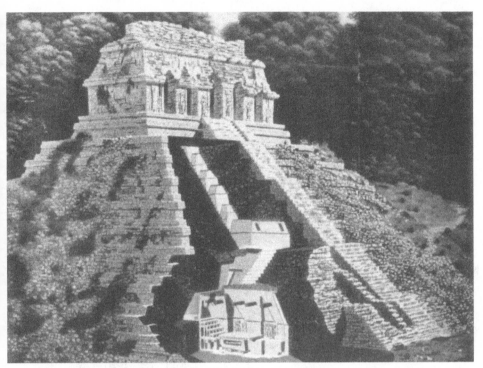

Figure 6.2. Cutaway view of cavelike tomb location in Palenque's Temple of Inscriptions. Copyright 1962, 1975, 1984, 1990 by George Kubler. First published 1962 by Penguin Books Ltd.; third edition reprinted with additional bibliography 1990; new impression 1993 by Yale University Press.

adjoining patio areas serve as family mountains for subfloor and chultun burials (for example, Brady and Ashmore 1999; Geller 2001). In Michael Coe's words, "The great Maya temple-pyramids were house-sepulchers writ large" (Coe 1988:235).

Susan Gillespie extends the social and spatial symbolism of house burial even further. In Lévi-Straussian terms, she points to the Maya "house" as signifying both a physical structure and the multifamily social group that occupies the structure (Gillespie 2000:142–143). She also describes nested scales for expression of "house"-ness, from the human body through domiciles, communities, and the cosmos (Gillespie 2000:159). Each of these scales replicates the proper spatial order of the Maya world, and what animates and ensouls all are the properly localized spirits of the revered dead (compare Gillespie 2002).

Specific burial location relative to landscape and settlement can carry additional social and cosmological significance. For example, the Early Classic royal necropolis of Tikal has supported multiple interpretations involving cosmological meaning (figure 6.3). Its position on the north edge of a principal Late Classic

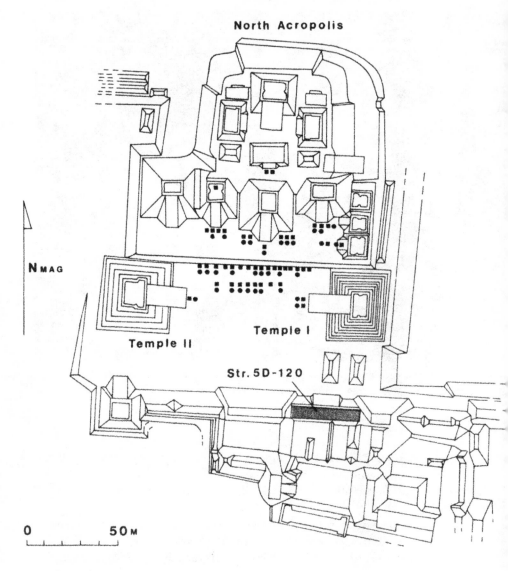

Figure 6.3. Plan of North Acropolis–Great Plaza area of Tikal (after Ashmore 1991: Figure 2).

public plaza complex may situate this "North Acropolis" simultaneously in the celestial and underworld realms of the Mayan universe (for example, Ashmore 1989). Diane Chase and Arlen Chase (1998:326) suggest further that particular cardinally positioned caches in that architectural complex ritually center the place, identifying it as the conceptual core of the city. In this manner as well, the burials constitute and materialize the center of the community (compare Buikstra and Charles 1999; Charles and Buikstra 2002).

Moreover, superimposition of royal burials and their shrines may define a particular spot within Tikal's North Acropolis as a specific *axis mundi*. Copán's acropolis likewise represents a royal burial ground and axis mundi, with superimposition of 400 years of royal shrines and temples commemorating the fifth-century A.D. burial spot of the dynastic founder, Yax K'uk' Mo', and his queen (Bell et al. 1999, 2004; Sharer et al. 1999). Sequential interments within commoners' domestic compounds may embody similar kinds of meanings, although differences in social class, formality of social identities, security of land tenure, elaboration of mortuary display, and likely mortuary ritual (for example, Coe 1988) have hampered our ability to elicit specific, detailed inferences from commoner Maya cases (compare Hodder 1984, 1990). Several authors have discussed these and related issues in *Space and Place of Death,* edited by Helaine Silverman and David Small (2002).

Mortuary remains may also define horizontal alignments with social and worldview significance. At Copán, for example, a line extended a kilometer north from the ninth-century tomb of the sixteenth ruler, Yax Pasah, in Structure 10L-18 of the acropolis, intersects the location of another tomb, in Group 8L-10 (figure 6.4). The latter tomb is provisionally identified as having been commissioned by Yax Pasah to commemorate the thirteenth ruler, 18 Rabbit or Waxaklahuun Ubah K'awil, a century after that earlier king's infamous assassination in a faraway act of secession from the realm (for example, Ashmore 1991; Carrelli 1990). The argument has been made that north–south horizontal axes are conceptually equivalent, for the Maya, to the vertical line of an axis mundi linking cosmic layers, such that northern position in one equates with celestial position in the other (for example, Ashmore 1989, 1991; Coggins 1980). Just as the vertical superimposition of Copán's acropolis tombs marks both dynastic and architectural continuity from the founder Yax K'uk' Mo', so too may the kilometer-long horizontal alignment that links rulers sixteen (Yax Pasah) and thirteen (18 Rabbit) materialize the last great dynast's reverence for his slain predecessor (compare Stuart et al. 1989).

Mayan Space: Placement within Interments

We turn now to formal orientation and arrangement of individual interments, briefly illustrating three aspects: orientation of chamber and decedent; position of the deceased; and arrangement of mortuary accoutrements.

There is no single orientation for Maya dead; consistency of orientation, as well as specific orientation, varies within communities, regions, time periods, social class, and sometimes with individual identity (for example, Golden 1997; McAnany et al. 1999; Welsh 1988:52–63). Consistency of body-alignment azimuth may relate to formality of mortuary ritual and belief according to class, as

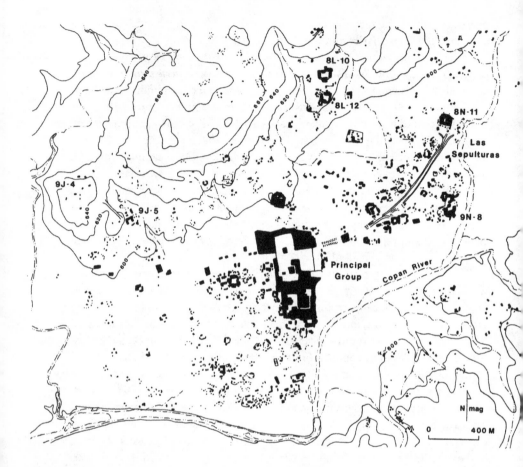

Figure 6.4. Map of Copán valley (after Ashmore 1991:Figure 4).

well as to regional customs. These possibilities need expanded review at a regional scale, in light of expanding information sets.

Some specific interments, however, are intriguingly suggestive of symbolic alignments. At the interment of Palenque's Pacal the Great in A.D. 683 (see figure 6.2), his remains were laid out with his head to the north, a position repeated by the World Tree emblazoned on his sarcophagus lid (figure 6.5). In life, kings individually embodied the World Tree, which reaches from its roots in the underworld to its crown in the heavens (for example, Bartlett and McAnany 2000:110; Schele and Freidel 1990:66).

The World Tree is also sometimes seen as the route of ancestral emergence (for example, Gillespie 2000:145). Elsewhere, public architectural materialization of a north–south alignment has been argued to assert the strength of dynastic continuity and authority (Ashmore 2005), and earlier in this chapter, tombs of two

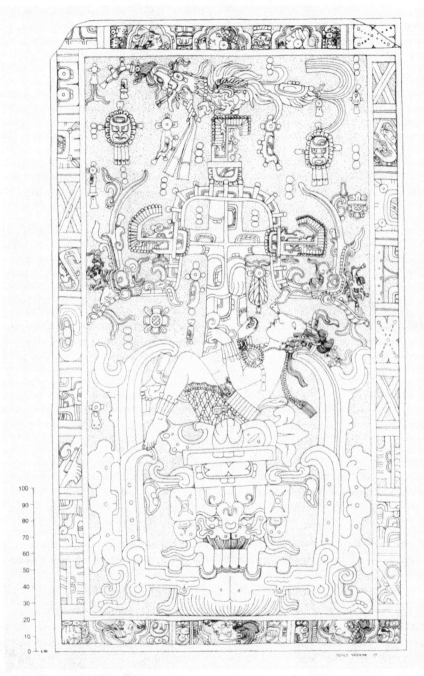

Figure 6.5. The sarcophagus lid of Palenque's Pacal the Great. Copyright 1973 by Merle Green Robertson, reprinted with permission.

Late Classic Copán kings were inferred as placing the ancestral dynasts meta-phorically in the heavens, on the north. Based on these inferences about Mayan directional symbolism, and because kings embodied the World Tree, it seems fitting that both the sarcophagus tree image and the king himself should be posi-tioned with crown or head in the north—again metaphorically in the heavens. Certainly Pacal's tomb and its surmounting temple-pyramid at Palenque consti-tute a mortuary, sculptural, and architectural program aimed in large measure at underscoring the authority of his line (for example, Schele and Freidel 1990; compare Gillespie 2000).

Arrangement and placement of mortuary accompaniments likewise varies. Specific positions of some elements suggest symbolic expression; items take on specific meanings by dint of where they were placed. For example, Robin (1989:127), McAnany, and others have interpreted bowls or plates inverted over the face as protective head coverings. McAnany and colleagues (1999:137) al-lude to the head as the "locus of strength in the ancestor guardians" among modern-day Chol Maya, a characterization those authors see as consistent with identification of ancient head coverings, particularly when the burial is not in a constructed open-air chamber.

Other items may describe collectively a meaningful formal arrangement, as an assemblage. Because such a situation is linked to numbers and elaboration of burial contents, it is therefore observable more frequently in graves of royal and noble classes. Three Copán burials highlight deliberate structure in spatial place-ment of multiple occupants, perhaps none of whom were themselves the subject of veneration. Their placement and arrangement may be clues to social identity. At Copán's Group 8L-10, two rectangular masonry crypts each housed paired interments of a woman and man, in each case with the woman to the north of the man (figure 6.6). Elsewhere these pairs have been interpreted as embodying complementary supernatural agents of resurrection, and they may have been sacrificed for interment together, to honor 18 Rabbit, the long-deceased thir-teenth Copanec king cited earlier in the chapter (Ashmore 1991, 2002:237–238; Carrelli 1990). One of the pairs, in Burial XLII-5, may even attend the actual skull fragments of the assassinated king (Carrelli 1990:184). If so, the treatment and placement of his weathered and broken remains illustrates some of the com-plex ambiguity of postmortem veneration and violation discussed by Duncan (this volume).

Indeed, if speculative identification of those skull fragments is correct, the royal ancestor's head would mark the ancestral-north end of the aforementioned alignment with the tomb of his reverent successor, Yax Pasah. This recalls the description of Pacal at Palenque and the placement of his head to the north within his sarcophagus. At Copán, Yax Pasah could plausibly have recovered the thir-teenth ruler's skull early in the ninth century, as he was on good terms with the king of Quiriguá, the once-rebellious center whose earlier king had beheaded 18 Rabbit in A.D. 738 (for example, Looper 1999:277–278; Sharer 1978). Although

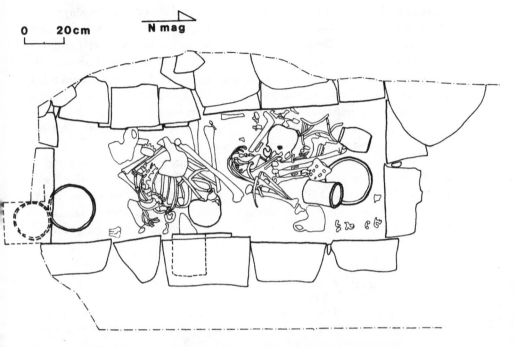

Figure 6.6. Burial XLII-5, Group 8L-10, Copán (after Ashmore 1991:Figure 9). The tomb's occupants are an adult woman (on the north) and an adult man (on the south), with fragments of a third skull that may be the remains of an assassinated Copán king.

Yax Pasah likely commissioned both the tomb for Copán Burial XLII-5 and the building group in which it was set, the actual interment must date to after A.D. 830 and therefore after Yax Pasah's own death (Ashmore 1991:214).

In the compound immediately south, Group 8L-12, excavation yielded another interment in which the skeletons of two individuals were packed tightly amid a series of paired stone slabs. Although the precise significance of this burial is not yet clear, its creators clearly invested great deliberation in its multiple symmetries and complementary pairs. In each case, the individuals coupled in death do not seem to have been treated as ancestors, but by the nature of their arrangement in mortuary space, they were clearly critical to defining the meaning of the place (for example, Ashmore 1991; Becker 1988, 1992; Carrelli 1990; Duncan, this volume).

Discussion and Conclusions

The deliberation that lay behind the interment of the dead encodes social meaning in spatial order. The cases described in this chapter only hint at the range of meanings archaeologists can now discern. Our examples stem from but a small fraction of the research that has been accomplished thus far in the Maya area alone, and they favor heavily the more emphatically formalized spaces of royal and noble decedents. Despite important efforts to broaden the social range of decedents involved, we still know less about the variation in location, orientation, and arrangement of Maya commoners' gravesites. In short, we need fuller examination and comparison of mortuary space across social class, gender, age, and other social signifiers. And we need to look further at how these co-vary with location across the full range of the anciently recognized landscape. This bespeaks a regional approach, crosscut by examining dimensions of time and social identity. Colleagues working in other cultural contexts are exploring some of these aspects quite fully (for example, Beck 1995; Buikstra 1981; Buikstra and Charles 1999; Meskell 1999; Silverman and Small 2002). Wherever we work, archaeologists have quite a few important clues to expanding the social dimensions of mortuary space, and the future of these analyses is as promising as it will be challenging.

Acknowledgments

The original version of this chapter was prepared for the 66th Annual Meeting of the Society for American Archaeology, for the symposium on "Archaeology of Death," organized by Gordon Rakita and Jane Buikstra. We are grateful to them for the invitation to participate in the symposium and to all of the editors of the current volume for their encouragement and helpful critique. Norman Hammond and Cynthia Robin have expressed generous enthusiasm for Geller's (1998, 2000) reconsideration of the extraordinary Cuello mortuary record. In the Programme for Belize, Fred Valdez, Frank Saul, and Julie Saul have offered invaluable support and guidance for Geller's ongoing research. Ashmore is grateful to the members of the Copán North Group Project, especially Christine Carrelli, for collaboration in study of burials from Groups 8L-10 and 8L-12 at Copán, and to Julie Miller for insightful conversations about them in 1992. Both authors thank Tom Patterson and the volume editors for critical reading of earlier drafts of this chapter.

II

Bodies and Souls

Gordon F. M. Rakita and Jane E. Buikstra

The chapters in this section focus attention upon the body of the deceased. By examining the way corpses are treated, curated, or disposed of, new insights are gleaned in the role of the deceased's soul in the lives of the living. Rakita and Buikstra reexamine and reevaluate Hertz's (1907) classic perspective that cremation and mummification can be interpreted as simply inconsequential variants of more elaborate secondary funerary processes. They use case studies from two American archaeological contexts, the U.S. Southwest and the Andes (Inca royal mummies), to explore the theoretical implications of two forms of secondary treatment—cremation and mummification—in relationship to Hertz's model, published nearly a century before. Contrary to Hertz's more one-dimensional view of cremation and mummification, Rakita and Buikstra argue that considering these processes in terms of ongoing negotiations and interactions between the dead and the living is essential to understanding mortuary practices in these two regions. This chapter demonstrates the importance of contextually sensitive studies and the limitations of generalizations made on the basis of a single case as well as the complexity of "secondary burials" noted by many of the other chapters.

Oakdale's contribution scrutinizes contemporary rituals that close a period of mourning among a Brazilian Amazonian people called the Kayabi. Jawosi rituals (including songs and dancing) and commentary on cosmology are discussed in relation to mortuary practices to show how, in this tradition, dead ancestors are encouraged to fade from memory rather than to become memorialized. Drawing inspiration from the theoretical traditions of both Hertz and Bloch, Oakdale is able to examine the universalistic characterization of a "quasi-universal" structure existing at the core of the ritual process that offers an explanation for the symbolism of violence present in a ritual like the Kayabi's Jawosi.

Building upon the warnings of Brown (1981, 1995), Byers questions the assumption that archaeologically recovered burials represent the final stage in the mortuary rites of passage. Specifically, Byers presents a complex model of extended funerary processing for some members of Ohio Hopewell society. He argues for an Ohio Hopewell "laying-in" crypt model as part of a complex funerary– mourning–spirit release–world renewal ritual that was truncated at the Hopewell and Turner sites, where extended interments dominate the mortuary records. This model posits a Hopewellian ethos characterizing the world as immanently sacred, a place where human material interventions into the natural order have profound implications for the maintenance of cosmological balance and continuity. This study is a reminder that mortuary data must be interpreted within the setting of a dynamic culture system.

Guillén presents a description and typology for the world's oldest artificial mummies, found in the coastal regions of the south central Andes. She contextualizes the Chinchorro example in a broader consideration of Andean mummies, develops a typology of mummification practices, and also discusses the meaning of this long-term Andean tradition. She further suggests that the elaborate nature of these mummies is related to ongoing relations between the living and the dead of the Chinchorro society. The role of these mummies in a complex ancestor cult is discussed and highlights yet another theme of this volume, the often complex and enduring relations between ancestors and those still living.

In an innovative approach that (like Byers' chapter) draws inspiration from James Brown's work, Beck links bioarchaeological knowledge of cremation practices and their effect upon bone to ethnographic and ethnohistoric documents from the American Southwest. Her goal is to explore the enigmatic nature of Hohokam cremation practices from prehistoric southern Arizona. Beck's data suggest that previous interpretations of archaeologically recovered cremations may be incorrect because they were incompletely contextualized. A more parsimonious interpretation of cremation features would involve the existence of a secondary burial program that involved the reburning of cremated remains in a memorial ceremony. Beck argues that this model "better fits the combined archaeological, osteological, and ethnohistoric data sets than prior interpretations."

Weiss-Krejci also underscores the complexity that must be appreciated to understand so-called secondary burials. By examining various postmortem handling of members of the Babenberg and Habsburg dynasties in Medieval Germany, she is able to demonstrate that not all secondary treatment is related to ancestor cults (or even the initial mortuary rites). Indeed, some multistage burial programs may simply be related to political, economic, or biological circumstances unrelated to the deceased individual's social status. Indeed,

Weiss-Krejci's observations clearly demonstrate that in some cases, elite status can *not* be decoded on the basis of mortuary treatments.

Also from a European context, Naji scrutinizes interments from the abbey of Saint-Jean-des-Vignes, established around A.D. 1076 on a hill overlooking the medieval town of Soissons, France. These interments led Naji to examine changing burial practices and conceptions of the dead and the deceased's soul in Medieval France. An examination of the historical literature demonstrates a complexity to mortuary behavior and religious orthodoxy that is not often recognized. Fear of the contamination afforded by dead bodies is shown as important, tempering the treatment of the corpse and the location of its interment. The importance of interment *ad santos* is also explored. Finally, recent excavations at the eleventh-century abbey provide an example of this complexity. By focusing on the burials from the cloister and chapter room, Naji considers how medieval people viewed the bodies of the dead and how remembrance of the dead was manifested, particularly through prayers. The obvious disturbance of graves and the seemingly cavalier treatment of bones is explained in terms of a belief system that placed emphasis upon the soul rather than the material remains of the dead.

The final chapter in this section, by Malville, explores Tibetan Buddhist mortuary procedures and treatment of the formerly dead. Tibetan Buddhists have extremely complex beliefs and practices involving the dead. Celestial ("sky") burial (exposure and cleansing of bones by vultures) and cremation are the preferred modes, with undesirable individuals buried in water or in the ground. An alternative treatment, preserving with salt, is normally accorded only a few high-ranking lamas. Malville's chapter examines these practices with an eye toward how they might be interpreted archaeologically.

7

Corrupting Flesh

Reexamining Hertz's Perspective on Mummification and Cremation

Gordon F. M. Rakita and Jane E. Buikstra

Death is surely as much a cultural process as it is a biological one. In modern Western society, death is most often viewed as an instantaneous event. However, in other societies throughout the world and through history and prehistory, death was or is viewed as a transition—oftentimes a slow one—to another existential state. This fact has been no better understood than by Robert Hertz in his classic (1960 [1907]) study of secondary burial treatments.

Hertz's Model

The primary concern of Hertz's 1907 work was to offer a generalized explanation for the variety of temporary or secondary burial practices found cross-culturally. In point of fact, Hertz argued that the specific forms of secondary treatment are irrelevant. What was most important was the end result of any extended processing of the corpse—namely, the separation of the corrupting effects of the rotting flesh from the permanent, dry, and pure bones. Moreover, Hertz made use of the "rites of passage" analytic framework soon to be published by Arnold van Gennep (1960 [1908]). Following van Gennep, rites of passage, among them funerals, are organized into three distinct phases. In the first, the rite of separation, the deceased is socially removed from society. Often this is initiated by the biological death of the individual. In the second, the deceased passes through a transitory or liminal period. A reincorporation rite follows, in which the deceased is introduced into the afterworld. In his study, Hertz emphasized the liminal or transition stage of rites of passage. Indeed, it was this stage that van Gennep suggested was most often elaborated in funerary contexts (van Gennep 1960:146 [1908]).

However, Hertz embellished van Gennep's framework. Specifically, Hertz suggested that during secondary burial treatments the corpse's rite of passage was mirrored or paralleled by rites of passage for the soul of the deceased as well as

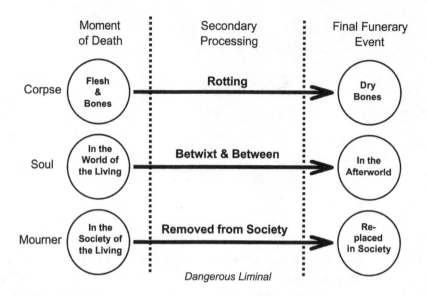

Figure 7.1. Hertz's model of secondary burial.

the mourners. Furthermore, he argued that the physical condition of the corpse represented the metaphysical condition of the soul and the social condition of the mourners. But the corpse's decomposition does more than represent these transitions, it is fundamental to the process. As Metcalf and Huntington (1991:35) have noted, Hertz expressly relied upon the framework of Hubert and Mauss' (1964 [1899]) assumption about sacrifice—namely, that for an item to enter the otherworld it must be destroyed in this world. Hertz's tripartite parallelism is illustrated in figure 7.1.

Here we can see that at the moment of death, the body is composed of flesh and bones, the soul is in the world of the living, and the mourners are within their proper social roles. After death, however, the corpse begins to putrefy, and the soul becomes liminal. It is neither of this world nor of the afterworld, and the mourners are removed from society because of their bereavement and kinship obligations to the deceased. Finally, all three are reintegrated into new roles or statuses. The clean, dry bones are placed within permanent facilities, the soul is installed within the realm of the ancestors, and the mourners reassume their roles—or new ones—within society.

Cremation and Mummification

Thus Hertz left us with a rather tidy interpretive framework for secondary funerary practices. However, a complication remains. How does his framework explain both mummification and cremation? In neither case is the corpse allowed to decompose by natural means. Hertz's response was to simply equate these forms of treatment with other secondary burial practices: "the aim of embalmment is precisely to prevent the corruption of the flesh and the transformation of the body into a skeleton; cremation on the other hand forestalls the spontaneous alteration of the corpse with a rapid and almost complete destruction. We believe that these artificial ways of disposal do not differ essentially from the temporary ways that we have listed" (Hertz 1960:41 [1907]). Thus, in the case of cremation, the dangerous liminal period of corpse decomposition is hastened by the incineration of the rotting flesh. The calcined remains are thus essentially equivalent to pure skeletal remains. In mummification, the protracted period of putrefaction is avoided and the embalmed or desiccated corpse is commensurate with clean, dry bone.

Our view is that Hertz overstated his case. By extending his model to include both mummification and cremation—or more accurately, by attempting to force mummification and cremation into the framework of his model—he neglected to consider the interpretive value of considering these two treatments as meaningful "exceptions to the rule." We would further suggest that by examining the ways in which mummification and cremation differ from other secondary burial processes, we can arrive at richer explanations of mortuary behavior. We turn now to our contrastive examples.

Andean Mummification

Buikstra has elsewhere (Buikstra and Nystrom 2003) referred to the Andean practice of mummification as an "embedded" tradition. And indeed, the practice seems to have been a fundamental aspect of mortuary behavior in the region for over seven millennia. Initially, mummification may have been simply a fortuitous result of life and death in one of the world's driest desert regions. However, by approximately 5000 B.C. the coastal regions of southern Peru and northern Chile were the center of a burgeoning intentional mummification tradition associated with the Chinchorro culture. Of the various mummification styles known to have been practiced until around 2000 B.C., the most complex were the so-called black mummies (Arriaza 1995). Arriaza and colleagues describe them thusly:

> After defleshing and evisceration, the mortician used sticks and grass ropes for internal reinforcement of the major joints of the skeleton. The volume and body contour were regained, although not to exact anatomical proportions, using a gray soil paste. Often the skin was replaced and painted black with a manganese pigment, hence the name black mummies. . . . On the head, the mortician added a short human hair wig and a facial mask of gray soil paste. The facial skin, which was skillfully put back in place, was coated with a paste of manganese and the facial features were insinuated. The sexual organs were modeled also. (Arriaza et al. 1998:191–192)

Many of the Chinchorro mummies predate—perhaps by several thousand years—the more well-known mummies of ancient Egypt.

After these early complex mummification patterns, there followed a period in which Andean mummies occurred frequently—though these were perhaps less elaborately constructed. Treatment of the corpse took advantage, either intentionally or not, of natural conditions encouraging desiccation and preservation. However, despite the less elaborate nature of patterns of corpse treatment, concern with ongoing relations between the living and the dead continued. Intermediate-period mortuary patterns range from relatively simple collared tombs that were utilized as final resting locales for single descent groups to more monumental *chulpas,* or burial towers, used by more inclusive *ayllu* groups.

The ultimate expression of Andean mummification is, of course, the classic royal Inca mummy bundles. Upon the death of an Inca elite, the corpse was carefully embalmed and wrapped in the finest cloths available. These mummy bundles were made to look as much as possible as the deceased looked in life. And far from being entombed and abandoned, the bundled individuals were accorded much the same treatment they had received in life. They were fed fine foods and drinks, accompanied by caretakers, and afforded all the respect and authority they had commanded before their death. In effect, rather than serving as a preparation for their future life in the afterworld, mummification made permanent their place in the world of the living.

However, Incan royalty were not the only individuals accorded such treatment. As recent discoveries in the Chachapoyas region of northern Peru have demonstrated, the practice of mummification was geographically extensive as well as having crosscut ethnic groupings. Over 200 mummies have been discovered in small chulpas constructed in caves in cliff faces. Although modern looters have disturbed many, the remains display an interesting mix of ethnic markers. The chulpas show architectural affinity with Chachapoya culture. However, some of the ceramics recovered are clearly Incan. The mummy bundles show a similar mix of ethnic affiliation. Many are the bundled remains of Chachapoyas, though some are clearly Inca in origin.

Cremation in the U.S. Southwest

Our second example is drawn from the U.S. Southwest. While cremations are perhaps less embedded within the prehistoric cultures of the Southwest than mummification is in Andean traditions, cremation nonetheless represents an important pattern of corpse processing. Hohokam cremation practices are presented in greater detail in another chapter of this volume (by Beck). However, we will note that cremations in the core Hohokam region of central and southern Arizona represent some of the earliest discovered in the Southwest. At least by the Vahki phase (dating from approximately A.D. 300 to 500), cremations in pits or trenches had begun to replace simple flexed inhumations (Crown 1991; Haury

1976). Certainly by A.D. 600 to 700, during the Sweetwater phase, cremations had become the dominant mode of corpse disposal. Funerary practices for the next 200 to 300 years seem to involve cremation areas associated with specific courtyard groups and involving deposition of cremated remains within simple pits and subsequently within ceramic vessels. Inhumations reappear in the Hohokam sequence by approximately A.D. 975–1150 and become increasingly popular throughout the Classic and post-Classic periods but never entirely replace cremations. During the Classic period, new ceremonial patterns (including platform mounds that replaced existing ballcourt ritual networks) evolved; these may have been related to sweeping changes in ceremonial life seen throughout the Southwest (Wilcox 1991).

We focus here on the cremations from regions to the north and east—frequently referred to as the Puebloan Southwest—including the Little Colorado–Zuni region, the Point of Pines and Mimbres areas of the Mogollon tradition, and the Rio Abajo region centered in New Mexico (table 7.1). The earliest known cremations from these areas were uncovered at the Cienega Creek site in the Point of Pines region. In 1955–1956, Emil Haury excavated 47 pit cremations at the site. The features included evidence of adults and subadults as well as 37 projectile points and other lithic artifacts. Forty of the cremation pits were located within a larger pit feature measuring 1.3 meters deep and 3 meters wide. An associated radiocarbon assay dated the feature to 575 ± 300 B.C. (Haury 1957). Haury suggested that these features—the earliest known cremations from the entire Southwest—could be considered to be culturally ancestral to the later cremation practice in the Hohokam and Mogollon regions. However, there is at least an 800-year hiatus before evidence of cremation is again seen in the Puebloan world.

The next time cremations appear in the Southwest is during the sixth century A.D. in the Mimbres region. Thirteen cremations were recovered from Late Pit House phase contexts in this area; they probably date from A.D. 550–1000. By A.D. 850, there is evidence of cremations again in the Point of Pines region. Both of these regions maintained a constant yet fairly rare tradition of cremation through at least the sixteenth century A.D. Many of the early cremations in the Mimbres region contained projectile points in a similar fashion to those associated with the remains from Cienega Creek. The greatest majority of cremations, however, come from the A.D. 1200 to 1400 period, with over 200 cremations recovered at the Point of Pines Ruin site alone. By A.D. 1350 the practice of cremating the deceased had spread to two more regions in the Pueblo world. In the Zuni or Little Colorado region, over 300 cremations were recovered from the ancestral Zuni village of Hawikuh, which dates from A.D. 1300 to the time of Spanish contact. In the Rio Abajo area, cremations are known—most notably from Gran Quivira, where approximately 150 were found, but also from the nearby Pueblo Pardo and Quarai Pueblo. These post–A.D. 1350 cremations in the Zuni and Rio Abajo areas were often associated with what appear to be offerings

Table 7.1. Cremations Found in the Pueblo Region

Region Site	Period	No. of cremations	Citation
Mimbres			
Galaz, Harris, Lee, NAN Ranch, Swarts, Wind Mountain	A.D. 550–1000 (Late Pit House phase)	13	Creel 1989
Galaz, NAN Ranch, Swarts, Heron, Mattocks, Old Town, Perrault, Rock House, Saige-McFarland, Talbert, Treasure Hill, Woodward	A.D. 1000–1150 (Classic period)	35	Creel 1989
Galaz, Swarts, LA 18342, McDonald, Montoya, Powe, Walsh	A.D. 1150–1350 (Black Mountain phase)	20	Creel 1989
Ormand Village	A.D. 1350–1450 (Cliff phase)	35	Creel 1989
Galaz, Old Town, Perrault, LA 18342, Cameron Creek, Red Rock, Upton, Watson Site 92	*Unknown age between A.D. 550 and 1450*	11	Creel 1989
Rio Abajo			
Gran Quivira	A.D. 1550–1672	149 (possibly 154)	Hayes et al. 1981
Pueblo Pardo	A.D. 1300–1630	7 (possibly 13)	Toulouse 1944; Toulouse and Stephenson 1960
Quarai Pueblo	A.D. 1315–1425	1	*Burial forms on deposit at the LA, Santa Fe, NM*

Point of Pines

Cienega site (Arizona W:10:112)	875–275 B.C. (Cochise)	47	Haury 1957; Robinson and Sprague 1965
Arizona W:10:37	A.D. 850–1050 (Reserve phase)	2	Robinson and Sprague 1965
Arizona W:10:56	A.D. 850–1050 (Reserve phase)	1	Robinson and Sprague 1965
Arizona W:10:65	A.D. 1050–1350 (Tularosa phase)	3	Robinson and Sprague 1965
Arizona W:10:78	A.D. 1050–1350 (Tularosa phase)	27	Robinson and Sprague 1965
Point of Pines Ruin (Arizona W:10:50)	A.D. 1200–1450 (Tularosa, Pinedale, and Canyon Creek phases)	212	Robinson and Sprague 1965
Arizona W:10:47	A.D. 1350–1500 (Point of Pines phase)	19	Robinson and Sprague 1965
Arizona W:10:52	A.D. 1350–1500 (Point of Pines phase)	10	Robinson and Sprague 1965

Upper Little Colorado–Zuni Region

Hawikuh	A.D. 1300–1400	11	Smith et al. 1966
Hawikuh	A.D. 1350–1475	13	Smith et al. 1966
Hawikuh	A.D. 1475–1650	88	Smith et al. 1966
Hawikuh	Probably A.D. 1300–1650	205	Smith et al. 1966
Kechipauan	*Unknown*	*Unknown*	Hodge 1920

Guadalupe Mountains

Burnet Cave, Cremation Cave, "a cave near Guadalupe Point," "another [cave] in South Three Forks Canyon," Williams Cave	*Unknown*	*Unknown*	Toulouse 1944

of corn as well as personal adornments, clothing, and ceramics. Not surprisingly, this expansion in the frequency of cremation occurs concurrently with the development of Kachina societies in both these regions (Adams 1994; Schaafsma 1994).

Hertz's Model (Re)examined

How then do we make use of Hertz's framework in understanding the practices of mummification and cremation in our two examples? We would suggest that Hertz's quick dismissal of cremation and mummification neglects significant insights into both practices that can be gained by considering each within his model.

Cremation, Hertz stated, is simply an accelerated method of reducing the decomposing corpse to clean, pure remains. However, it does rather more than that. Unlike traditional secondary corpse processing, the final remains from a cremation are often quite difficult to equate with human remains. That is, while the clean, dry skeleton of a corpse is easily recognized as the final remains of an individual, a pile of calcined bone is not. Indeed, the identification of cremations archaeologically is often extremely difficult, as Hayes and colleagues note about some of the cremations from Gran Quivira (Hayes et al. 1981:174). In at least five cases, no human bones were identifiable from within the ashes. Similarly, Hodge noted complete incineration for the cremations at Hawikuh (Smith et al. 1966:203). It seems reasonable therefore to conclude that the purpose behind cremation was not necessarily simply to transform the corpse but to remove it from this world altogether. As noted earlier, Hertz's model falls back upon Hubert and Mauss' (1964 [1899]) ideas concerning sacrifices. Items must be destroyed in this world to be able to proceed across to the afterworld. We believe that changes in how the ancestors were perceived led to the increasing frequency of cremation. In the case of Puebloan mortuary practices, it is during the development of the Kachina societies—especially at Zuni and the Rio Abajo—that cremation practices become most frequent.

Ruth Bunzel outlined the principles behind the Kachina societies: "The Katcina [sic] cult is built upon the worship, principally through impersonation, of a group of supernaturals. . . . [These supernaturals] . . . live in a lake . . . west of Zuni. . . . Here they spend their time singing and dancing, and occasionally they come to Zuni to dance for their 'daylight' fathers. . . . By origin and later association they are identified with the dead. Mortals on death join the katcinas at katcina village and become like them" (Bunzel 1930:843–844). Among the most important ceremonial acts within Kachina societies are those occasions when living members don masks and costumes and impersonate the part of the ancestors when they return and dance in the village. There are thus imperatives to the cremation of the deceased in communities with Kachina societies. These involve the removal of both the soul and the body from the world of the living. These entities are thus able to completely transition to the world of the supernaturals. Moreover, they are free to engage in cyclical revisits to the world of the living.

That is to say, in this case, the role of the ancestral beings is to repeatedly travel to and from this world and the supernatural one. In so doing, they periodically reinfuse this world with sacred forces—be they directed toward agricultural fertility, social cohesion, or moral proscriptions. In fact, according to Dennis Tedlock (1979:507), these ancestral spirits "stand before" or in front of the living kachina impersonators. However, they typically are not recognized or acknowledged as individuals or by specific names. These returning ancestors are grouped together in prayers as the generalized dead of the society.

To return to the Inca, Hertz would have us interpret the Andean mummification procedure as simply another secondary process by which the rotting corpse is transformed into dry, hard, durable bones and flesh. Moreover, he would suggest that the period of time required for this process to be completed is mirrored by liminal periods for the soul of the deceased as well as the mourners' relationship to the rest of society. We would, however, disagree—at least insofar as the royal Inca mummy bundles are concerned. As noted earlier, the completion of the mummification process is not marked by the final removal of the corpse from the world of the living. Neither are the mourners reinstalled in society in new configurations. Indeed, both mourners and deceased maintain their former roles despite the physical death of the individual. We prefer to view mummification as a method for sustaining the position of the soul in the liminal phase. Hertz is correct that the condition of the corpse mirrors the situation of the mourners and the deceased's soul. However, in this case the permanence and immutable nature of the corpse—both there as in the world of the living, but not there as during life—is representative of the liminality of the deceased's soul. Furthermore, once mummification is complete, the mourners are returned to their original social statuses as if they had never left them. For the Andeans, death as a culturally defined event simply did not exist for some individuals.

Indeed, far from representing the finality of death, Inca mummies were powerful social and ritual forces in ancient Andean society. Their power derived from the fact that they not only anchored the social structures of Andean communities but also empowered the Inca state. Ancestor cults have appeared many times in human history, but the influence of the Andean mummies appears inordinate. Recognizing the Andean propensity for multivocality and metaphorical meanings, we find it hard to escape the arrested liminality that the durable mummies represent. Even with the departure of the spirit and the flesh, these hardened images stand in an arrested and perilous transitional state, their bodies suspended between the living world and the generative cycles that produce new lives. Thus they were both dangerous and powerful.

Here we are left with a situation in which the ancestors never entirely *leave* this world but are nevertheless not quite *of* this world. Drawing upon Turner's (1995 [1969]) conceptualization of liminal periods, we would argue that Inca mummies represent an example of extended or permanent liminality. As such they are infused with considerable sacred power. If Turner's formulation is carried further, the power of these ancestors is derived from their continued state of *communitas* with both the society of the living and the realm of the dead. They thus act as important conduits in the living community's ongoing relations with the ancestors.

Conclusion

Thus in one case the power of the ancestors returns—albeit only periodically—in living supernaturals. Their identities generalized, these ancestors are the quintessential powerful "Other" (*sensu* Helms 1998). They momentarily provide a connection with the sacred forces of the afterworld, only to ultimately return there when their stay in this world is done. Cremation allows for the complete transition to this state of the Other. In the Inca case, the ancestors remain—both body and soul—among the living, acquiring power from their incomplete transition via mummification—their extended liminal state. However, in this example, ancestorhood does not involve a loss of identity within this world. Thus they bridge in a uninterrupted way the divide between the world of the living and the afterworld and continue to structure the lives of their descendents. They do so by denying the decomposition of social structure that death brings, by denying biological decomposition. In each of our cases, death is defined culturally in a specific and unusual manner—irrespective of the fact of biological death.

Bloch and Parry (1982:3) once criticized Hertz's model for being "somewhat over narrowly related to the particular ethnographic material with which he started." We would agree that to a certain extent—at least in the case of mummification and cremation—Hertz's reliance upon the funerary practices of Borneo as support for his model constricted his ability to interpret alternative forms of secondary treatment. We would certainly not presume that the interpretations of Andean mummification and Puebloan cremation that we have offered represent a complete account of the meaning of these practices in these disparate regions. However, we do feel that our examples provide alternative insights into both cases and do justice to Hertz's framework, while simultaneously expanding upon it.

8

Forgetting the Dead, Remembering Enemies

Suzanne Oakdale

In his essay "The Collective Representation of Death," Robert Hertz (1960 [1907]) treats the series of rites concerning the remains of the deceased as "rites of passage" and observes that the final burial rites complete the separation of the dead from the living as well as usher the soul of the dead into a new group, the community of ancestors. In this chapter, I focus on the first part of this process: how the living and the dead become separated. I look at this process in one Amazonian tradition, that of the Kayabi of central Brazil. The Kayabi celebrate a ritual, called Jawosi, several months after a death has occurred, explicitly to help the bereaved definitively cut their ties with their dead relative. In Kayabi phrasing, Jawosi rituals help people forget about their dead.

Kayabi practices are not unusual in Amazonia, for rites that separate the dead from the living often center on the process of forgetting. As Anne Christine Taylor has observed, this focus is in keeping with the fact that Amazonian traditions are known for having shallow genealogical memories as well as little that resembles ancestor cults (1993:653). Much like the traditions that Hertz surveys, several Amazonian traditions manipulate or use imagery of the corpse to facilitate the process of separation or forgetting. The Ecuadorian Achuar, for example, sing funeral laments describing the decomposition of the face of the deceased to encourage mourners to forget this person as an individual with distinctive features and to think of him or her in less visualized terms (Taylor 1993). Other traditions, such as the Wari' of northwestern Brazil, traditionally relied upon mortuary cannibalism to transform the memory of the deceased (Conklin 2001). Through butchering, roasting, and consumption, the deceased was transformed in the eyes of the mourners from a human individual to a more generic animal or meatlike state (Conklin 2001). These kinds of procedures, as Taylor (1993) and Conklin (2001) both observe, rest upon manipulating the image of the deceased held by the mourners. The body of the deceased moves from being thought of as a well-loved living person to decomposed, cut apart, or burned flesh, and with this transformation mourners are better able to let go of their dead and cope with their loss.

For the Kayabi, forgetting also involves focusing on the fate of a body, but rather than the fate of the body of the deceased relative, it concerns the bodies and death experiences of enemies. Jawosi rituals feature songs recounting the death of non-Kayabi at the hands of Kayabi warriors. They also at times involve a focus on actual or symbolic representations of enemy bodies. Through Jawosi rituals, the bereaved are supposed to end their communication and sympathy with their own dead, to understand their own dead as "other."[1] I argue that it is through meditating on dead who truly are other (that is, enemy dead) that they accomplish this end. The dead with whom the Kayabi interact in Jawosi are, therefore, not their own, but the dead of other peoples.

Maurice Bloch has formulated a "quasi-universal" structure existing at the core of the ritual process that offers an explanation for the symbolism of violence present in a ritual like the Kayabi Jawosi. According to this model, the biological fact that living beings go through a process of birth, growth, reproduction, aging, and death is perceived by people in all societies, in one way or another (1992:3). Despite this biological fact, or rather because of this biological fact, human societies represent life in a ritual context in an inverted way, as occurring within a permanent framework that transcends this natural, universally perceived process (Bloch 1992:4).[2] The first phase of the ritual process, then, involves participants transcending biological life. "The social and political significance of such a passage is that by entering into a world beyond process, through the passage of reversal, one can then be an entity beyond process, for example, a member of a descent group" (Bloch 1992:4). The final phase involves returning to this world once again with this transcendence in tow. At this phase "the vital here and now" is transformed by the presence of a "conquered vitality obtained from outside beings" (Bloch 1992:5). "It is through this substitution that an image is created in which humans can leave this life and join the transcendental, yet still not be alienated from the here and now. They become part of permanent institutions, and as superior beings they can reincorporate the present life through the idiom of conquest or consumption" (Bloch 1992:5).

Drawing on regionally specific theories about the role of enemies and the dead in other Amazonian societies, I argue that if enemy dead provide the living with a substance such as "a conquered vitality" to be "consumed," this "substance" is most productively understood metaphorically, more as a position of alterity than an actual substance per se (Viveiros de Castro 1992:286). As Taylor has observed for Amazonia in general, the dead (and I would add, especially the enemy dead) engage interest as "paradigms of sociological foreignness" (Taylor 1993:654).

After introducing the Kayabi and the Jawosi ritual, I turn to how meditating on the enemy dead encourages Kayabi mourners to see their own dead as enemies, that is, how the ritual works rhetorically, how (in Clifford Geertz's phrasing) the ritual has a dramatic force that causes people to "surrender and be changed," at least with respect to their connection to their own dead (1983:30).

Finally, I turn to why the position of enmity is important in lowland cosmologies and conceptualizations of vitality.

The Kayabi

The Kayabi are a contemporary riverine, Tupian-speaking, Amazonian people who practice hunting, gathering, and extensive slash-and-burn agriculture. Earlier in the twentieth century they lived predominantly in extended family homesteads led by senior family headmen. A headman's authority over other family members was, and still is, tied to a postmarriage period of bride-service. Newly married men live with and provide labor for their in-laws for several years. After the period of bride-service is complete, residence can either continue to be uxorilocal, change to patrilocal, or shift between the two. In the past, disparate households would gather together mainly during Jawosi festivals or shamanic curing ceremonies. Over the course of the past twenty years, as many Kayabi families have moved into a reservation, the Xingu Indigenous Park, many of these independent extended families have started to settle together in larger multifamily villages. Senior family headmen continue to lead their own extended family households, but villages as a whole are run by young leaders proficient in Portuguese and other aspects of contemporary life.

My research concerns Kayabi communities within the Xingu Indigenous Park reservation located on the Xingu River in central Brazil. Families moved to the Xingu Park from areas located farther to the west and northwest, along the Tapajos and Peixes rivers, beginning in the 1950s.[3] They relocated in response to pressure from miners, ranchers, and rubber tappers, who have been moving into Kayabi territories over the course of the twentieth century. Within the Xingu, Kayabi individuals have managed to work successfully with members of the other ethnic groups who also reside in the park despite the fact that in the past, before moving to the park, they had long-standing hostilities with some of these same groups. Kayabi men have, for example, been leaders at posts that serve several indigenous communities in the north of the park. They have also worked with many non-Kayabi, both indigenous and nonindigenous, at higher levels in the park administration, serving as chiefs and assistant chiefs of the park as a whole. Thus, despite the frequent use of images of enmity in Jawosi songs, contemporary Kayabi people live quite productively within the interethnic society of the park.

Because the park was established in explicit contrast to the dominant government policy of acculturation of indigenous peoples, residents were and still are encouraged to practice traditional customs and rituals (Davis 1977:50). Kayabi Jawosi rituals have therefore been encouraged by nonindigenous park directors over the years, and currently they occur relatively frequently in Xinguan Kayabi villages. The park founders and subsequent park administrations have, however, at the same time, made a concerted effort to discourage traditional warfare between park residents. Because Jawosi rituals focus on the bodies and fates of enemies, one might well wonder how they have continued to be practiced with the cessation of warfare. The answer is that Jawosi rituals, including those of past epochs, are based on previous generations' battle experiences as much as, or possibly more than, they are on the current generations' experiences. Memories and songs about these past battle experiences are passed down through the generations and are creatively adapted to new kinds of contemporary encounters with enemies.

Jawosi in the Context of Mourning

The Kayabi Jawosi rituals that I saw performed to help mourners were also held for other reasons as well, such as to celebrate hunters' successful return from collective hunting trips or to celebrate the arrival of a visitor from a distant local group. In the past, Jawosi also took place when Kayabi warriors returned from battle—a function that has led several anthropologists to label them "war rituals" (Grünberg 1970:127; Travassos 1993). They were also part of initiating boys into manhood when such initiation was still performed. In addition, they may have been done as seasonal rituals—held at the harvesting of green corn (Travassos 1993:461) or once during the wet season and once during the dry season (Grünberg 1970:164). Kayabis say that Jawosi rituals, no matter why they are performed, always help to make people happy, to make them forget about their dead. The role Jawosi rituals play in attenuating mourning therefore appears to be salient in a variety of contexts.

While no Jawosi should be performed in the months directly after a death, Kayabi people say that after three or four months the mourners are greatly helped by having one celebrated. Kayabi understand Jawosi rituals and the forgetting they encourage during these months to be necessary because bereaved families are overly interconnected with their deceased relative at this point in time. Because of their meditation on and longing for the deceased, mourners are believed to run a very real risk of following the deceased into death. Mourners' connection to their dead begins with their intense physical interaction with the dead body. Relatives spend days holding and caressing the body before burial, during the time that other relatives are being summoned to come and pay their respects. Much as in other traditions, members of the family also publicly recount the life of the deceased during this time. This is done in the form of angry accusations at other families for slights or wrongs they committed against the deceased while he or she was alive (see Briggs 1992, 1993 for a similar example of anger in funeral laments). During burial, contact with the body is equally intense as particularly close mourners such as children or spouses allow themselves to be partially buried as a show of their sorrow. After burial, one of these individuals may also hang his or her hammock over the grave and sleep directly over the deceased's buried body.

During the following months, mourners' interaction and identification with the dead is paired with a distance from other living people. Female mourners, for example, carry on extended communication with the soul (*'ang*) of their deceased loved one: at sunrise and sunset, they "call out" to the deceased through high-pitched keening as the soul makes its way across the sky. At the same time, however, they and male mourners almost completely stop speaking with other living people. Members of a mourning household do not visit other households and do not even speak very much among themselves for extended periods of time. When they do, they speak in whispers. In my experience, a mourning household is eerily devoid of sound, as if in sympathy with the silence of the dead. This kind of isolation among mourners is not unusual in the Amazon. Peter Gow, for example, has observed that the Piro of the Peruvian Amazon also mourn alone rather than collectively (2000:48).

According to Kayabis, mourners cannot distance themselves from their dead on their own. Rather, they need the help of others. After the initial period of mourning, lasting several months, affines and cross-cousins of the bereaved have the obligation to try to help the bereaved stop thinking about their loss, to forget, and to fully rejoin the community of the living. They wash the bereaved with sweet-smelling leaves to remove the "soul of the corpse" (*'angjang irirewat*), which is understood to cling to the bodies of the bereaved from their intense contact with the corpse and grave. The relatives then paint the bereaved with red annatto (*Bixa orellana*) body paint, give them gifts, make them food, and point out the dangers of mourning. It is at this point that relatives should also hold a Jawosi ritual and encourage mourners to participate.

Jawosi rituals consist mainly of singing and dancing in Jawosi style. Jawosi singing takes place over the course of several days and can last for weeks or more. Singing consists of a group of women, the majority of whom are unmarried, asking each of the married men in a local group to sing for them. The women serve as a chorus for each singer and collectively repeat each of the lines the male soloist sings first, along with a repeating refrain. In contrast to high-pitched keening, women try to imitate the low-pitched male voices. Singing begins in the late afternoon as people are resting in their hammocks. In Xinguan villages, the women's chorus goes to each house and asks the most senior men in each to sing first. These men are usually reclining in their hammocks and sing from this position. Eventually as more people finish their daily activities and afternoon bathing, the chorus will ask some of the younger adult men to sing for them as well. As night falls, the singing increases in intensity, and the women's chorus attracts more members, including young mothers and little girls. After dark, the women continue to walk from house to house and ideally ask each of the married men in each of the households to sing for them. After several hours of singing, the women eventually go to their homes to go to sleep.

The last few nights of a Jawosi are the most festive. While I witnessed 19 nights of Jawosi singing, most of the periods of singing I witnessed were cut short

by other deaths or sicknesses.[4] During the Jawosi that I saw performed to completion, people gathered in one of the more traditional-style longhouses, large structures that are rectangular and spacious in contrast to the newer houses, which are
smaller and oval. Families came with their hammocks and pieces of meat to roast
over small fires as they lounged, visited, and participated in the singing. Families
hung their hammocks together in clusters, and parents and their young children
sat together. On these last nights, only the most senior men (that is, men who
were grandfathers) were asked to sing. They began in their hammocks but after
a few lines got up to dance.

In Jawosi-style dancing, each male soloist dances up and down the central
corridor of the house, taking several steps forward and a few steps back. The
women's chorus follows in one or two rows behind the soloist. The women dance
side by side with their arms around each other's waists and shoulders, alternately.
Men carry weapons or hunting implements such as bows and arrows, fishing
poles, clubs, or shotguns. On these last days of singing, men are also painted with
designs in red annatto and black charcoal representing enemies or game animals.
Others are painted solid red. On these last few nights, the singing and dancing
lasts until a few hours before dawn and ends with a blast from a jaguar bone
flute.

The Jawosi ritual is only one of several practices that are supposed to encourage mourners to forget their deceased relatives. After a person dies, their possessions are either buried with them or destroyed—both actions are described as
helping the living erase the dead from memory as well as a means for the "souls"
('ang) of the destroyed or buried objects to accompany the soul of the dead.
Personal effects such as clothing, hammocks, and jewelry are buried with the
deceased. Baskets are often destroyed; gourds, broken; photographs, burned;
and large items such as shotguns, thrown into the river.[5] The name of the deceased is also not supposed to be used after death.[6] And while Kayabi say it is
avoided so as not to call the deceased back to the living in the form of a ghost, not
uttering the name of the deceased would also seem to facilitate putting them out
of mind. Finally, many months after death, the house where the dead person lived
and is buried is often burnt down and a new house built.[7] In the past, the death
of a family headman caused not only the destruction of his house, but also the
complete dispersal of the local group.[8] Once the house was burned, the resident
nuclear families would each attach themselves to other local groups or live on
their own for a while. These practices too are associated with forgetting. For
other Amazonian peoples, the reordering of place through burning and sweeping
is an important technique used to restructure and erase the mourners' memories
of the dead (Conklin 2001:172–174). For the Kayabi, Jawosi celebrations were
traditionally held in conjunction with the construction of a new house (for one
example, see Travassos 1993:480).

The Role of the Enemy in Mourning

Clearly one of the key aspects of Jawosi festivals that helps mourners distance themselves from their dead and reconnect with the living is simply their social nature. In fact, with a similar logic in mind, one Kayabi community held two Brazilian-style parties in the hope of helping one family end their mourning. I was told that in 1991, two Brazilian *farró* dances were held at Christmas and New Year's Day to help a family forget the loss of their son. These two parties, however, were reported to have had, on the contrary, a negative affect, making the deceased boy's father even more disconsolate than before. A series of Jawosi rituals were finally held and were gradually effective for this family. I argue that the efficacy of Jawosi rituals, in addition to their social nature, lies in the fact that they provide powerful models for turning the dead into enemies rather than consociates. To do this they use imagery and the remains of actual enemies.

Jawosi rituals feature enemies in several ways. Jawosi songs are considered to have been emitted from the bones of dead enemies. Enemies are, therefore, the authors of Jawosi songs. This resonates with the beliefs of other Tupian peoples concerning similar genres: for the Tupian Arawete the dead enemies are considered to be "song teachers" (Viveiros de Castro 1992:241); for the Tupian Parakanã, songs are gifts from enemies appearing in dreams (Fausto 1999:940). After encountering enemy bones while walking in the forest or during battle, the Kayabi warrior "hears" a Jawosi song in an internal way, repeats it to himself, and then, after much repetition, sings it publicly in a Jawosi ritual. In the case of inherited songs, the singer learns a song from a paternal relative, who, of course, may also have learned it from a relative of the previous generation rather than directly from the bones of a dead enemy.

Songs describe interactions in which a single Kayabi warrior encounters a single enemy. Most are about moments of battle when the enemy was killed or kidnapped by the Kayabi warrior. Many feature the words and thoughts of the dead individual as the enemy interacts with the warrior at the moment of his or her demise. The Kayabi warrior featured is frequently understood by most listeners to be the singer himself. Paradoxically this is the case even in inherited songs (see Oakdale 2002). Singers, in some sense, come to "own" the dead they sing about. For example, even in a song that clearly makes reference to being about an elder's brother's victim, the dead enemy is sung about as the singer's own, as a type of inheritance passed down from elder to younger. These songs are, therefore, understood as if they were always autobiographical accounts of battle experiences, recounted from the perspective of a defeated enemy.

Jawosi songs are also supposed to call the souls of deceased enemies who authored them back from the dead and into the present social gathering. The dead enemies are described as "guests," much like the other living Kayabi who may come to the ritual from other local groups.[9] The souls of these enemies are controlled through their songs: the songs bring or call the dead to the event.

Many songs also use the enemy's proper name—presumably, in light of the Kayabi avoidance of the names of the dead, as a more powerful means to call the dead enemy. In one song, for example, the soloist, speaking as the enemy, recounts,

> I went to get my fish trap.
> Like this I told it. Like this I told it.
> The fish were splashing, I went, and my assassin shot me with an arrow.
> . . . I was a "Stone-Ax-Person" [an ethnic identification].
> . . . I was a short enemy.
> . . . I shot your son, various times.
> . . . My name was "Tattooed-Face."[10]

When enemy names are used they are not used with the proper suffix ('i) denoting that the individual is deceased, adding to the sense that these enemy dead have come back to life.[11]

With their focus on one interpersonal encounter between a warrior and an enemy, Jawosi songs provide models for how the living should relate to their own dead family members. The enemy is in a parallel position to the recently deceased, and by extension the mourners should come to see themselves in the position of the Kayabi warrior. While the songs describe interactions that took place when the enemy was alive, during the course of the song, the enemy is clearly understood to be dead. One song begins, for example, with a description of the enemy in his grave: "I sing from my hammock all covered with dirt." Much like recently deceased family members, these dead enemies want to establish sociable relations with the living Kayabi. Dead relatives, especially in the first few months of their new existence, are conceptualized as missing their living families desperately. They can appear as a ghost around their house and grave or beckon their family to come join them in death. In Jawosi songs, the dead enemy's desire for sociability is often expressed through the idiom of food sharing. For Kayabi, food sharing is one of the most sociable acts. Hospitality during intergroup visits often involves food sharing, and collective meals are held to make amends after an argument. In Jawosi songs, enemies beg for food from Kayabi warriors or plead with the warrior to come eat a meal that they have prepared. One song, for example, describes, from the victim's point of view, how he tries to befriend his Kayabi killer by making a meal for him. A few lines of this song are as follows:

> Just like this I always wander about.
> I make food for the one who comes for me [my assassin].
> The one who comes for me, foresees my death.
> I try to make him forget me. To no avail.
> I try to pacify him. To no avail.

In others, captive enemy children beg and cry for food. In one a little girl begs for some honey as her captor runs with her through the forest. The Kayabi warriors described in these songs refuse to share food or relate in any sociable way, much as mourners are encouraged to do with respect to their own dead relatives. The unwavering enmity and emotional detachment of the Kayabi warriors toward the dead enemies featured in these songs provides a model for the living to emotionally dissociate themselves from their own dead.

Singers who have killed the enemies they sing about provide a particularly powerful image of individuals who have been intimately connected to the dead but have been able to separate themselves. Warriors who have taken a life come to have a very close relationship with their victim for a period of time: the blood of the victim fills the killer's stomach and necessitates a special diet and seclusion "to change blood" (see Conklin 2001:202; Viveiros de Castro 1992:240 for similar beliefs in other Amazonian societies). During Jawosi, this same type of bodily communication may be revisited in a brief and controlled manner. For the Arawete, who hold a similar type of ritual, the enemy soul can take over the body of the singer and make him deranged while he sings (Viveiros de Castro 1992:245). In any event, Kayabi killers are individuals who, like mourners, have had a close identification with the dead. The fact that they are alive and singing Jawosi implies that they were also able to separate themselves, for those who do not are understood to die from the unpurged blood of their victim.

While many songs depict in detail the relationship of enmity and estrangement between a Kayabi warrior and a non-Kayabi, others focus on the decay and destruction of the enemy's body. Much as in Achuar mortuary songs (Taylor 1993), these Jawosi songs present images of transformation and decomposition. Unlike Achuar songs, in which the naturalistic process of bodily decay is featured, these kinds of Jawosi songs describe the disintegration of humans in a way that is once removed. They use a series of well-known metaphorical equivalents.[12] In the medium of Jawosi songs, I was told, enemy bones can, and often do, sing about themselves through metaphor. They sing about themselves and their former person as if they were animals, trees, arrow points, or a porridgelike broth. Each of these objects metaphorically relates to a different part of the previously living enemy. When bones sing about themselves as broth, they are singing about their previous flesh. When they sing about themselves as animals, they are singing about their former hair. And when they sing about themselves as trees, they are singing about the entirety of their former body. Most of these Jawosi songs describe how the body parts of the enemy are destroyed or transformed. Some, like those about making a porridge, use the metaphor of cooking: they describe metaphorically how the flesh of the enemy or the flesh of the head is boiled into a porridgelike liquid called in Kayabi kãwi. Kãwi made with starches such as corn or manioc is a staple of the Kayabi diet.[13] A white porridge in Jawosi songs refers to the flesh of an enemy that did not have the tradition of wearing red body paint; a red porridge, to one that did; a hot porridge, to a savage enemy; and a cold porridge, to a less hostile enemy or one who was already dead when encountered. Those songs that make reference to a bitter broth refer to an enemy body whose flesh had already begun to putrefy (Travassos 1993:472). Songs featuring the metaphor of trees also involve images of transformation: they describe how trees are cut down and chopped up by a Kayabi warrior. The soloist's lines of one (which, while originally emitted from the bones of a dead enemy, are sung from the perspective of the Kayabi warrior) are as follows:

> Like this I felled trees.
> I almost lost the handle of my ax.
> I felled redwood.
> Up river, I cut, I cut up the tree that I felled.
> I was yelling
> while I was cutting.
> It was redwood that I felled.
> The name of the tree was Juporyta [an ethnic group].
> It was redwood that I felled.

Images of destruction, such as wood being chopped, or transformation, such as flesh being boiled into broth, may help the bereaved see their own deceased family member as a destroyed body too. In light of Achuar and Wari' ideas about the role their mortuary practices play in making their dead into impersonal or generic entities though images of decay and butchering, Kayabi metaphors in which nonhuman items are used to talk about dead enemies may also work to move mourners from thinking of the dead as persons to conceptualizing them as nonhuman objects that are being chopped and boiled.

As well as employing enemy songs, Jawosi rituals often utilize enemy body parts. During those Jawosi held directly after battles, enemy heads were a featured part of the ritual. One man described for me how when warriors returned home with trophy heads in the 1920s, in the midst of the Brazilian government's attempt to control Kayabi territories, the Kayabi women waiting for them immediately began to sing Jawosi. Others report that in earlier points in time, a warrior gave a head to the sponsor of a Jawosi ritual in exchange for gaining the sponsor's daughter in marriage (Travassos 1993:461). Traditionally, at Jawosi rituals held for the initiation of boys into manhood, enemy bones were also necessary (Grünberg 1970:128; Travassos 1993:459). Craniums were featured in Jawosi rituals not necessarily directly connected to warfare as well. In the 1950s, according to the diaries of a Catholic priest who had a mission in Kayabi areas, a human cranium and a painted jaguar cranium were used in a Jawosi ritual (Travassos 1993:463). Two singers each placed their respective skulls on their shoulders as they sang (Travassos 1993:463). Often human craniums were decorated with cotton string (Grünberg 1970:128). Parts of craniums are still supposedly used at various moments, though I have never been present when this has occurred (for a similar observation see Travassos 1993). One elderly man, for example, was reported to have used a cranium given to him by someone who had found it in the forest during a government-sponsored expedition to "pacify" a more remote indigenous group. The Kayabi (like other indigenous people) functioned as guides and translators on many of these sorts of expeditions. As one man explained, now, mostly old bones are used in these rituals since warfare is prohibited.

On some occasions a fiber doll, representing the body of an enemy—either a specific human enemy or a mythic monster who persecuted the Kayabi in a past epoch—is part of the event as well. There are two kinds of dolls: one is made only of fiber (Cowell 1974:152; Ribeiro 1979:257; Travassos 1993:462), and another is made of the actual bones of an enemy, tied together with cotton string (Travassos 1993:462).

While ethnographic material on the role of enemy bones in these rituals is limited, one consistent feature in that which does exist seems to be that they too are used to present images of enmity and destruction. In rituals in which the fiber doll representing an enemy is used, it is shot full of arrows at the conclusion of the ritual. I was told that the arrows are given to the sponsor of the Jawosi. During men's initiations, enemy craniums were broken into small pieces and distributed, first to men and then to women (Grünberg 1970:128). I was told that a warrior would bring bones to the festival and the group of boys who were being initiated would hit them, presumably breaking them into pieces, this being the first time they touched the remains of a corpse. The pieces of the craniums were then discarded, with the teeth being saved to string onto necklaces. When heads were taken in battle, I was told by some that Jawosi singing was correlated with the moment that the teeth began to loosen from the skull.

Amazonian Notions of Vitality

It is tempting to interpret the enemies' role in these rituals as Maurice Bloch might, as a kind of "positive predation," a means of capturing generative power or vitality from enemy bodies, in the form of heads, bones, teeth, blood, or souls (Bloch 1982:229, 1992). Much as in other funerary rituals (Bloch and Parry, eds. 1982), these Kayabi rituals are also infused with images of fertility. As Carlos Fausto has observed, in South America, destruction and consumption are necessary parts of the productive process of constructing new persons and bodies (1999:937). For example, when the bones of the enemy are used to make an effigy of the victim, the model is suggestively called the "image or model of a child" (Travassos 1993:462). Furthermore, in the past when Jawosi rituals were done to initiate boys, it was the sign that they could legitimately father a child. However, in the Kayabi case, if vitality is being canalized from enemies it is not understood so much as an objectified substance as it is a perspective or position. While substances of the enemy—such as the enemy's blood (in the body of the killer), bones, or cranium—are incorporated, at least for a short time, they are purged quickly or broken and, for the most part, thrown away. The most lasting aspect of the enemy, the part that is passed down through the generations, is his or her song, the musical description of the position of enmity.[14] Countering previous interpretations of sixteenth-century Tupinambá cannibalism, which argued that the motivation for eating enemies was the desire to incorporate the qualities of the victim, Viveiros de Castro has observed that the "quality" that was incorporated was the enemy position, not the substance of the enemy (1992:286). He sees this capacity to see oneself as the enemy as the key to Tupi-Guarani-speaking peoples' cannibalism more generally (1992:249). Given that Jawosi rituals are supposed to make the living forget about their dead, to turn the dead into non-Kayabi of a sort, the position of enmity is likely one of the most salient qualities gained from the Tupian Kayabi's Jawosi songs as well.[15]

Viveiros de Castro (1998) has further argued that in the Amazon, perspective is linked to the body—that is, a particular worldview comes from having a certain kind of body, either animal or human or the body characteristic of one ethnic group or another. A killer's temporary incorporation of the blood of his victim may therefore be a necessary step in accessing the enemy's perspective. The blood of the victim is not, however, where the vitality is located. Rather, vitality (understood as the power to live) is associated with the process of movement back and forth between perspectives. Conklin has observed that for the Amazonian Wari', agency and "productive relationships are generated by crossing, transcending, and reversing boundaries, including especially the boundaries between predator and prey" (2001:203). One could extend this observation and comment that for the Kayabi, it is generated by crossing back and forth between enemy and Kayabi perspectives, which the above excerpts from Jawosi songs show are essentially perspectives of predator and prey.

The power of the sung images for Kayabi mourners is very likely found in these perspectival shifts. The most prestigious songs, those that listeners say are the most pleasing to hear, dramatize these changes in perspective by adding a further elaboration. They switch midway from the enemy's perspective to the warrior's perspective and then back again to the enemy's before the song finishes and the Kayabi warrior returns to his own persona. In these songs, for one or two lines, the singer breaks out of the persona of the enemy and sings as a Kayabi warrior. In one example of such a song, the soloist begins by singing from the perspective of an enemy girl:

My killer was a person of renown.
I cried to my killer, to my killer.

Then, at the midpoint of the song he shifts to the perspective of the girl's relatives and describes their quiet anguish about their loss. In the following passage "my killer" becomes "your killer" and "I" becomes "her." My translators explained that these lines were sung as if they had been uttered by the Kayabi warrior who abducted the girl to the girl's relatives.

You all were quiet
when your killer of renown brought her.

After these two lines, the singer shifts again to the perspective of the little girl:

The first time he grabbed me I cried.
My killer was a person of renown.

Finally, after the song is complete, the singer returns to his Kayabi identity.

The frequent use of metaphor in Jawosi songs also fosters a focus on perspectival changes. If a warrior sings as if he were an enemy and the enemy sings about himself as if he were an animal or an inanimate object such as broth or a tree, there is a similar kind of emphasis on changing one's point of view. As Viveiros de Castro (1998:470) has observed for Amazonian perspectivism more generally, "The way humans perceive animals and other subjectivities that inhabit the world—gods, spirits of the dead, inhabitants of other cosmic levels, meteorological phenomena, plants and even objects and artifacts—differs profoundly from the way in which these beings see humans and see themselves." These other beings see themselves as anthropomorphic humans and their own behavior and habits as a "form of culture" (Viveiros de Castro 1998:470). "They see their bodily attributes (fur feathers claws beaks etc.) as body decorations or cultural instruments" (Viveiros de Castro 1998:470). From this perspective, humans, by contrast, are the "others," the nonpersons, the animals to be preyed upon. The use of metaphor in Jawosi songs gives the impression of seeing the world from a new point of view, of seeing the world as if at one moment one were human and then at the next, when the metaphorical references become understood, as if one were a tree, an animal, or a spirit inhabitant of an "other" domain, who sees trees, animals, or inanimate objects as fellow anthropomorphic persons.

The emphasis on changes in perspective found in Jawosi songs makes sense in light of Kayabi ideas about fertility and regeneration. For the Kayabi, like so many other Amazonians (Conklin 2001; Descola 1992, 1996; Lorrain 2000; Pollock 1993), new life comes from a kind of cycling between humans and non-human domains. For Kayabis, human souls, prior to being born, are kept by animal-like spirits, spirits whose primary charge is to take care of the animals in the forests and rivers. Sickness and ultimately the moment of human death is also caused by these same animal spirits as retribution for the animals humans kill in the hunt.[16] For other Amazonians, there is a similar kind of reciprocity between animal and human domains. These others, however, put more of a positive emphasis on what it is that is exchanged: for the Wari' and the Kulina, dead humans, directly after their bodies are destroyed by fire or decay, are reborn as white-lipped peccaries who present their bodies as food to their former human relations (Conklin 2001; Lorrain 2000; Pollock 1993). In these cosmologies, once the deceased is free of his or her human body, he or she can take on other perspectives and other kinds of bodies to benefit the living. With respect to this cosmic reciprocity, Conklin observes for the Wari' that while empowerment comes from appropriating various items and substances, this incorporation never establishes domination over the other. Rather, "the flow of life is generated through exchange. To be a predator, one must sometimes be prey" (Conklin 2001:204).

While the Kayabi do not explicitly draw a connection between changing perspective (and body) and the process of forgetting, other Amazonians do. The Ecuadorian Achuar, for example, explicitly state with respect to their mortuary songs that only when the dead are forgotten as persons with a distinctive face can new babies be born, life being a limited resource (Taylor 1993:659). Given the similar emphasis on forgetting in Kayabi Jawosi rituals and similar ideas about the movement of souls from human to nonhuman domains and then back again, one can conclude that not forgetting, giving the deceased a kind of permanence, is a fate fit only for enemies. Remembering the dead holds an individual apart from the reciprocity between domains. It could be seen as an unusual kind of example of Bloch's "negative predation"—unusual in the sense that rather than Jawosi being an act that stops the enemy from performing rituals to ensure that the dead will "continue uncorrupted in memory for ever, as they wish their state to remain" (as in the case of the Greeks and the Trojans), it is a ritual that stops the enemy from being forgotten and entering fully into process (Bloch 1982:228). While Kayabis did not make explicit to me exactly where in the cosmos the souls of enemies reside that are sung about in Jawosi, it seems clear that they are in a kind of stasis, since they can be remembered and "called back" through their songs generation after generation. Similarly, for the Achuar, victims of headhunting raids were also given a kind of postdeath permanence for a period of time, a fate that was the antithesis of what was done for relatives. In contrast to the forgetting of facial features encouraged by Achuar funeral laments, the facial features of enemies were preserved through a process of shrinking, molding, and drying the facial skin to produce a realistic portraiture of the dead (Taylor 1993:672).

For the Achuar, the enemy (in the form of the shrunken head) was then turned into a kinsman, executed a second time, and buried and mourned as a kinsmen, that is, forgotten as one's own relative would be. Taylor argues that this process was linked to stealing the enemies' capabilities for existence and increasing the stock of individuals and faces to be reborn to one's own group (1993:672–674). A similar argument could be made for the Kayabi, given that they in the past (like their fellow Tupi speakers, the sixteenth-century Tupinambá) also adopted enemies, though they did this while the enemies were alive, only to kill their adopted kinsmen later (Carneiro da Cunha and Viveiros de Castro 1985; Viveiros de Castro 1992). These adopted enemies of the past, however, have not been forgotten like those among the Achuar. For Kayabi these adopted enemies are still sung about just as are more recent enemies; their souls are still called back through

Jawosi songs. They are, therefore, still in a position of stasis and have not entered back into life through new Kayabi births. Unlike the Achuar, it would seem that for the Kayabi, the issue is not so much stealing the life force of enemies to be used as one's own, but holding onto the position of enmity in a permanent fashion to use it when need be, when, for example, Kayabi mourners need to distance themselves from their own dead. In other words, giving the enemy a type of transcendence over time and the cycling of life allows one's own dead to be fully forgotten and to be reborn, to be immersed in process.

Conclusion

Enemies hold a central place in Kayabi rituals that help mourners close a period of mourning. They author the songs sung at these rituals, are guests at these events, and, at times particularly in the past, have their bones displayed and destroyed during these moments. Following regionally specific understandings of mortuary rituals (and rituals involving enemies), I have tried to give a more regionally and culturally specific account of one of the functions of such a ritual, namely, in the words of one Kayabi man, the way it encourages people to "breathe deeply and forget." I argue that during these events, if something is being canalized from enemies, it is best understood as a type of perspective or position of enmity and that vitality is understood as an ability to switch or move through different cosmological perspectives. Jawosi rituals—which, like many mortuary rituals, emphasize regeneration—celebrate warriors' and participants' abilities to change perspective from Kayabi to enemy, from human to animal, or from animate to inanimate. It is, in fact, the ability to take on the position of enmity toward one's own dead that ultimately leads to personal and collective regeneration after the loss of a loved one. Given that life is seen as a limited resource, with souls moving back and forth between human and nonhuman domains, and that forgetting is the means by which this movement takes place, Jawosi songs hold the enemy dead in a kind of permanent and undesirable stasis. In this way, they stand outside of the process of life and become a kind of fixed resource for mourners to use when need be. In a cosmological system like that of the Amazonian Kayabi, permanence and transcendence is only an ideal destiny for one's enemies.

Acknowledgments

The field research on which this chapter was based took place between the years 1991 and 1993 and was funded by an IIE Fulbright Grant for Doctoral Dissertation Research Abroad, a Predoctoral Grant (no. 5372) from the Wenner-Gren Foundation for Anthropological Research, and a Travel Grant from the Center for Latin American Studies at the University of Chicago. I am also grateful to the Museu Nacional in Rio and to Eduardo Viveiros de Castro, my Brazilian sponsor during this period. The archival research (done during 2000) on which this chapter was based was funded by a Resource Allocation Committee Grant from the University of New Mexico and a Field Research Grant from the Latin American and Iberian Institute, also at the University of New Mexico. I am grateful to all these institutions.

Notes

1. The dead are often understood as "other" or "nonhuman" in Amazonian cosmologies (see Carneiro da Cunha 1978; Viveiros de Castro 1992:482).

2. In Bloch's earlier work (1982) this seems to be an issue only for certain types of systems, "those like the Merina, whose ideological representation implies an unchanging permanent organization" (1982:223). In his later formulations (1992) this is a "quasiuniversal" goal.

3. Some Kayabi people continue to live outside the park in these areas.

4. Jawosi rituals cannot be held if other deaths have subsequently occurred or if people are sick.

5. Recently, many families have begun to choose not to destroy large consumer items. One family also conducted a long discussion about whether photographs of the deceased should be destroyed or kept.

6. The taboo on using a name is not maintained if a story is being told about the person but is maintained if the name is simply asked to be uttered by a speaker.

7. In the burial I witnessed, the deceased was buried under the place where he had hung his hammock. Others consistently commented, however, that the dead are buried next to the central house posts.

8. Moving away from the house of the deceased is a common practice in the lowlands, especially among Tupian peoples (Kracke 1978:54, 1981; Fausto 2001:407) but also among groups in the Guiana region (Riviere 2000:260).

9. The same term, *pareawa*, is used to refer to these dead enemies as is used to refer to the living Kayabi guests who have been invited to a Jawosi from other local groups. Pareawa is also used to refer to the relatives that travel from other local groups to pay their respects before a burial. Living Kayabi guests are often treated in jest during the invitation process as if they too were enemies (Travassos 1993:464). The notion that the dead become guests at some other type of being's festivals is common throughout Amazonia, though usually this "other type of being" is not human (see Conklin 2001).

10. For one other example see Travassos 1993:473.

11. The names of enemies are always in Kayabi, so they most likely could not have been the name the victim used in his or her own community.

12. Taylor's (1993) examples of Achuar songs also rely upon similar metaphors, but she does not address this aspect of them.

13. Kayabis negate any suggestion that they actually ate the bodies of enemies.

14. The enemies' names and souls are also linked to these songs. Kayabis change their names frequently throughout their life, and warriors often take on the name of their slain enemies as their own. Whether or not they pass these names down to their children is unclear. If they do, the name of the enemy may also therefore be "incorporated" in a permanent manner. Songs call the enemies' souls back to the living, so in a sense, enemy

souls may be passed down through the generations as well. I am uncertain what happens to the enemies' teeth that are made into a necklace. Presumably these would be buried with the Kayabi warrior when he dies.

15. Viveiros de Castro (1998) has also argued that in the Amazon, perspective is linked to having a certain kind of body. A killer's temporary incorporation of the blood of his victim may therefore be a necessary step in accessing the enemy's perspective.

16. I, like other researchers of the Kayabi, have very little information on the Kayabi afterlife. From shamans' accounts of sicknesses and death, it would seem that human souls spend some time as pets, children, or spouses of the animal spirits. The soul also makes its way across the sky after death, according to some. What life is like for those who have died, however, is unclear and not a subject of much elaboration, with the exception of the fate of the shaman. Shamans go to live with their spirit familiars after death and have a life much like their life on earth. Living shamans visit the dead shamans in dreams and report upon their activities.

The Mortuary "Laying-In" Crypts
of the Hopewell Site

Beyond the Funerary Paradigm

A. Martin Byers

Archaeologists have characterized the mortuary aspects of regional and transregional material cultural complexes such as the Adena, Red Ochre, Glacial Kame, and Hopewell as cults of the dead (Cunningham 1948; Dragoo 1963; Sanger 1973). While these phenomena are commonly discussed in terms of religion and cosmology, articulations between these "cults" and living communities remain only vaguely defined.

Since the groundbreaking work of Binford (1971) and Brown (1971b), this question of articulation has become paramount in prehistoric mortuary studies. However, using mortuary data to reconstruct social systems has been limited by the assumption that most mortuary deposits mark the termination of funerary events. A commonly accepted axiom is that mortuary treatment is a measure of the social position of the deceased at the time of death. Therefore, variation in mortuary treatment within a given burial population is used to map the social articulations of the living. I will call this the funerary paradigm (Binford 1971; Braun 1979; Brown 1971b, 1979, 1981; Greber 1976, 1979a, 1979b; Tainter 1977b, 1978).

While critiques of the funerary paradigm have appeared (for example, Hodder 1982a; Shanks and Tilley 1987; Parker Pearson 1999), these have generally centered on the presentation of counterexamples that focus upon social and political behavior. None has considered issues relating to concepts of the soul and its relationship to real and symbolic bodies in the context of corpse disposal. Thus, the funerary paradigm and its critics have developed arguments largely premised on the Judeo-Christian-Muslim worldview that the individual is a singular spiritual subject embodied in a corporeal unity, a sort of unitary body/spirit dualism. However, if cultures define a human individual as possessing multiple spirits embodied in different components of the body, each of which requires different mortuary treatment, a complex range of postmortem manipulation and variable burial treatments would be expected. These could make the social standing of the deceased at the time of death irrelevant, thereby obscuring the possible social structures of the responsible community. This perspective further reinforces the complexity of the relationship between social structure and the mortuary record, but it also offers us powerful tools for investigating that relationship.

William Mills (1922) was one of the first archaeologists to promote the funerary paradigm for Ohio Hopewell. He strongly argued against Squier and Davis's interpretation that emphasized human sacrifice, probably derived from Mesoamerica (Squier and Davis 1848:143–160). Mills proposed that such mortuary data were simply the outcome of the funerary practices characteristic of the Ohio Hopewell complex:

> [T]he idea of human sacrifice was in no way borne out by our investigations. The sites of the Mound City group were found to be similar in every way to that of the Tremper mound, on the lower Scioto, where the sacred structure, with its crematories and depositories was used solely for the cremation and burial of the dead, and for the attendant funereal ceremonies. This present conclusion regarding the surmise as to human sacrifice automatically answers that as to relationship with the southern culture groups. (Mills 1922:561)

Mills' position effectively banned the use of those terms favored by Squier and Davis when describing the mortuary data, such as sacrificial mound and sacrificial altar, and replaced them with terms from his own cultural background. Thus, mortuary features became burial mounds, burial platforms, crematory basins, tombs, and graves. Mills' reduction of Ohio Hopewell complexity to a prehistoric version of the twentieth-century Euro-American funerary complex has continued. For example, the dispersed hamlet/vacant center model (Dancey and Pacheco 1997; Pacheco 1989, 1993, 1996, 1997; Prufer 1964, 1965, 1997) follows Mills' lead by interpreting the mortuary contents associated with such major earthworks as the Hopewell site, Mound City, Seip, and Liberty Works in funerary terms. Thus, largely predetermined by the social premises of this paradigm, the broad range of mortuary artifacts, their variable distribution across the burial populations, and the variation in the forms of postmortem manipulation of the deceased, as well as in the burial facilities, are interpreted as marking a hierarchically ranked social system (Greber 1976, 1979a, 1979b, 1983; Mills 1916, 1922; Shetrone 1926).

Despite these arguments, no adequate justification has been offered for applying the funerary paradigm to Ohio Hopewell mortuary data. Furthermore, if mortuary complexity is a true measure of the varied range of mortuary events, then little can be given. This paper, therefore, will present an alternative model of Ohio Hopewell mortuary practices, grounded in a generalized conception of historic Native American worldview. This view characterized the world as immanently sacred, a place where human material interventions into the natural order have grave implications for the maintenance of cosmological balance and continuity. Humans believed they possessed multiple souls that animated the different components of their bodies. The living were expected to carry out mortuary rituals that released these souls in a manner that would ensure personal, social, and cosmic renewal.

Robert Hall (1979, 1997) has argued convincingly that historically known Native American mortuary practices incorporated a series of rites that had both strong funerary and world renewal components. Typically, the death of a person initiated rites of death and burial, often to be followed later with an incremental series of separate mortuary rites: mourning, spirit release, memorial, name adoption, reincarnation, and world renewal rites. Each required progressive transformation of the body. Several months following burial, the remains were disinterred and the bones were cleaned, bundled, stored, and reburied. Then another disinterment would be carried out, followed possibly by cremation, and then reburial. Each step progressively distanced the funerary mortuary aspect and emphasized rebirth and world renewal. Hall gives historical depth to these practices, arguing that certain material components required by these different stages can be traced back to the symbolic aspect of the Early, Middle, and Late Woodland mortuary practices.

> The sods in the Cheyenne and Arapaho Sun Dances explicitly represent lumps of mud brought from beneath the primordial sea by mythical Earth Divers and have explicit associations with toes.[1] The importance in northern Midwestern Woodland burial mound architecture of mud and sediments from watery environments implies that Woodland mound ceremonialism may have had a hitherto unrecognized relationship to World Renewal ritual. These mortuary and World Renewal connections lead in several directions. . . . [The] Cheyenne and Arapaho Sun Dance altars relate as well to certain symbolic earth entrances represented two thousand years ago in Hopewell art and ritual structures; some in the form of a bear paw, others more explicitly sexual.[2] What is a grave but a portal to the netherworld by which one returns to the womb of the Earth Mother? (Hall 1997:22–23)

Based on a number of recent analyses of the embankment earthworks (Byers 1987, 1998; Romain 1994, 1996, 2000), there are convincing empirical reasons to postulate that those who were responsible for these monumental works experienced them as embodying the essential sacred powers of the cosmos and therefore constructed them as monumental iconic symbols of the cosmos. Because the living thus participated in constituting the essential nature of the world, the earthwork construction was also a means by which mortuary activities were transformed into world renewal rituals. The Ohio Hopewell earthworks consequently served as the media by which the deceased were subjected to a complex incremental series of mortuary/world renewal rites. This complex mortuary series can be generally termed the funerary–mourning–spirit release–world renewal ritual process. To clarify this, a brief theoretical discussion is required concerning how material culture mediates social activities, particularly mortuary events.

The Constituting of Mortuary Events

The court warrant is a useful analogy to illustrate the constitutive dimension of the stylistics of material culture (Byers 1999). Warrants are documents that constitute their legitimate bearers as officers of the court, such as bailiffs or sheriffs. With the appropriate warrant a sheriff seizing and handcuffing a person constitutes a legal arrest. In the absence of the warrant, this same behavior might be better characterized as an assault. Thus, warranting is important to ensure that relevant persons recognize both the intentions and the social position of the doers, thereby constituting their intended behavior into the type of social action that it is. This is well illustrated by the court warrant. Part of performing the act of arresting a person is to carry out the physical behavior so that it is understood as an arrest, and using the warrant is critically important. It is also conventional. Therefore, it is a critical symbolic component of the behavior by which it is made to be the action intended. For this reason, warranting, or more properly, the instruments of warranting, are always symbolic in nature.

If material warranting is a necessary part of contemporary life, we may assume that it was in the past, as well. In a world without writing, and therefore without written warrants and other forms of authoritative documentation, material items may have served this purpose. Archaeologists recognize that the symbolic aspect of material culture is carried by style. Thus, it is postulated that material cultural style has symbolic powers equivalent to those mediated in modern societies by authoritative documentation, such as warrants, licenses, money, stamps, passports, and visas, not to mention military and police badges, insignias, uniforms, and so on (Douglas 1982). This means that in nonliterate societies, warranting is a symbolic material process that is built into the use of the artifacts mediating particular practices. We can even speak of warranting as the symbolic pragmatics of behavior—*pragmatics* being used in the action sense.

Therefore, for nonindustrial societies, material cultural items bearing different styles can be termed action warrants, symbolic warrants, symbolic pragmatic devices, and so on. These terms are essentially synonyms. For example, in a typical foraging society, anyone who carries out predatory behaviors would use tools displaying the local hunting styles. In this way he or she ensures being perceived as a hunter. Implicated in this, of course, is the opposite. Those who use hunting gear bearing unfamiliar styles will be treated as "strangers." To be perceived as a stranger may be tantamount to being perceived as an actual or potential "poacher" by the local population, even though the predatory behaviors these strangers were to perform would be no different objectively from those performed by local people using tools bearing recognized hunting styles. Thus, by bearing appropriate styles, both ordinary and not-so-ordinary artifacts serve as different types of action warrants, symbolic pragmatic devices, or simply warrants by which the "raw" behaviors they typically mediate are constituted as the appropriate types of social activities their doers intend.

The term *focal position* is used to refer to social positions that define the action nature of events. Persons occupying such positions are considered focal participants. It is therefore appropriate to speak of focal warrants, material cultural items that symbolically constitute their legitimate users as occupants of focal positions.

In these terms, mortuary events constitute one type of performative social event. The participants' intentions are signaled by the use of the appropriate material cultural warrants. A mortuary event is also unique in that two warranting conditions must be met. One condition constitutes it as a mortuary event per se, and the second condition constitutes it as a particular type of mortuary event.[3] The first condition is satisfied by having the deceased present in some state (as a full body, as a bundle of bones, as cremated ashes) or, if no tangible bodily form or part is available, in some symbolic form (for example, a picture of the deceased or some closely associated artifact). The second condition is satisfied largely by the nature of the mortuary treatment accorded to the deceased. This treatment constitutes the particular action nature of the event, that is, a funeral, a mourning rite, a name-adoption rite, and so on. A critical aspect of mortuary treatment can be the form and degree of the postmortem manipulation to which the deceased were subjected.

Thus, the funerary event takes on its general mortuary character by virtue of the deceased being present, and it takes on its particular mortuary character by the treatment of the deceased. A tension arises over a choice between treating the deceased in terms of his or her focal or other social position and the treatment of the deceased as a symbolic warrant that mediates the behaviors of the living participants. Since the humanity of the deceased defines the event as mortuary, the deceased may be treated as a participant, with his or her social position assuming primacy. Alternatively, since the deceased is inert, much like other material objects, the remains may be treated as a symbolic warrant of behaviors by the participants.

This ambiguity may arise from a recognition that while death brings about changes in the social standing of deceased persons, it does not eliminate their action capacity. Of course, deceased individuals cannot behave in the same manner as they did when they were living. However, they typically are still recognized as having action capacities—and in many cases, very special capacities. For example, death did not eliminate the powerful action capacities of the royal Inca, ruler of Tawantinsuyu. The mummy of the deceased ruler continued to exercise the royal will by being regularly and ritually consulted on political and economic matters vital to the future of the Inca state (Conrad and Demarest 1984:113–116).

Hence, the presence of the deceased is necessary to define the event as mortuary in nature. Yet it is the form of postmortem corpse treatment that constitutes the pragmatic meaning of the mortuary event, and this treatment realizes the symbolic warranting or action-constitutive moment. If the mode of postmortem treatment is such that the deceased are being presented in the manner in which they would have presented themselves publicly when living, then the deceased can be interpreted as the focal participants of the mortuary event, as virtual "hosts" or "honored guests." Since the host position determines the type of event that is occurring, then, in this case, it is appropriate to characterize the mortuary event as a funeral.

If we use this deceased-as-in-life presentation as the baseline, it follows that each increment of postmortem manipulation diminishes the focal participant aspect of the deceased and increases the symbolic warranting aspect. A complex series of postmortem transformations might lead to a symbolic warranting state that constitutes a sacrificial ritual. In short, the deceased or selected elements of the deceased might serve as sacrificial offerings. As offerings, then, the mortuary events could be characterized as different types of postmortem sacrifice.

The term *postmortem human sacrifice* is presented in deliberate contrast to *lethal human sacrifice*. A lethal human sacrifice is the type of initiatory mortuary event postulated by Squier and Davis (1848:143–160) for Ohio Hopewell. A postmortem human sacrifice is constructed by deliberate manipulation of the deceased and is linked to renewal rites. Different forms and degrees of manipulation constitute different types of sacrificial renewal rites, such as ancestral renewal, clan renewal, tribal renewal, sodality renewal, and minor to major world renewal. Typically, the postmortem manipulation of the deceased systematically deconstructs their corporeal unity and thereby transforms their social identity. The differential weighting of these two opposing roles played by the deceased, as mapped in variable mortuary treatment, is what I will call the focal participant–symbolic warrant continuum. The participant extreme, in which the symbolic warranting aspect is subsumed under the focal participant role, is most clearly articulated in a mortuary event that we term a funeral. The symbolic warranting extreme, which subsumes the participant aspect and effectively eliminates funerary content, is most fully realized in the postmortem sacrificial mortuary aspect. In an important sense, as a type of postmortem sacrifice, cremation may be the ultimate form by which the deceased as symbolic warranting capital are invested in world renewal.

Methodologically, the following analysis assumes that broad variation in postmortem manipulation is frequently associated with a range of types of mortuary activities, from funerals to sacrificial rituals. The probability that this variation involves an incremental shift from funerary to postmortem sacrificial ritual is increased when specially prepared mortuary contexts are present. As stipulated earlier, since the Ohio Hopewell embankment earthworks were built to embody and present the essential sacred nature of the cosmos (Byers 1987, 1998; Romain

2000), they would be excellent examples of world renewal ritual locales, suggesting that the mortuary practices performed in their context were forms of postmortem sacrifice constituting world renewal rituals.

The "Laying-In" Crypt Model of the Hopewell Site

In his overview of the mortuary data of Mound City, Seip, Liberty Works, Tremper, Hopewell, and Turner, Shetrone (1926) noted that Turner and Hopewell contrasted with other major Ohio Hopewell sites. While the vast majority of the remains recovered from Mound City, Seip, Liberty Works, and Tremper involved cremation, 70 percent of the burials at Hopewell were extended interments (Lloyd 1999, 2000), and about the same proportion was reported for Turner.

If the goal of all Ohio Hopewell burial programs was an incremental series of postmortem sacrificial rites leading to cremation, why does this disparity exist? The explanation proposed here involves the "laying-in" crypt model, as developed for the Hopewell site. This model specifies that the mortuary data of the Hopewell site are the result of a complex funerary–mourning–spirit release–world renewal ritual process that was abruptly truncated, possibly twice, the first accounting for Mound 25 and the second accounting for Mound 23 (figure 9.1).

A significant component of the mortuary program for Mound 25 is the vaulted chamber feature. Both Moorehead (1922) and Shetrone (1926) commented that encountering a large arch or vaulting of loose earth while excavating would lead to encountering an entombed, extended skeleton. (This was also the case for Mound 23.) The "most common type of tomb recorded by both surveys [of Shetrone and Moorehead] appears to have been constructed of logs placed about a 'platform' and supporting a bark or timber roof. Such tombs . . . are associated with the characteristic easily recognized 'arch' of loosened earth which results from the roof's collapse. None of these typical log tombs were found outside these three burial groups" under Mound 25 (Greber and Ruhl 1989:52–54). Although some of these "vaulted" chambers may have been only a little over 1 meter high, as Shetrone commented, a number reached almost to the top of the primary mound and its gravel cover. "A good illustration of the caving down of earth above a grave following the decay of the enclosing timber structure is shown in [Burial 12]. The archlike opening in this was 7 feet long and 4 1/2 feet wide, extending 6 feet above the floor level. It was not unusual to find this loose arched condition extending practically to the top of the mound, in some instances, more than 10 feet above the base" (Shetrone 1926:72).

As illustrated by both of the above quotations, the terms *grave* and *tomb* were consistently used to label such features. This terminology predisposes the reader to identify the whole mortuary process as reflecting funerary events. However, as pointed out by James Brown (1979), any extended mortuary period involving postmortem manipulation would have required a substantially constructed, easily accessible mortuary facility. This facility would constitute an important sym-

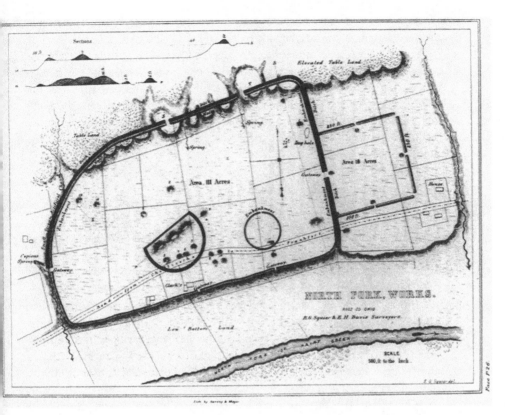

Figure 9.1. Map of the Hopewell site by Ephraim Squier and Edwin Davis (1848) titled "North Fork, Works."

bolic warrant of the mortuary rites that it mediated. Therefore, the laying-in crypt model postulates that these vaulted chambers served as "laying-in" crypts. The period during which they were used to process the corpse is termed the "laying-in" period.

Robert Mainfort (1989; also see Clay 1992) accounted for a structurally equivalent Adena mortuary facility in similar terms when he argued that large centrally located "tombs" served as crypts in collective mortuary ritual cycles. In his view, individuals archaeologically recovered from these crypts represented final interments that were left in place rather than being removed and buried elsewhere, as were their predecessors. He concluded, "It is inappropriate . . . to equate the status of a particular individual found within a crypt with the effort expended in construction of the facility, as Shryock (1987) has done. Nevertheless, the postmortem manipulation of corpses processed through crypts appears to represent greater effort than that accorded individuals buried in smaller peripheral graves" (Mainfort 1989:168). By extension, he argued that it was a mistake to take the variable Adena mortuary treatment as indexing a simple chiefdom system, a point also made by Clay (1991, 1992, 1998).

There is a significant difference, however, between the postulated laying-in crypts of the Hopewell site and the typical Adena crypt. While only one or two Adena crypts were available for use at one time, many and perhaps all of the Hopewell site crypts were used simultaneously. If this was the case, then the many extended burials would reflect a truncated interment sequence caught up in the ritual abandonment of the mortuary features and facilities on the floor of this mound.

Demonstration

Thus, the laying-in crypt model rests on the claim that the Hopewell mortuary data resulted from a truncated funerary–mourning–spirit release–world renewal ritual process. It is important, therefore, to spell out the possible mortuary steps to which the deceased would have been subjected and then to predict empirical expectations that can be used to verify the model. First, following the initial death rites, the deceased would have been placed in an appropriate crypt to initiate her or his laying-in period. During the first "half" of the period, incrementally staged mourning, spirit release, and other such rites would have been performed. Since these would have involved a series of gatherings of kin and companions, artifacts appropriate to each ritual stage would have been cumulatively deposited with the deceased in the laying-in crypt.

It is postulated that these artifacts would be emically classified into four broad categories: laying-in warrants; personalty; mourning gifts; and custodial regalia. The laying-in warrants would be artifacts that were specific to and partly consti- tutive of the laying-in period, materially distinguishing it from the prior funerary and subsequent post-laying-in periods. The latter is postulated as focusing heavily on the postmortem sacrificial moment critical to world renewal rituals. Personalty artifacts would be those artifacts accumulated by the deceased during her or his active social lifetime. This set would have accompanied the deceased from one stage to the next.

Mourning gifts—a generic term implicating mourning, spirit adoption, and spirit release—would be artifacts contributed by companions and kin during the incremental stages of the laying-in period. Because of the incremental nature of the rites during this period and because both close and distant kin and compan- ions would participate, the mourning gift category may be resolved into at least two subcategories: formal mourning gifts and personalty-mourning gifts. The former would have been contributed by those who held a more distant relation with the deceased, while the latter would have been given by closer kin and companions.

The fourth set includes artifact types constituting custodial regalia. These would be artifact types directly associated with Ohio Hopewell, such as copper plates, headdresses, and "trophy skulls." Because of their importance as focal warrants of ritual positions, they would have constituted their users as custodial officers endowed with the power of these artifacts. Such power would have enabled the warranted users to conduct the rituals with which the regalia were associated, primarily world renewal in nature. They would also have been accumulated during her or his lifetime and would have accompanied the deceased during the total process.

As stated above, these are postulated as emically real categories. However, the personalty and mourning gift categories would have overlapping artifact types. Closely related kin and companions might have contributed as mourning gifts some of their own treasured personalty items, such as copper ear spools, a valued shell necklace, and so on, thereby making up the personalty-mourning gift subcategory. These would be identical to the same artifact types making up the deceased's personalty assemblage, but they would have emic meaning as mourning gifts. Because of the overlap of personalty and personalty-mourning gift artifact types, it is expected that many such artifact types would have accumulated during the laying-in period.

With the termination of the laying-in period, the deceased was removed from the laying-in crypt and transferred to the next ritual stage, in this case, constituted by rites having significant world renewal content. This transfer would have involved sorting the accumulated laying-in period artifacts according to category. Some would have accompanied the deceased to the next stage. Others would have been removed (as being inappropriate for that stage), and they would have been curated for later use. Thus, laying-in warrants and mourning gifts, both personalty and formal subcategories, would have been curated for later collective memorial/world renewal rites. The deceased—along with his or her own personalty and custodial regalia, if any—would then have been moved to the post-laying-in stage. The termination of the process would not have involved crypt burial, as the body either was left in the terminal ritual locale as an extended burial or it was transformed through cremation, depending largely on whether the deceased had custodial regalia status. Cremated burials would mark the deceased as a mediator of sacrificial rites for lesser world renewal rituals, while the extended burials with custodial regalia would mark the deceased as accompanying the regalia, constituting the total as a sacrificial offering mediating major world renewal rites.

However, truncating the funerary–mourning–spirit release–world renewal ritual process would "freeze" the distribution of all four artifact categories, generating three major deposit contexts: the crypt burial context, the noncrypt burial context, and the burnt deposit context. The mix of category types would be unique to each deposit context. The crypt burial context (A) would be the set of laying-in crypts on the floors of the two mounds, Mounds 23 and 25. These would have been interpreted archaeologically as "tombs," as they would contain the deceased in a state that was "frozen" partway through the laying-in period.

This burial context would include the range of warranting artifacts that would have been accumulated during that period. The noncrypt burial context (B) would be the burials marking the normal set of post-laying-in period terminal world renewal rites. The burnt deposit context (C) would be the result of the use of the curated laying-in warrants and mourning gifts.

Hall (1997) argues that memorial rites were significant mortuary events in historic Native American practices. The laying-in crypt model postulates that the accumulated laying-in warrants and mourning gifts would be excellent candidates for this purpose, ensuring that these artifacts were appropriately used both as warrants of collective memorial rites for the deceased and as memorial/sacrificial offerings, thereby enhancing the world renewal aspect of the mortuary rituals. Therefore, these accumulated artifacts would have been used as sacrificial media for collective memorial/world renewal rites, and the mode of such sacrifice would have been via massive burning in a ritual context.

Given this ritual cycle, it follows that there should be observable and specifiable differences in the distribution of the four categories of artifact types across the three deposit contexts. This patterning is postulated in table 9.1. Since the laying-in period in the crypts was the time when all four categories would have been accumulated with the deceased, crypt burial contexts should display artifact types from all four categories. Being the result of the post-laying-in period, noncrypt burial contexts should be characterized by an absence of artifacts belonging to the laying-in warrant and mourning gift categories, the latter having been removed and curated following the laying-in periods of their respective deceased. Burnt deposit contexts should lack the personalty and the custodial regalia that would have accompanied the deceased to the post-laying-in period ritual, while being rich in the residue of mourning gifts, both personalty and formal types, and laying-in warrants.

Identification of mourning gift and personalty artifact types cannot be determined just from this postulated distribution across the three contexts, since some mourning gifts could have been the donor's own personalty, thereby constituting the personalty-mourning gift subtype. However, it is relatively easy to identify the formal mourning gift types. Since these would have been removed from the laying-in crypt for final deposition in the burnt deposit context, only items suitable as personalty and custodial regalia should be associated with the noncrypt burial context (that is, no formal mourning gift items and no laying-in warrants). Therefore, the only artifact types that are common to all three contexts are personalty types.[4] By subtracting the custodial regalia from the noncrypt burial context, the remaining artifact types make up the personalty type artifacts. Because all four categories are represented in the crypt burial context, by subtracting the personalty type artifacts, the laying-in warrant type artifacts, and the custodial regalia type artifacts from this context, the remaining types make up the formal mourning gift category.

However, as table 9.1 indicates, there is still a problem. What would count as

Table 9.1. Artifact Patterning across the Three Artifact Contexts

Artifact category	Depository context		
	Crypt burial	Noncrypt burial	Burnt deposit
"Laying-in" warrants	Present	Absent	Present
Mourning gifts	Present	Absent	Present
Personalty	Present	Present	Absent
Custodial regalia	Present	Present	Absent

laying-in warrants? Both formal mourning gifts and laying-in warrants would have the same cross-context pattern, namely, being absent from (or rare in) the noncrypt burial context and present in both the crypt burial and burnt deposit contexts. This may not be a significant problem, since the notions of mourning gift and laying-in warrant define real artifacts that are related in noncontradictory warranting terms. Laying-in warrants would be artifacts that would constitute the total spread of incremental events making up the laying-in period. Mourning gifts would have the effect of defining only some of the stages of this process (for example, name-adoption or spirit release or mourning rituals). Thus, mourning gifts would not contradict the warranting effect of the laying-in warrants and, indeed, might enhance the impact of the mortuary event. Therefore, the laying-in warrant would tend to be rather standardized while the formal mourning gift would be variable. For this reason, these two categories can be sorted through a careful contextual analysis of the actual artifact types.

Finally, since burials making up the noncrypt burial context would have occurred after the laying-in period, the overall richness of artifact association, in terms of both number of categories and quantities of artifacts, should distinctly favor the crypt burial context over the noncrypt burial context. To control for variation that might be a result of differential prestige among the deceased, comparison will include only those burials that are accompanied by artifacts that fall under the custodial regalia category. The null hypothesis is that there should be no significant quantitative or qualitative differences between crypt and noncrypt burials associated with custodial regalia in the overall and individual distribution of those artifacts falling under the other three categories of laying-in warrant, personalty, and mourning gifts.

Distribution of Mortuary Artifacts

Table 9.2 summarizes the distribution of 17 artifact types across all three contexts: crypt burial, noncrypt burial, and burnt deposit. The expected patterning for the four categories as stipulated in table 9.1 occurred. As shown in table 9.2, there were 4 (possibly 5) types of artifacts that were absent from the burnt deposit context that were associated with both crypt and noncrypt burial contexts.

Table 9.2. Distribution of Selected Artifact Types of Four Categories across the Three Artifact Contexts

Artifact type	Crypt burial context	Noncrypt burial context	Burnt offering context
Custodial regalia category			
Copper plates	Yes	Yes	No
Headdresses	Yes	Yes	No
"Trophy skulls"	Yes	Yes	No
Ocean shell	Yes	Yes	No
Copper celts	Yes	Rare	No
Formal mourning gift category			
Stone celts	Yes	Rare	Yes
Platform pipes	Yes	Rare	Yes
Flint bifaces	Yes	Rare	Yes
Obsidian bifaces	Yes	No	Yes
Mica effigies	Yes	No	Yes
Bone effigies	Yes	No	Yes
"Laying-in" warrant category			
Cones	Yes	No	Yes
Buttons	Yes	No	Yes
Personalty category and personalty-mourning gift subcategory			
Ear spools	Yes	Yes	Yes
Shell beads	Yes	Yes	Yes
Pearl beads	Yes	Yes	Yes
Bear canines	Yes	Yes	Yes

These include copper plates, copper headdresses, "trophy skulls," and ocean shell containers (and possibly copper celts), which are considered custodial regalia. Equally important, table 9.2 isolates 4 artifact types that were found in all three contexts: ear spools, shell beads, pearl beads, and bear canine teeth. As discussed above, these would be candidates for both personalty and personalty-mourning gifts. Six categories are shared by the crypt burial context and the burnt deposit context, while absent from (or rare in) the noncrypt burial context. These include stone celts, platform pipes, flint and obsidian bifaces, and mica and bone effigies; these artifact types appear to be (formal) mourning gifts because ear spools, pearl and shell beads, and bear canines were common to all three contexts. The distribution of the latter across all contexts indicates that they served as mortuary artifacts under both personalty and personalty-mourning gift categories.

These conclusions can be confirmed by a comparative analysis of the crypt burial and noncrypt burial contexts (and, as suggested above, controlling for variation in social standing by comparing only those extended burials associated with custodial regalia). These comparative data are summarized in table 9.3, which lists crypt burials with one or more custodial regalia artifacts from the floor of Mound 25. Table 9.4 lists noncrypt burials with one or more items of custodial regalia. A review of column 3 in table 9.3 shows that it was not unusual

Table 9.3. Crypt Burials from the Floor of Mound 25 with at Least One Item of Custodial Regalia

Burial number	Custodial regalia	Other
Burial 6	3 copper plates	100s pearl beads; 50+ buttons of stone, clay, wood (copper covered); 2 copper ear spools; 6 bear canines at neck; 2 copper "skewers"; copper nose
Burial 7	2 copper plates	50+ ear spools, 100s pearl beads, many copper-covered buttons encircle burial; 2 copper bracelets, 2 copper "skewers," copper nose
Burial 11	ocean shell, 2 copper plates, copper headdress	8 bone deer awls, 4 copper ear spools, 6 bear incisors, numerous pearl beads
Burial 12	2 copper plates	seed pearl beads at neck, copper pan flute
Burial 13	2 copper head plates	bead bracelets
Burial 22 (double)	No. 1: copper headdress, 2 copper plates; No. 2: none	100s pearl and shell beads, 4 grizzly bear canines, large biface, 22 split bear canines, 2 ear spools, cannel coal celt; No. 2: shell and pearl beads
Burial 23 (double)	South: crescent copper plate; North: none	4 bear canines at neck, 2 ear spools, pearl beads, bladelet
Burial 24	2 copper plates, ocean shell	2 copper ear spools, numerous pearl beads, mountain lion jaw, 4 bear canines
Burial 34	trophy skull, copper plate	wildcat jaw, many bear canines, 100s shell and pearl beads, human maxillary (worked), 4 large and 12 small bear canines, 4 copper ear spools, 3 mica effigy spear heads, headless female mica effigy
Burial 35	trophy skull, 2 copper plates, copper headdress	wildcat jaw, shell beads at wrist, 2 copper ear spools, bear canine necklace, cremation
Burial 41 (triple)	Skeleton 1, south: copper plate; Skeleton 2, middle: trophy skull; Skeleton 3, north: none	limestone cone between knees, 14 bone imitation bear canines at hips and neck, 4 bear canines, pendant of barracuda jaw, shell and pearl beads, curved bone needle, human maxillary and mandible—worked, raccoon teeth, 25+ bear claws, shell and pearl beads, 4 bladelets, 3 bone awls, large hollow antler tine, numerous shell beads, black steatite pulley-shaped ear ring

(continued)

Table 9.3—*Continued*

Burial number	Custodial regalia	Other
Burial 47 (double)	South: ocean shell; North: none	several bone needles, pearl and shell beads, 2 copper axes, mica effigy eagle foot-claw with 3 toes, large biface, mica effigy human hand, 2 shield-shaped mica items, mica effigy eagle foot-claw with 4 toes, 2 mica circles, curved mica figure, 2 copper ear spools, number of shell beads
Burials 242 and 243 (double on single platform)	242: none; 243: copper plate	large pile of pearl and shell beads, copper spoon ornament, 1 ear spool, numerous beads, copper spoon ornament
Burial 248	3 copper plates, copper headdress	platform pipe, large biface, spool-shaped ornaments, copper-covered buttons, bear teeth, garment (neck to knees) with 1000s pearl and shell beads
Burials 260 and 261 (double on single platform)	66 copper celts, 23 copper plates, copper head ornament, ocean shell	large jaw, many pearls, shell beads, engraved human bones, worked copper, mica effigies, meteoric iron, etc.
Burials 265 and 266 (double)	266: none; 265: copper headdress	—
Burial 270	copper axe, copper plate	200 shell and pearl beads, cut mica ornaments, bear canines
Burial 277	copper plate	—
Burial 279	ocean shell	3 mica sheets, 3 lumps galena
Burial 281	3 copper plates, copper headdress	copper ear spools, copper-covered clay beads, copper beads, carved human femur, tortoise-shell ornament, otter or beaver and bird effigies

to find custodial regalia crypt burials associated with multiple types of artifacts under the personalty, mourning gift, and laying-in warrant categories. Large numbers of each type—including shell, bear canine teeth, and pearl beads, one or more bifaces, copper celts, mica cut-outs, and copper cones and buttons—were distributed across and around the bodies in both linear and broadcast patterns. The linear pattern probably marks bracelets and necklaces, indicating personalty and personalty-mourning gift categories, and the broadcast pattern probably marks blankets or shrouds that were decorated with these minor items, particu-

Table 9.4. Summary of Noncrypt Burials with at Least One Item of Custodial Regalia

Burial number	Custodial regalia	Other
Mound 2		
Burial 1	copper headdress plate	2 copper ear spools
Burial 3	ocean shell, 2 copper plates	1000s shell beads, 2 copper ear spools, small copper axe
Burial 4	copper plate, ocean shell	2 copper ear spools, many shell beads, a few pearl beads
Burial 5	ocean shell container, copper plate, trophy skull, copper headdress	2 copper ear spools, many shell beads, shell spoon, small mica plate
Mound 4		
Burial 6	ocean shell	—
Mound 26		
Burial 6	copper headdress, copper plate, ocean shell, trophy skull	large pearls, platform pipe, many shell beads and shell disks

larly buttons and cones, and placed over and also possibly under the deceased during the laying-in period. These latter items would constitute laying-in warrants. There are two exceptionally rich examples of laying-in artifacts: Burials 260 and 261 had the single largest deposit of copper plates known for Ohio Hopewell. The other example is the abundance of copper ear spools, 50+ pairs, associated with Burial 7.

As indicated by column 3 in table 9.4, noncrypt custodial regalia burials stand in striking contrast to crypt custodial regalia burials. The noncrypt burials had no bone or mica effigies and, with very few exceptions, lacked bifaces, platform pipes, and celts. In effect, they lacked formal mourning gifts, as predicted by the model. Furthermore, while these noncrypt extended custodial regalia burials displayed the linear pattern indicating necklaces of shell and pearl beads and bear canine teeth bracelets, they lacked the broadcast patterns of copper, shell and bone beads, buttons, and cones characteristic of the crypt burial contexts. This absence strongly supports the prediction that noncrypt burials lacked laying-in warrants, particularly the shrouds or blankets elaborately decorated with copper, shell and bone beads, buttons, and cones. In sum, the crypt and noncrypt burials systematically differed in ways that correspond to the expectations of the laying-in crypt model.

Given the above findings, the null hypothesis can be rejected. Thus, the presence of many of the deceased in the crypts probably resulted from a rather abrupt truncation of the mortuary process, thereby "freezing" the process that was typical of the laying-in period. Many of these crypts became tombs, as defined by twentieth-century archaeologists. This analysis supports the claim that the noncrypt extended burials and the cremated burials were the result of postmortem sacrificial rites of world renewal following the normal laying-in period.

This is an incomplete demonstration since it lacks an empirically grounded demonstration that the materials making up the burnt deposit context mark collective memorial/world renewal mortuary rites. Space precludes pursuing this aspect postulated by the laying-in crypt model, although it is considered in full detail elsewhere (Byers 2004:chapters 16 and 17).

Conclusion

It seems appropriate to close this discussion by reflecting upon the apparent contradiction posed by the contrastive Ohio Hopewell burial programs. The Hopewell and Turner sites have more extended than cremated interments, while Mound City, Tremper, Seip, and Liberty Works are characterized by cremations. If all these earthwork locales were the outcome of the same mortuary process as postulated under the laying-in crypt model, how can this discrepancy be accounted for? In fact, it is rather easily explained.

Greber (1976, 1979a, 1979b, 1983) has convincingly argued that the Seip-Pricer, Seip-Conjoined, and Edwin Harness Great Houses were two-tiered structures, each having an upper timber-supported floor and a lower earthen floor. Almost all of the mortuary deposits are found on the earthen floors. It is reasonable to assume that the upper floors of these great houses would have been largely reserved for the incremental series of laying-in period rituals, and the lower earthen floors, for the post-laying-in period world renewal rituals terminating in cremation-mediated postmortem sacrifice. Therefore, laying-in crypts would have occupied the upper floors. Then, prior to the ritual burning of the great houses at the time of their abandonment, the crypts would have been progressively emptied and the deceased would have been subjected to post-laying-in period mortuary rites and finally deposited as cremated sacrificial offerings in the log-crib crypts found on the lower floors. The crypts on the upper floors were destroyed with the burning of the great houses. It seems reasonable to conclude that different stages of the same mourning/world renewal mortuary process are reflected in the burial deposits of these two different groupings of sites. For the most part, the crypt burials on the floors of Mounds 23 and 25 of the Hopewell site mark the rites of the laying-in period, while the cremated burials on the floors of Seip-Pricer, Seip-Conjoined, and Edwin Harness, as well as those on the floors of the mounds of Mound City and Tremper, mark post-laying-in period, postmortem sacrificial rites.

Notes

1. The five sods represent the mud carried under the five nails or claws of the Earth Divers. The Earth Diver is a mythical animal. Different animals are depicted in different versions of the creation story. The Earth Diver figures importantly in the world creation stories by going to the bottom of the primordial sea to gather mud that the Creator then

uses to "grow" the middle world, the earth on which humans stand (Hall 1997; Wright 1990).

2. There are vulviform gate entrances in some earthworks; Hall interprets these as the portals into Mother Earth. There are also engraved vulviform designs on several Adena and Hopewell artifacts associated with mound burials (Hall 1997).

3. One of the serious problems with the funerary view, of course, is that it largely but not absolutely precludes thinking of mortuary events as being of different types. In the funerary view, funerals are the only legitimate mortuary event, and other events involving the dead either are simply different aspects of a complex funerary practice or are treated as atypical or even illegitimate.

4. To be perfectly clear on this point, it is important to note that because personalty and personalty-mourning gifts would be identical, the same type of artifacts would be found in all three contexts. But those found in the burnt deposit context would be there because they were emically identified as belonging to the mourning gift category (personalty subtype).

10

Mummies, Cults, and Ancestors

The Chinchorro Mummies of the South Central Andes

Sonia E. Guillén

The two most ancient traditions for artificial mummification in the Old and New World occur in dry environmental settings. Here, however, similarities end, as Pharaonic Egypt contrasts with the Archaic Chinchorro cultures of the south central Andes, from Ilo in Peru nearly to Antofagasta in Chile.

The earliest Egyptian examples date to the Fourth Dynasty (2613–2494 B.C.), including cases in which the internal organs of the deceased were removed and preserved outside the body. Not until the New Kingdom (1550–1086 B.C.) was mummification standardized and broadly applied (Quirke and Spencer 1992). As part of an extended sequence of funerary behavior, procedures for artificial mummification occupied the liminal space between the time the soul left the body, immediately after death, and when the *sem* priest breathed life into the mummy's mouth and thus restored soul to body (Smith and Dawson 1924; Strouhal 1992). The individual, once more complete, then traveled west to the afterworld. There was no worldly reincarnation, no cycle of regenerated human life. While the ancestors had received ongoing attention from their immediate descendants, ancestral intervention among the living was not significant. In contrast to Chinchorro ancestor cults, the Egyptian practice of artificial mummification serves as an example of an elaborate cult of the dead (*sensu* Fortes 1945) or funerary ritual (*sensu* Morris 1991).

However, the world's oldest artificial mummies are found not in ancient Egypt but in dry coastal environments of the south central Andes in Peru and Chile. Small groups of Archaic fishers and hunters, termed today Chinchorro, began elaborate procedures during the sixth millennium B.C. that prepared bodies for long term display. Though considerable variation occurred over the several thousands of years that the Chinchorro culture persisted, fundamental body treatments for a significant portion of the deceased involved defleshing, cleaning, and wrapping the bones with fiber, subsequently replacing the skin. The artificial body thus created was frequently covered with clay and painted with pigment, and there is evidence for display of some Chinchorro mummies for an extended period prior to final, casual disposal. It is argued here that prior to final deposition, the ancestors continued to play an active role in the economic and ritual lives of the living Chinchorro, thus conforming to our definitions of ancestor cult (*sensu* Fortes, Morris).

In this chapter, I first contextualize the Chinchorro example in a broader consideration of Andean mummies. I also develop a typology of mummification practices, based on these cases but useful beyond the Andean world. I then focus upon the Chinchorro, closing with a discussion of meaning for this long-term Andean tradition.

Andean Mummies

Most pre-Hispanic Andean mummy remains have been recovered from coastal environments. Arid conditions are beneficial for soft tissue preservation and were enhanced by cultural practices, such as sealing tombs and wrapping bodies in textiles and thus creating a microenvironment conducive to preservation. Mummified remains from the highlands and jungle areas have been restricted to cases where the bodies were protected in bundles and deposited in dry contexts: caves, rockshelters, or permanently snow-capped mountains. Elsewhere, drastic changes in temperature and humidity did not permit the preservation of soft tissue.

The earliest Andean mummy has been recovered from Acha 2, a Chinchorro site in northern Chile (Aufderheide et al. 1993). This naturally mummified body was dated at approximately 9000 B.P. The most ancient artificial mummy was also associated with a Chinchorro context (7810 B.P.; Allison et al. 1984). Overall, the best combination of factors for preservation of fragile human tissues occurs on the north coast of Chile.

After preceramic times, the number of mummified bodies increased. Previous, intensive debates focused on the remains from Paracas (400 B.C.–A.D. 300). Tello (1926) discovered more than 50 boot-shaped tombs at the Cerro Grande site. Each tomb contained 30–60 bodies of different ages at death and both sexes, filling the structure to the top of its circular entrance. Tello (1926) also reported funerary structures at the nearby Paracas site of Cabezas Largas. Tello inferred that artificial mummification had been practiced in these Paracas sites. He believed that the bundles showed carbonization, beginning at the lowest levels and extending upward. He interpreted this as the result of incineration that did not affect soft tissues, bones, or hair, while producing carbonized masses inside body cavities. Tello argued that artificial preservation had been produced by smoke, heat, and chemicals. Cloth rigidity of external wrappings was the result of the salty seawater sprinkled over the bundles while exposed to heat. He concluded (1926) that all body cavities had been eviscerated and that in certain cases the extremities had also been defleshed.

As Vreeland and Cockburn (1980) indicate, Tello confused the effects of natural body decomposition with those of heat. Studies of Paracas mummies and bones (Allison and Pezzia 1973; Rivero de la Calle 1975; Weiss 1932) have *not* provided evidence of artificial preservation procedures. Vreeland and Cockburn (1980:140) suggest that the leathery consistency and dark brown skin color indicate intentional desiccation; they based this conclusion on microscopic studies of tissues from a small bundle that were burned in some parts and associated with charcoal. Manipulation of the eyes and nose suggested to these authors that although evisceration had not occurred, external methods might have been used to preserve the body. Further study is needed, however, to convincingly resolve the issue of artificial mummification in the Paracas example. The leathery consistency and dark skin color could have resulted from natural degenerative processes following burial or alterations in conditions after disinterment. Similar conditions have been observed in prehistoric mummies from northern Chile and Ica and even in modern autopsies of recently buried bodies (M. Allison, personal communication April 1992). In several examples, all recognizable organs were transformed into leathery, soft, gummy masses. Chemical studies (Sullivan and Schram 1989) suggest that this soft tissue condition could be caused by putrefaction pigments such as indican or bilrubinoid, but the exact cause is not known. Exposure after excavation might initiate or accelerate incipient enzymatic decay, as suggested by the considerable number of amino acids observed in chromatograms of mummified tissues from northern Chile.

Few mummies from the Peruvian north coast have been encountered despite the hot and dry environmental conditions there. Three mummies were recovered by Ubbelohde-Doering (1966) at Pacatnamú, and a mummy from the Lambayeque valley is displayed at the Brunning Museum in Lambayeque. All the bodies were in the extended position typical of the region prior to the Late Intermediate period. Mummy bundles from later periods are usually characterized by poorly preserved textiles and skeletonized human bodies (Heyerdahl et al. 1996).

Mummies from the Middle Horizon (A.D. 600–1000) and the Late Intermediate period (A.D. 900–1476) have been reported from the central and south coasts of Peru and from northern Chile. Some of the best-illustrated cases are those found in Ancón (Reiss and Stubel 1880–1887). All subsequent observations have confirmed that these were natural mummies, although external procedures may have been introduced to desiccate the body (Allison et al. 1974, 1977, 1978).

There are several cases of human sacrifices on snow-capped mountains, where frozen bodies have been preserved. The examples reported for Cerro Aconcagua in Chile and Cerro el Toro in Argentina (Schobinger 1991), Cerro El Plomo in Chile (Mostny 1957), Cerro Esmeralda in Chile (Checura 1977), Pichu Picchu in Peru (Besom 1991; Reinhard 1992; Schobinger 1966), and Ampato in Peru and Llullaillaco in Argentina (Reinhard 1997, 1999) involve the deposition of young individuals as offerings at Inca mountain sanctuaries, associated with other offerings. These sacrifices had been elaborately dressed and deposited in specially prepared mountain-peak shrines, with metal and shell statues. The child recovered from El Plomo had died of hypothermia, as evidenced by the findings that the body had been freeze-dried and the deeper soft tissue layers transformed into adipocere (Besom 1991).

Ponce Sanginés and Linares Iturralde (1966) studied ten Late Horizon mummies from the Bolivian province of Carangas. Three showed abdominal incisions—evidence for evisceration. These observations confirm ethnohistorical references about mummification procedures used by the altiplano Pacaqes (Jiménez de la Espada 1965:339). These sources reported that Pacaqes of the Titicaca basin eviscerated their dead, interring the viscera in jars adjacent to the bodies.

Ethnohistoric documents indicate that artificial mummification was an Andean practice during Late Horizon times, apparently restricted to the upper class. No artificially prepared royal Inca mummies are known because all were destroyed by the extirpation of the idolatries or otherwise lost (Acosta 1954 [1590]; Cobo 1964 [1653]; Garcilaso de la Vega 1987 [1609]; Guáman Poma de Ayala 1956 [c.1613]; Polo de Ondegardo 1916 [1585]; Sancho de la Hoz 1917 [c.1525]; Valera 1945 [c.1590]).

Garcilaso de la Vega (1987:306 [1609]) described the process of preservation for bodies of the royal Incas, who were worshipped as gods after death. He reported that he saw the body of Inca Viracocha in 1560 at the house of Licentiate Polo de Ondegardo, the *corregidor* of the city of Cuzco. The corregidor had transported five bodies of the royal Inca from Cuzco to Lima. The other male bodies were said to belong to Túpac Inca Yupanqui and Huayna Capac. Women included Mama Runtu (wife of Inca Viracocha) and Mam Oclly (mother of Huayna Capac). He recalled that the bodies were perfectly preserved, with all their hair in place (Garcilaso de la Vega (1987:307 [1609]). Garcilaso quoted the chronicler Acosta, who had also seen them and said, "The body was so complete and so well preserved with a certain bitumen that they [*sic*] appear to be alive. Its eyes were made of cloth of the gold, and so well fitted that one did not notice the loss of the real ones" (307). He also indicated that Acosta mentioned that Viceroy Marqués de Cañete had ordered the mummies to be removed from the places where they were kept and destroyed as part of the efforts to extirpate idolatry. Garcilaso had been very impressed with the perfect and beautiful complexion of the bodies after so many years had transpired. The bodies had been in Lima for 20 years before Acosta saw them, and Garcilaso marveled at the fact that they were still preserved at his viewing, despite different climatic conditions on the coast. He suggested that the bodies had been preserved by taking them first up to the snow line of the mountains and thus freeze-drying the flesh. These observations were based on the common altiplano practice of dehydrating meat outdoors (Garcilaso de la Vega 1987 [1609]).

More recently, discoveries at La Laguna de los Cóndores in Peru has facilitated our understanding of the Inca mummification process (see Buikstra and Nystrom 2003). An emergency project allowed the recovery of over 200 mummies at a site originally built by the Chachapoya people in a remote cliff over-looking a lake. The site was found by looters, but prompt archaeological work recovered unique evidence from the cloud forest and from the time when the Inca conquered the Chachapoya people. A complex process of artificial mummification, including evisceration through the anus and tanning of the skin replaced the previous local burial pattern that involved defleshing and the burial of skeleton-ized parts of the body. The Inca emptied the Chachapoya mausoleums and filled them with the mummies of the members of a new Chachapoya-Inca society (Guillén 1998).

Classification of Mummies

Just as there are problems in defining the term *secondary interment,* the defini-tion of *mummy* is not straightforward. The issue is complicated by problems in differentiating between natural mummies and various artificial preservation methods. As a baseline, I define mummies as preserved corpses that include some soft tissue.

Natural Mummies

The category of natural mummies includes those corpses that are preserved as a result of favorable environmental conditions. Aside from burial in conditions that promote spontaneous mummification, bodies have been preserved after ca-tastrophes and abandonment in appropriate environmental conditions. Ex-amples include bog bodies from Europe, freeze-dried bodies from Qilakitsog in Greenland, and the Alpine Tyrol mummy (Hart Hansen 1985).

In most cases, a combination of factors promotes body preservation. For ex-ample, the central and north coasts of South America are both hot and dry, yet bodies do not preserve there as they do on the south coast. Each area must be considered individually to identify environmental factors that encourage tissue preservation.

In northern Chile, environmental conditions favored spontaneous natural mummification from preceramic times until the present. Thus, the northern desert of Chile has special soil conditions, very rich in nitrates that when com-bined with other factors ensure organic preservation. Salts arrest bacterial growth; the hot, dry conditions facilitate rapid desiccation. Soft tissues dry before they decay.

Preservation patterns are also related to gravity. If the body is seated in a flexed position, the body fluids drain downward so that enzyme action destroys the organs, especially those in the lower part of the body. Preservation of the extremities depends on their position relative to the autolytic decomposition of the organs.

The "natural mummification" category would also include instances when agents such as copper, arsenic, or similar chemicals have "accidentally" produced soft tissue preservation. Adipocere also stimulates soft tissue preservation inadvertently (Cotton et al. 1987; Micozzi 1991). Adipocere is a postmortem chemical alteration that transforms normal adipose tissue to a grayish white and waxlike consistency. At the beginning of the process, changes are superficial, including the lower dermis and subcutaneous tissue; later, deeper adipose deposits may be involved. Once formed, adipocere is relatively resistant to chemical and temporal effects.

Artificial Mummies

This category includes examples in which some organic or inorganic substance has been used to enhance body preservation. Three subcategories can be distinguished.

Externally Prepared Mummies

In these cases intentional artificial preservation is achieved through the use of substances applied directly to the body—for example, lime (*cal viva*), balsam, honey, juices, and sand. The body is not manipulated internally.

Internally Prepared Mummies

Corpses are manipulated to ensure that all remaining body parts are preserved. All or most of the body cavities are emptied and filled with materials designed to enhance preservation. Some embalming procedures introduce chemicals into the arteries (such as with the preservation of Lenin and Eva Perón). More ancient examples include the Inca and the Egyptian Pharaohs. In all cases, evisceration occurred and tissues were treated to prevent decay.

Reconstructed Mummies

In addition to internal manipulation, bodies may be disassembled and then reconstructed. Elimination of viscera is followed by defleshing. A variety of materials may be used to reconstruct body shape, followed by the refleshing of the body. A key example of this category is the Chinchorro tradition.

The Chinchorro

As noted above, the Chinchorro mummies are the most ancient examples of artificial mummification in the world. Some, though not all, Chinchorro corpses were defleshed, the bones cleansed and wrapped in fibers, and refleshed. The application of artificial substances, including pigment and animal fur, completed the artificially reconstructed body. In beginning an analysis of Chinchorro mummification forms, the development of a typology is useful.

The first typology for Chinchorro mummies was developed by Uhle (1919,

1922, 1974). He defined three types, including naturally preserved bodies as Type 1, artificially prepared bodies with evisceration and reconstruction as Type 2, and bodies preserved through the application of mud as Type 3. Allison and colleagues (1984) have revised this typology; their categories combine features related to body treatment with disposal activities and personal attributes. This categorization is difficult to apply, as it combines important and minor technical features without defining their level of importance in the preparation. The result is an extended number of types that are cumbersome for practical use.

By contrast, the typology offered by Arriaza (1995) defines three subtypes for the prepared mummies: black, red, and bandage mummies. He proposes stylistic and temporal differences for these categories. Considering the extended distribution of the mummies and the customarily poor provenience for the finds, the use of external appearance and finishing details as the main criteria for differentiation become a forced system rather than a technical tool to use in the study of mummies. I offer the following categorization based on the typologies proposed by Uhle (1919) and Allison et al. (1984). The categories are based on experience gained through the study of the mummies from the site Morro 1–5 (Guillén 1992), where almost all the technical features used in prepared Chinchorro mummies were present.

Type 1: naturally desiccated mummies. This category includes partially or completely painted bodies.

Type 2: mummies that show both internal and external processing. Filling type varies, as does the manner in which body cavities and the extremities were altered.

Type 3: external application of mud. Mummification was attained by the exclusive use of a layer of sand or mud.

Type 4: desiccation through application of heat. In addition to heat, evisceration might also be involved, but there was no internal or external reconstruction.

Type 5: partial defleshing, with partial or complete evisceration. Bodies were partially or completely defleshed, usually through posterior cuts, with efforts focused on rough external reconstruction. Lumps of dense layers of unfired red clay were used to reconstruct body volume, mainly in the anterior chest and abdominal regions.

Type 6: Chinchorro figurines. Often mistaken for artifacts, this category includes human or animal bones encased with unfired clay, with the final product resembling clay figurines.

Conclusions

Artificial mummification developed and reached its greatest sophistication in both Egypt and the south central Andean coast, places where natural conditions favor corpse desiccation. This phenomenon was apparently observed by ancient settlers, and in each example, they attempted to replicate and enhance natural corpse preservation. Why might this have been?

Historic documentation from Egypt suggests that increasing efforts were placed upon preserving a body that when united with the spirit or soul following mummification would persist as a whole individual in the afterlife. Intact ascent to the afterlife became an increasing preoccupation of both elites and commoners. This pattern conforms to definitions of cults of the dead (Fortes 1945).

The Chinchorro example is more enigmatic. We have no written record, only a long-standing coastal tradition for funerary ostentation (Buikstra 1995). In addition, such complex disposal forms may be unexpected in prestate societies. Ethnographically, however, we know that artificial mummification is not restricted to complex societies, as in the ancient Egyptian example. One compelling explanatory argument follows upon theories of interment behavior (Charles and Buikstra 1983; Goldstein 1981; Saxe 1970) that link funerary ritual and disposal facilities to ancestrally validated rights to the control of significant, scarce resources. Rights to fresh water or specially productive fishing loci could be among those considered economically significant, though as cultural beings we must realize that importance need not be judged on a strictly economic basis. Clearly, at one level the Chinchorro mummification procedure represents a unique, complex disposal form, while at another this is yet another way to engage the ancestors in the lives of their descendants, thus constituting an ancestor cult, a common feature of sedentary Archaic groups.

11

Secondary Burial Practices in Hohokam Cremations

Lane A. Beck

Previous studies of archaeologically recovered Hohokam cremations from southern Arizona have often reported exceedingly small bone quantities (for example, Merbs 1967; Birkby 1976). Average weights are less than one-tenth of that normally expected when an adult human corpse is incinerated (Mays 1998). Furthermore, there are differences between Hohokam cremations and those from other parts of the Southwest. Bone texture in Hohokam contexts often differs from archaeological cremations elsewhere in the United States and in Europe. Thoroughly burnt human bone should become calcined and hardened (Baby 1954; Mays 1998). By contrast, bone from Hohokam cremations is often powdery and soft. Since burnt bone is more stable than unburnt bone (Mays 1998:209), diagenesis is an unlikely explanation. Although the warpage and fragmentation patterns are unremarkable for Hohokam cremations, average fragment size is much smaller than is typical for cremation events in preindustrial societies.

In the 1976 publication on Snaketown, Haury and Birkby each proposed that the observed low bone volume of Hohokam cremations might be explained through the division of the cremated remains into multiple deposits. Both researchers cited Spier (1933:303, 305–307) as documenting this practice ethnologically. I therefore consulted Spier's work and other ethnohistoric reports for California and the greater Southwest.

The literature I examined reported that there was tremendous similarity in fundamental aspects of the cremation process. Near the time of death, a shallow, oblong pit was dug; a new pit was dug for each cremation. The pit was located either near the house of the deceased or in the cremation grounds for the village. The pyre was built up from this pit. Long logs were placed in or over the pit, spanning the long axis. In some cases, poles were upended in the ground in or adjacent to the pit to provide stability and support for the pile of logs. The corpse was placed extended or slightly flexed on the pyre with logs below, above, and on both sides of the body. In all cases that referenced burning intervals, the firing episode is reported to have lasted no longer than half a day (evening to dawn or dawn to evening; for examples, see Davis 1921:96; Strong 1929:300; Forde 1931:211; Spier 1933:303).

Following incineration, two general disposal patterns are reported for the cremated remains. Among some groups, the larger pieces of wood were first removed, allowing all other materials to drop into the shallow pit beneath the pyre. Additional soil was then added to fill the pit. In these cases the cremation locus became the burial site. Among other groups, during the day following the cremation a member of the family or someone designated for this task sifted through the ashes to gather up the remains. The remains were then placed in a basket or bowl. Another pit was dug in an appropriate burial location, and the container of cremated bones was placed in the deepest portion of this feature. In some cases additional sweepings from the cremation locus were gathered and added as a layer above the cremated remains (Davis 1921:96–97).

There is a third pattern of interment reported in the literature. It entailed the division of remains, as cited by Haury (1976), and is considered an exception to the usual disposal pathways reported for cremations in the Southwest. All describe this process as occurring only among the Maricopa. The practice is described by Spier as follows: "When the fire had burned out, four holes were dug close to the heap of ashes, two on the south side, two on the north. Then the fire tender, starting at the west end of the heap, scraped the ashes alternatively to the north and south of the center line. He then divided these two piles to the west and east, so as to form four piles. Each was put in its respective hole and covered with dirt" (Spier 1933:303). This division of cremated remains into four closely spaced but separate piles resulted in each deposit being largely restricted to a quadrant of the body. In other words, the legs and lower body were localized in two locations near the foot of the pyre while remains from the head and shoulders were located in the two deposits at the other end of the fire pit. This pattern of body part distribution would be expected unless the fire was stirred or the original arrangement of the corpse on the pyre was not in a extended supine or prone position.

Mourning ceremonies are generally reported to have been held at irregular intervals after the cremation event. According to reports made early in the twentieth century, this ritual may have either celebrated individual deaths or commemorated all who have died since the most recent ceremony. Intervals between cremation and the mourning ceremony varied from one to several years.

Most reports state that the mourning ceremonies were a symbolic reenactment of the earlier cremation event with objects and/or images of the deceased being burnt, often on or near the location in which the cremated remains were buried. In most cases, residues were buried in a manner similar to that for debris from the prior cremation. Two reports (Loeb 1924; Strong 1929) state that the mourning ceremony was not merely symbolic but also included a reburning of the cremated remains.

Interpretation of Cremation Deposits

Several patterns emerge from the ethnohistoric literature. First, cremation fires were built in shallow oblong pits. They lasted approximately 12 hours. The features in which cremations occurred were each used only once, so remains from multiple individuals generally would not be anticipated in cremation features. Remains were either left in situ or gathered into a container and placed within a smaller pit. If division of remains into multiple deposits occurred, body parts would be differentially distributed. Mourning ceremonies either should have produced greater reduction and disorganization of the remains through reburning and redeposition or should have created a layered deposit with the cremated remains deep in a pit and remains from the associated burning ceremony positioned above. Sweepings from a cremation event should include a mixture of very small fragments of bone, ash, and other debris. Remains from a mourning ceremony should include portions of burnt offerings with no bone present if the remains themselves were not subjected to a second cremation.

Basing my expectations on these ethnohistoric reports, I evaluated archaeological field records, published analyses, and cremated remains for over 500 cremations from Hohokam sites located in the Tucson and Phoenix basins. Several sites had been excavated by members of my lab during fieldwork over three years; others include collections curated at the Arizona State Museum or described in publications (Beck 2000). Most cremation deposits were located near house clusters but not within the immediate vicinity of the houses. They tended to be grouped nearer to one another than to the houses. These cremation clusters could each be considered a cemetery.

Sherds are the most abundant artifacts recovered from cremation features. They range in size from fragments smaller than 5 square centimeters to fully reconstructible vessels. In most cremation features, sherds were scattered throughout the pit fill with larger sherds concentrated in proximity to the osseous remains. Departures from this pattern are elaborated on later.

The first issue I examined was the potential division of the cremated remains of an individual into multiple deposits. Although bone quantity is low, there is no evidence to suggest division of the remains of an individual as reported by Spier. Even low-volume deposits often include skeletal elements from all portions of the body.

Additionally, cremation deposits are not spatially clustered, as described by Spier. Given the absence of these patterns, I see no evidence for division of individual remains into multiple deposits at any of the sites I examined.

In reviewing osteological data against feature content and structure, I identified three modes that appear to correspond to the expectations for (1) primary cremation loci where incineration occurred, (2) initial deposits of remains from cremations, and (3) redeposits of remains from potential mourning ceremonies.

The first category consists of locations where corpses were burned. These primary cremation loci—shallow subrectangular or oblong pits—were present at most sites. Although size varied, most were approximately 1 meter wide and 2 meters long. Bone quantity ranged from less than 10 grams to approximately 100 grams. This is consistent with the idea that most cremated remains were removed from primary cremation loci after burning.

Very few artifacts were recovered from these primary cremation features. Sherds varied in number and tended to be rather small in size. Feature fill usually included ash, with bone and artifact fragments occasionally recovered along feature bases, which were usually ashy. Oxidation and other evidence of burning were commonly noted at the feature base and on the sides.

The presence of cremation pits from which the majority of the human remains and artifacts had been removed suggests that remains had not usually been left within primary cremation sites. Initial deposits of cremated remains, as described in the ethnohistoric literature, should be characterized by greater quantities of bone, either in a durable container or clustered as if held by a perishable container. Sweepings from cremation pits may have been layered above the clustered deposits of bone. Such sweepings would be expected to contain small fragments of burnt bone and medium-to-large portions of artifacts. Features matching this pattern were found in each cemetery.

Features potentially identified as representing initial interments of cremated remains were shallow oval pits. Size varied, but most were roughly 1 meter in diameter. In many of these pits a deeper area or alcove served as the repository for most of the osseous remains. These clusters were often surrounded by larger sherds or, in some cases, reconstructible vessels. Interior depressions that contained large bone fragments were often covered with deposits containing sherds mixed with small fragments of bone. This pattern most closely resembles that expected for an initial (re)deposition of bone from a site of primary cremation, with the deposit closed by debris collected as the pit was cleaned. The presence of small human bone fragments within the sherd scatter suggests that this does not represent a symbolic cremation from a mourning ceremony.

The quantity of bone in these features varies between 10 grams and 1,500 grams. The larger weight is consistent with the amount of bone expected following an open-fire incineration of an adult human corpse (Mays 1998). While the fragments recovered from the cremation loci tended to be less than 3 centimeters in length, fragments from large-quantity deposits in these features were somewhat larger, perhaps averaging as much as 5 to 10 centimeters in their greatest dimensions.

Artifacts were more abundant in these features than they were in the cremation pits. Most reconstructible vessels were recovered from such contexts. Similarly, many lithic artifacts were found within these initial cremation deposits.

The third category of cremation deposits are interpreted as secondary deposits from mourning ceremonies. If mourning ceremonies did involve reburning remains, bone quantity should have been further reduced, both from the second burning and from a second removal from the site of burning. Artifact abundance should have been greater than that for the primary cremation pits but possibly less than that found in initial deposits. Artifact quantity would have been dependent upon the addition of durable offerings at the time of reburning. If no materials were added, it is likely that the original objects would have been further fragmented. Potential secondary deposits resulting from recremation during mourning ceremonies were tentatively identified in each cemetery. These features were shallow, oval pits ranging in size from roughly 0.25 meters to approximately 1 meter in diameter, with a modal diameter of 0.50 meter. Cremated bone quantity for these pits is very low, varying from less than 10 grams to approximately 50 grams. In general, bone fragment size was smaller than that for initial interments. Artifact quantities were greater than in the primary cremation pits but less than in the initial interments. Very few reconstructible vessels were recovered.

Summary

Using ethnohistoric and ethnographic information about mortuary behavior to generate expectations for archaeological and osteological data has enriched this study of Hohokam mortuary behavior. Hohokam sites throughout the Phoenix and Tucson basins exhibit similar cremation sequences, which may be explained by the existence of a secondary burial program that involved the reburning of cremated remains in a memorial ceremony. This interpretation better fits the combined archaeological, osteological, and ethnohistorical data sets than did prior interpretations. The peoples of southern Arizona, who are strong candidates for cultural affiliation with the Hohokam, are reported to hold memorial ceremonies on an annual basis (Underhill 1939; personal communications from various tribal representatives). This study provides additional support for continuity between these tribes and the Hohokam.

In general, patterns are similar for all sites and cemeteries. However, cremation features within each cemetery are more similar to one another than they are to those from other cemeteries within the same site. The ethnohistoric literature most often identifies immediate family members as being responsible for gathering and burying cremated remains. The greater similarity among cremations within each cemetery meshes nicely with the proposal that these house clusters are diachronic composites of courtyard groups. One might expect minor differences in mortuary treatment to be more visible between rather than within households.

The current mortuary analysis suggests widespread continuity among communities within the Hohokam area with the family or lineage—the courtyard group—assuming a major role in cremation and funerary rituals. This study further reinforces the need for nuanced reading of ethnohistoric reports to develop models for traditions that transcend time and thus link living American Indians with their ancestors.

12

Excarnation, Evisceration, and Exhumation in Medieval and Post-Medieval Europe

Estella Weiss-Krejci

Human bones may enter the archaeological record as articulated, disarticulated, or cremated deposits. The archaeologist must explain the differences in the physical remains of the dead and determine the causes that are responsible for variability in the mortuary record. One first step to accomplish such a goal is to decide whether deposits with human remains represent expressions of funerary behavior or result from other processes. This is not an easy task. Human remains from funeral rituals, for example, may end up in nonfunerary contexts. Bones and artifacts from river burials will be most likely found in nonfunerary contexts, if found at all (Bradley 1995). Bones in funerary contexts, by contrast, may be the product of various natural and cultural postdepositional processes (O'Shea 1984:25–26; Schiffer 1987) or may represent a phase in a program of mortuary treatment (Brown 1995b:16; Hutchinson and Aragon 2002).

When corpses are incomplete or disarticulated, it is difficult to evaluate the original burial mode. This may be one reason why archaeologists refer to such deposits as "secondary burials" without regard to their potential complex nature. There exists increasing awareness among mortuary specialists that the concept of "secondary burial" implies a wide range of rather unrelated mortuary practices (Houlbrooke 1998:372; Orschiedt 1997; Williams and Beck 2001). A term that does not allow researchers to distinguish between secondary rites in Indonesia (Hertz 1960 [1907]) and the relocation of bones into European charnel houses is bound to confuse any cross-cultural discussion of mortuary practices. Additionally, there is no commonly applied method to evaluate whether disarticulated remains result from human sacrifice, cannibalism, body processing, or reburial, and only a few studies have addressed the problem (for example, Murphy and Mallory 2000; Peter-Röcher 1997).

In the past I have discussed the complex potential scenarios of "secondary burial" formation using historical data from two European dynasties, the Babenbergs and the Habsburgs. I have shown that both multistage burial programs (body processing and temporary storage) and postdepositional processes (postfuneral relocation and disturbance) are responsible for a high percentage of disarticulated remains in elite mortuary contexts. Of a sample of 868 people who died between A.D. 994 and 1993, 40 percent of the remains had been tampered with in one way or the other. Three people were excarnated, and 32 had been temporarily stored and later reburied. Bones of 70 people had been moved from one country, town, or building into another after the funeral; 247 corpses had been relocated inside a building. Additionally, coffins of 226 individuals had been either renewed or opened. No specific intention can be made responsible for these manipulations. The reasons for "secondary burial" formation lie in a wide range of circumstantial and intentional, ritualistic and nonritualistic behavior (Weiss-Krejci 2001:778–779).

Such processes are not restricted to the burials of the Babenbergs and Habsburgs but occurred among many members of the European aristocracy. There exists a large body of literature on the treatment and whereabouts of corpses from a variety of other European dynasties (Boase 1972; Brown 1991; Daniell 1997; Dodson 1994; Ehlers et al. 1996; Kolmer 1997; Meyer 2000). This chapter discusses the formation of "secondary burial" in a wider European context and reveals multiple and complex factors that determined variability in mortuary behavior among Medieval and post-Medieval elites.

Variability in Mortuary Treatment

Before the nineteenth century the ideal burial mode in christianized Europe was deposition of a body in the flesh in consecrated grounds. This burial mode was born out of a deep concern with resurrection of the body. Cremation of the corpse was considered a heathen procedure, and burning was seen as destruction of the body and hence the soul, and therefore was used only as punishment for heretics (Finucane 1981:55–56; Naji this volume).

The considerable size of territories under the rule of kings, long-distance warfare, pilgrimages to Rome, interdynastic marriages, and the Crusades all resulted in kings, queens, and nobles leading very mobile lives (figure 12.1). Despite their mobility, aristocrats often chose, for a variety of reasons, a specific burial place. Many nobles wanted to be buried in their own territories, surrounded by other family members, to await resurrection there (Boase 1972:113; Daniell 1997:88; Schaller 1993:66). Especially with the foundation of new orders between the eleventh and the thirteenth century, monastic lineage burial places widely spread through Europe. Founders of religious houses could expect spiritual welfare for themselves and their family members in return for their donations. The most important new orders were Cartusians (founded in 1084), Cistercians (founded in 1098), Premonstratensians (founded in 1120), Franciscans (approved in 1209), and Dominicans (founded in 1214) (Bordua 1997; Dunn 1997).

Royal burial places were sometimes also established in newly acquired lands and served to tie the foreign dynasty to the new territory or to create a link to the

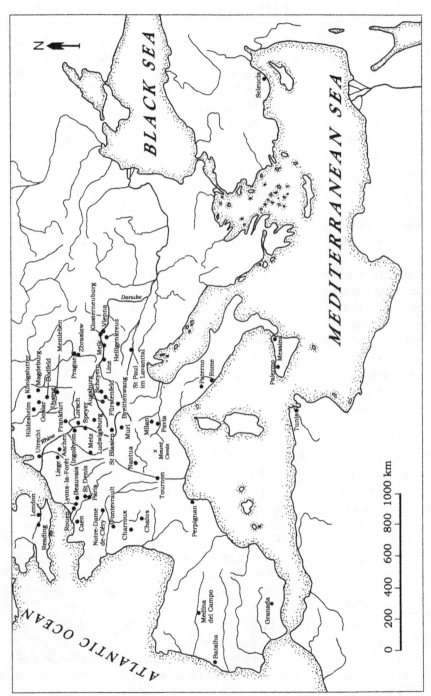

Figure 12.1. Part of Europe, showing sites mentioned in the text.

preceding dynasty (Schaller 1993:67). These political motivations explain the burials of Holy Roman Emperor Henry VI in Palermo (Staufen dynasty, died September 28, 1197, in Messina), Holy Roman Emperor Charles IV in Prague (House Luxembourg, died November 29, 1378, in Prague), and Castilian Queen Isabel "the Catholic" in Granada (House Trastámara, died November 26, 1504, in Medina del Campo). On the verge of death, Rudolph of Habsburg rode to Speyer to make sure that he would be buried in the cathedral among the emperors from the Salian dynasty. One day before his death, on July 14, 1291, he said: "On to Speyer, where more of my ancestors are, who have also been kings. And so that you don't have to bring me, I will ride there myself" (Meyer 2000:19 [my translation]).

As aristocrats traveled hundreds of kilometers per year over the European continent, death frequently occurred at a distance from the assigned burial place. If a person had expressed a wish to be buried at a specific place, the corpse had to be transported from the place of death to the place of burial. Such transport could either involve bodies in the flesh or only the bones (see also Naji, this volume). Bodies that were transported in the flesh were usually embalmed and eviscerated. To transport merely bones, two methods were possible: one was active excarnation (defleshing), the other consisted of temporary storage and later exhumation (a passive way of excarnation). Which of these three basic methods—evisceration, excarnation, or storage—was applied depended on the conditions at the place of death, distance from the burial place, the climate, and the projected time between death and burial.

Treatment of the Corpse

Evisceration

One way to delay putrefaction of corpses was evisceration and treatment with aromatics or salt. In Europe embalming was not highly efficient, and the technique was perfected only in seventeenth-century France and England (Dodson 1994:82; Giesey 1960:27). But it was sufficient for a short time, especially if death occurred during cold seasons and waterways could be used for transport. The earliest historical accounts on mortuary treatment in the Middle Ages relate to circumstances surrounding the death and burial of kings. Son of Emperor Charlemagne, Emperor Louis I "the Pious" (who died June 20, 840) was transported approximately 250 kilometers from Ingolheim to Metz, and grandson King Louis II "the German" was transferred from Frankfurt to Lorsch (70 kilometers) after his death on August 28, 876 (Schramm and Mütherich 1962:122–128). We do not know how their bodies were treated.

The first detailed historical account of evisceration relates to the circumstances surrounding the death and burial of Emperor Charles "the Bald," son of Louis I and half-brother of Louis II, in October 877. After passing Mount Cenis in the Alps, the king passed away in a mountain hut approximately 2,000 meters above sea level. The body was eviscerated and treated with spices and wine so that it could be taken to Saint-Denis. After carrying the corpse approximately 1,800 meters down in altitude and 250 kilometers in distance, a presumably exhausted burial party reached the flatlands. Though the body had been encased in a barrel, sealed with pitch, and surrounded by leather, the bad smell that emanated from inside urged them to bury the cask with the corpse at Nantua. The deceased's wish to be buried at Saint-Denis was granted seven years later (E. Brown 1981:226; Schäfer 1920:493–494).

To the reign of the German emperors, the Saxon kings (Ottone dynasty), and their successors the Franconian kings (Salian dynasty), we owe the first accounts of separate burial of intestines (with the heart) from the corpse. Otto I died on May 7, 973, in Memleben: his entrails were buried at the place of death, and the corpse was transported to Magdeburg and buried before two weeks had passed. Emperor Conrad II died on June 4, 1039, in Utrecht, where his entrails remained; the corpse was buried at Speyer Cathedral after 38 days. His son Emperor Henry III died at Bodfeld in 1056 and was buried at Speyer Cathedral after 23 days (Gerbert et al. 1772:62–63; Schäfer 1920:479–481). Henry III's entrails and heart were buried not at the place of his death but at Goslar, where his daughter Mathilda rested and where "his heart was" (E. Brown 1981:228).

Separate burial of entrails from the corpse was also practiced in the Norman Kingdom in Sicily at the end of the eleventh century (Giesey 1960:20). The first incidence of separate heart burial comes from France and is connected to the death of Robert of Abrissel in 1117, the founder of Fontevrault Abbey. His heart remained at the place of his death, Orsan, but the rest of his body was taken to Fontevrault (E. Brown 1981:228).

The first eviscerated English ruler is Henry I (House of Normandy), who died December 1, 1135, in Lyons-la-Forêt near Rouen and was buried at Reading Abbey four weeks later. His viscera, brain, and eyes were buried at Rouen, but the person who performed the embalming died from an infection and according to a chronicler became "the last of many whom Henry destroyed" (Boase 1972:113). As Henry's example shows, embalming was not particularly successful. After having been brought to Caen, Henry's corpse—though sewn into a bull's hide and filled with salt—leaked black liquid that was caught in vessels and discarded by the disgusted servants (Schäfer 1920:495). The practice of evisceration might have been directly brought to this English king through his daughter Mathilda (ancestress of the Plantagenet dynasty), whose first husband, German Emperor Henry V, had been eviscerated 10 years earlier.

From the Plantagenet dynasty we not only have evidence for evisceration, but also for the first time the corpse was buried at three separate places. Entrails, blood, and brain of King Richard "the Lion-Hearted" (who died 1199 at Chalus) were buried at Charroux, his heart at Rouen (where body parts of his great-grandfather Henry and the corpse of his grandmother Mathilda rested), and his corpse at Fontevrault with his parents and sister (Giesey 1960:20; Schäfer

1920:496). Among French royalty and nobility, evisceration and separate burial of body parts became a common practice in the thirteenth century.

While in the Middle Ages embalming flourished in France, England, and Scotland independent from a necessity to transport a corpse, in the German Empire the treatment remained predominantly functional (Meyer 2000:212). The establishment of two and three different burial places for one corpse developed between the sixteenth and seventeenth century in the Houses of Habsburg and Wittelsbach. Although the tradition ceased in the nineteenth century, it saw a revival in 1989, when the heart of the former empress Zita was buried in Muri, Switzerland (Hawlik–van de Water 1993:311).

Excarnation

To facilitate the transportation of bones, corpses had to be defleshed or temporarily stored and later exhumed. Active excarnation became known as *mos teutonicus* (the German custom). The bodies were eviscerated and cut into pieces, and the flesh was removed by boiling the body in water, wine, or vinegar. Flesh and intestines were usually buried at the place of death (sometimes cremated), while clean excarnated bones were wrapped in animal hides for their journey (Finucane 1981:46; Schäfer 1920:484).

The earliest historical account for dismemberment dates to A.D. 992, when the corpse of Bishop Gerdag of Hildesheim, who had died coming home from a pilgrimage to Rome, was cut into pieces and taken back to Germany in two containers (E. Brown 1981:226; Schäfer 1920:486). Emperor Otto III died January 1002 in Paterno, Italy. The chronicle reports that his intestines were taken back to Germany in two containers and buried at Augsburg, while the remaining body was buried at Aachen (Schäfer 1920:480). Although the chronicler mentions only *intestina,* the long distance (more than 1,000 kilometers) and the fact that the inner organs were transported in two containers may indicate that the corpse was defleshed.

Whether bodies of men who died in battle before the twelfth century were eviscerated or excarnated is also not clear from the historical record. In the battle at the Unstrut, many noblemen died in their fight against the rebellious Saxons in June 1075, and Emperor Henry IV ordered their transport home (Schäfer 1920:491). Among the dead was Babenberg Margrave Ernest, who was transported to Melk, Austria (approximately 550 kilometers away), where he still rests today. His bones were exhumed and reburied several times after the first deposition, and in 1735 they were deposited in a collective coffin together with other family members, all of whom had died in the eleventh century. In 1968 when the remains were investigated by physical anthropologists, the bones of 15 individuals were found. One skeleton was ascribed to Margrave Ernest based on sex, age, and four distinctive unhealed injuries inflicted by axe and sword, all interpreted as battle wounds. The collective coffin also held one scarred isolated humerus and an unidentified male skeleton, which also showed traces of burning and an unhealed injury. The burnt bones were ascribed to a fire that broke out in the monastery in 1297 (Jungwirth 1971:663–665). The issue of excarnation was not addressed at the time.

The first evidence that a body was boiled and defleshed is based on results from an investigation of the bones of Saxon King Lothar of Supplingenburg and two of his relatives. Through determination of aspartic acid racemization in bone samples and comparison with the ratios in the bones of two relatives, Bada and colleagues (1989) came to the conclusion that Lothar, who died in December 1137 near Breittenwang in the Alps, had been boiled for about six hours. The historical records are silent on that matter, and all we know is that it took 27 days to transport the body 500 kilometers from the Alps to Königslutter in Saxony (Schäfer 1920:482).

By the second half of the twelfth century, excarnation seems to have become well established. After dying in battle at Milan in 1158, Ekkebert of Puntten was excarnated in a nearby monastery. Fredrick of Altena was defleshed in Pavia in the same year. Henry of Liege was boiled also in Pavia in 1164. Many noblemen were killed in the summer of 1167 when the plague broke out in Rome in Frederick Barbarossa's army. The bodies were boiled and stripped of flesh and their clean bones brought back to their homelands (Schäfer 1920). Frederick Barbarossa was excarnated after he drowned at Seleucia during the Third Crusade on June 10, 1190 (Prutz 1879:30–33). Babenberg Duke Frederick I died April 16, 1198, during the Crusades and was treated in *more teutonico* (Lechner 1976:193). His remains were buried in the chapter house of the Cistercian monastery Heiligenkreuz (figure 12.2) in Coffin VIII. The eighteenth-century engraving displays a tightly packed bone bundle that differs from other secondary arrangements at the site, such as bones in Coffins I, II, and III that have been reburied from the monastery of Klosterneuburg in the thirteenth century (Koch 1976:194–196). It is generally accepted among historians that Coffin X from Heiligenkreuz (figure 12.2) holds the remains of Count Henry "the Cruel" (Koch 1976:198). The articulated state of his bones points to burial in the flesh and supports the assumption that differing corpse treatment is a result of distance and climatic conditions.[1] Count Henry met his fate in the autumn or winter of 1228 in Swabia. The much shorter distance (approximately 400 kilometers) and the colder time of the year did not require excarnation. The small urn that was found beside the left side of the body might have once held the intestines.

Excarnation was not restricted to the German Empire. French Capetian King Louis IX "the Saint" (who died in Tunis in 1270) and his son Philip III (who died in Perpignan in October 1285) were both eviscerated and boiled. The rulers' bones were buried at Saint-Denis, Louis' nine months and Philip's two months after death (E. Brown 1981:235–236; Vones 1996:192–193; Zotz 1996:201). English King Henry V, from the House of Lancaster, died in France in 1422 and was buried at Westminster Abbey in London two months after his death (Dodson 1994:77).

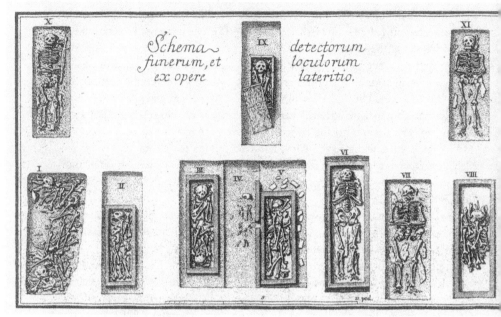

Figure 12.2. Chapter house of the Cistercian monastery Heiligenkreuz (Austria): the twelfth-century foundation became the final burial place of approximately 13 members of the Babenberg dynasty and 2 members of the house of Wittelsbach (from Gerbert et al. 1772:4(2):Table 6).

Regulation of Burial Practices

In the Middle Ages, monks who tended the dying and took care of their corpses often processed bodies. King John "Lackland" (who died in 1216), for example, was eviscerated by his father confessor, the abbot of Croxton (Dodson 1994:73). Despite being a clerical occupation and a benefit to the monasteries that received body parts, division of the corpse was banned in 1299 and again in 1300 by Pope Boniface VIII (Schäfer 1920:497; E. Brown 1981:221). The pope wanted to end the savage practice and ruled that if someone died in a Catholic country the body should be instead temporarily buried in or near the place of death. Nevertheless, privileges were granted to Philip the Fair in 1305 (when Clement V became pope), permitting him to determine "that his body should be eviscerated, boiled, split or divided in any other way and buried wholly or partly in as many churches as he wished" (E. Brown 1981:256). More licenses for separate burial of the corpse were obtained, and the difficulty of gaining papal permission made it an even more desirable practice, since it became a sure sign of status and distinction (E. Brown 1981:264). In the fourteenth century the Church gave way and the custom regained its former popularity.

In the aftermath of the ban, alternative techniques to chopping up bodies and boiling may have been sought. Meyer (2000:55) suspects that the treatment of German Emperor Henry VII (House of Luxembourg) may represent such a response. Henry died in Italy on August 24, 1313. According to some sources the body was roasted over a fire. When the sarcophagus was opened in 1727 the bones exhibited signs of burning.

Variability in Treatment of the Corpse

Body processing arose out of the necessity of transporting a corpse, and both excarnation and embalming were applied only to people of noble descent. A sample of 85 high-status individuals (76 males, 9 females) who died between 877 and 1493 partially reveals the motives for the choice of treatment. The sample—which draws data from the German Empire, Bohemia, France, and the British Isles—includes members from the Capetian (n=12), Plantagenet (n=11), Habsburg (n=6), Luxembourg (n=5), Babenberg (n=4), and Salian (n=4) dynasties as well as members of other houses (such as Przemyslide, Ottone, Staufen, Ludowingian, Valois, Bruce, Lancaster). Among them are kings and queens (41 individuals); princes, dukes, and margraves (30 individuals); and clerics (14 individuals). Of 85 treated individuals, 52 were eviscerated and 33 excarnated. Of the excarnated individuals only one was female. Over two-thirds of the excarnated people died during wars.

A direct comparison between the two methods of treatment shows that defleshing was applied if someone died far from home and the assigned burial place (figure 12.3), if death occurred in a warmer season or climate (figure 12.4), or if a long time period between death and burial was required. If bodies were defleshed, at least one of these three factors applied. If transport occurred over shorter distances and the time period between death and burial was shorter, bodies were usually eviscerated and embalmed. While excarnation remained predominantly functional and ceased after the fifteenth century, evisceration became gradually disconnected from any function. It is a status marker at all times, but at least in England the number of separate burials of different body parts dropped after Boniface VIII banned division of the corpse in 1299 (E. Brown 1981:253). Sometimes doctors refused to eviscerate corpses of people who displayed signs of communicable diseases. Such fate befell Bohemian and Hungarian King Ladislas Posthumus (Habsburg), who died in 1457 and whose symptoms of leukemia were confused with the plague (Bláhová 1997:104). Duke Albert VI (Habsburg) died in 1463 two days after black carbuncles had emerged on his body. The doctors interpreted them as plague-boils, and Albert's untreated corpse was temporarily buried in a plague pit (Mraz 1988:43). The doctors who cared for the son of Duke Christoph of Württemberg, Eberhard (who died in 1568), were afraid of infection from the festering ulcers that had obviously caused his death (Schukraft 1989:42).

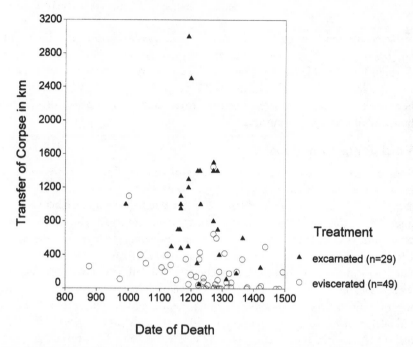

Figure 12.3. For 78 of 85 treated individuals in the sample, both death and burial places are known. The graph plots the relationship between the distance of corpse transport, evisceration, and excarnation over time in the Middle Ages.

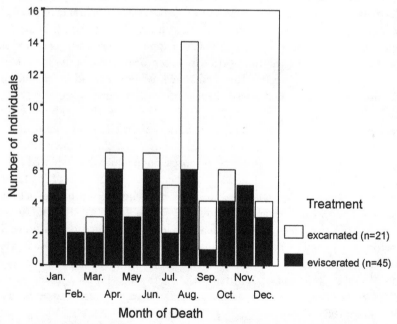

Figure 12.4. For 66 of 85 treated individuals in the sample, the month of death is known. The graph shows the relationship between evisceration, excarnation, and month of death from the ninth to the fifteenth century.

Deposition of the Corpse

Temporary Storage as Passive Excarnation

Pope Boniface VIII suggested temporary storage as an alternative to body processing when banning division of the corpse. This method had been used before 1299 when corpses had to be transported. The temporary burial of Charles "the Bald" at Nantua in 877 is an early example. But temporary storage required a possibility to recover the bones at some later point in time. The expansion of new monastic buildings all over Europe after the eleventh century promoted temporary storage and improved the conditions. If bodies could not be transported, there were many new ceremonial structures available for them to be stored in (Weiss-Krejci 2001:775).

Waiting for the Funeral

Temporary storage was not only a method to separate flesh from the bones; it was also applied for other reasons that were unrelated to transport of the corpse. Excommunicated people were sometimes stored. Such a ban on a person denied the right to burial in consecrated ground and thus seriously endangered the destiny of the soul (Schaller 1993:62). It was probably one of the most powerful— and therefore most frequently used—political instruments that a pope could direct against a ruler who did not follow his orders. Salian Emperor Henry IV died on August 7, 1106, in Liege while excommunicated. After four weeks he was transported to Speyer and buried in a nonconsecrated side chapel of the cathedral, where he remained for five years. When the ban was lifted, he was buried on August 7, 1111, beside his father, Henry III (Ohler 1990:147).

Storage could also take place when buildings, crypts, or tombs were not yet ready to house the mortal remains. Since death dates of family members often preceded the construction of tombs and crypts in which they are buried now, the implication is that they entered those places as "secondary burials." It is not always easy to determine whether these corpses were previously deposited with the intention of exhumation (temporary storage) or whether a decision to exhume and rebury was made at some later point in time (postfuneral relocation).

In 1263 Ludwig II of Bavaria (House of Wittelsbach) founded the monastery Fürstenfeld, to conciliate the execution of his first wife, Mary of Brabant. The Founder's Chapel became the burial place of Ludwig, his second and third wives, and several children. His second wife, Anne of Glogau (who died in 1271), and his daughter Agnes (who died in 1269) were most probably first buried in the Prince's Chapel at the monastery Scheyern, which was given up as a burial place for the Wittelsbach family at the end of the thirteenth century (List 1980:524, 527). King John I of Portugal, founder of the Avis dynasty (who died in 1433), and his wife, Philippa of Lancaster (who died in 1415), were both reburied into a double tomb in the Founder's Chapel at the monastery of Batalha in 1434 (Mosteiro da Batalha 1988).

In a few cases we can be sure that corpses of family members were simply stored to await burial with another family member. Two previously deceased young adult sons of French Valois King Francis I were included in his funeral and buried together with their father at Saint-Denis in 1547.[2] According to Giesey (1960:8), Francis had not buried the bodies of his sons when they died, since he wanted them to be buried together with him in his mausoleum.

Stored people were not always reburied. In the chapter house of Heiligenkreuz rest the remains of two members of the House of Wittelsbach. Rudolph and Heinrich in Grave IV are the children of Catherine of Habsburg (daughter of Rudolph of Habsburg) and Duke Otto III of Lower Bavaria (alias Bela V, King of Hungary) (Koch 1976:194). Niemetz (1974:23) thinks that their burial at Heiligenkreuz in 1280 was meant to be only a temporary solution until they could be transferred to the monastery of Tulln, which had been founded in the same year by Rudolph of Habsburg. But for unknown reasons the transport never took place, and the bones remained at Heiligenkreuz.

Deposition and Funeral

In Europe months could pass before a body was deposited, but deposition did not always imply that the funeral was completed. Disposal of the corpse and funeral rite in Europe could form distinct, temporally separated events that could be performed independently of each other. Such behavior has resulted in situations in which both primary and secondary burials can represent the remains of either incomplete or multiple funeral rites.

In post-Medieval Europe, corpses that were buried in dynastic crypts were enclosed in two coffins. A simple wooden coffin was usually used to deposit the corpse soon after death. Sometime later the first coffin was put into a larger outer coffin, which was made from wood, tin, or lead. In the House of Württemberg, burial was considered complete only when the inner coffin had been deposited in the outer one, but this had not always been the case. Duke Eberhard Ludwig (who had founded the crypt Ludwigsburg) lost his heir, Friedrich Ludwig, in 1731 and wanted his son's inner coffin to be enclosed in an outer elaborate tin coffin, as this had been the custom in the House of Württemberg since the seventeenth century. By 1733 court-tin founder Tambornino had made a cost calculation, draft, and model for the coffin, but when Duke Eberhard Ludwig died in the same year the coffin had not yet been commissioned. Since Eberhard Ludwig had died without heir, his cousin Carl Alexander inherited the duchy, a change in inheritance that also caused a religious shift, since Carl Alexander was Catholic in contrast to Eberhard Ludwig, who had been Protestant. Carl Alexander ordered two tin coffins (one for the duke and one for his son), but when the contract with Tambornino was signed the original plan and model could not be found and the project was cancelled. As a result, both Eberhard Ludwig's and Friedrich Ludwig's burial remained incomplete. Four years later, on March 12, 1737, Carl Alexander died. It took less than a month for Carl Alexander's outer coffin to be ready, and the new tradition using a simpler outer coffin was probably a direct result of the previous experiences. Carl Alexander's funeral took place in three stages. First his intestines were buried in the floor of the burial crypt five days after death. Then almost four weeks after death, the corpse was quietly deposited in the crypt on April 6 in a black-velvet-covered coffin. In the meantime an empty red-velvet-covered coffin was lying in state in the castle. Five weeks later the funeral was held. The empty consecrated red coffin was lowered into the crypt, and the black coffin was put inside. Similar procedures were conducted at the later burials of Dukes Carl Eugen, Ludwig Eugen, and Friedrich Eugen at the end of eighteenth century. On the occasion of Carl Alexander's funeral in 1737, the unnamed simple wooden caskets of Friedrich Ludwig and Eberhard Ludwig were walled in and the evidence for unfinished burial made invisible (Schukraft 1989:94–98).

Carl Alexander's funeral with an empty coffin indicates that funerals can be held independent from deposition of the corpse.[3] The example from Ludwigsburg further shows that too expensive or too elaborate projects may either inhibit complete burial or cause a major delay. The latter was the case with Habsburg Emperor Fredrick III (V), who received two funerals. Frederick III (V) died on August 19, 1493, in Linz and was immediately eviscerated and embalmed, his heart and intestines buried in a dignified ceremony in the City Parish Church of Linz (Meyer 2000:178). After burial of intestines and heart, Frederick's corpse was transported to Vienna. The summer weather instigated the need for rapid burial, and on August 28 the royal corpse was temporarily laid to rest at St. Stephen's Cathedral, accompanied by a "small" ceremony in which 6 bishops and 13 abbots and prelates were present (Lipburger 1997:132). The big funeral was scheduled to take place whenever the future emperor, Frederick's son Maximilian I, arrived, but this took a while. A few days after Frederick had been deposited, the Turks attacked Carinthia, and Maximilian was too busy to hold the funeral. When Maximilian finally arrived in Vienna, a pompous funeral was held on December 6 and 7, but there exist doubts whether the corpse was present during the funeral (Lipburger 1997:133). Thirty years before his death Frederick had commissioned a large marble monument in which he wanted to be buried (Hertlein 1997:139), but in 1493 the tomb was not ready. Another 20 years passed before the mortal remains could be moved to their final resting place. This last relocation in November 1513 was accompanied by yet another funerary ceremony, almost as splendid as the one of December 1493, but in the absence of Emperor Maximilian. From the records we know that this time the mortal remains were displayed for a few days (Lipburger 1997:134) before they were deposited in the marble monument at St. Stephen's Cathedral.

For political reasons French King Louis X also received two funerals. The king died suddenly and unexpectedly on June 5, 1316, in Paris and was buried two days later. His brother Philip of Poitier had missed the funeral, but since Louis did not have an heir, Philip was one of the potential successors. In missing his brother's funeral Philip had failed to perform one of the functions expected of a person destined to succeed to the throne. So Philip arranged a second funeral five weeks after the first and thus secured the regency and ultimately the crown of France. In the second funeral Louis X was not disinterred, but clothes were laid on his grave. According to Brown (1978:256), Philip clearly intended the ceremony to be seen as a second funeral, not an ordinary commemorative service.

The use of historical evidence from Europe underscores the problem of equating deposition of the corpse and funeral. Some stored corpses were never moved to their destined burial location, and some people did not receive the full funerary treatment, whereas others received more than just one funeral.

Postfuneral Processes

Disturbance

Once a body is finally buried, a series of other formation processes can change its state. Disturbance frequently occurred in burial crypts into which sequential interments were made. Bones were disturbed when coffins were opened during inspections. Artifacts were sometimes removed and bones taken. Charlemagne's grave, after having been hidden from the Normans in 882, was disturbed by Emperor Otto III in 1000 and Frederick Barbarossa in 1165. Otto III cut Charlemagne's nails, broke a tooth from the jaw, and took a golden cross and parts from the clothes. His deed was considered a sacrilege in his time, and Otto's death two years later was seen as a just punishment by one chronicler (Ohler 1990:142).

Postfuneral Relocation

While a disturbed corpse at least remains in its original mortuary context, postfuneral relocation poses a serious problem from the point of mortuary analysis. In Medieval and post-Medieval Europe, relocation could take place within a crypt or funeral chamber, within a building or building complex (internal relocation), or from one building, town, or country into another (external relocation). This happened for ritual and profane, friendly and hostile reasons (Weiss-Krejci 2001:775–778).

Postfuneral Long-distance Transport

Corpses were sometimes transported over hundreds of kilometers and hundreds of years after the funeral, with bones ending up in rather unexpected places. In 1770 Abbot Martin Gerbert exhumed 14 Habsburgs who had been buried in Switzerland between 1276 and 1386 and reburied them at his newly rebuilt monastery St. Blasien in the Black Forest. But only 36 years later the monastery was secularized, and the convent was forced to leave. In 1809 the monks took the bones to St. Paul im Lavanttal in Carinthia, where they were eventually buried in a small crypt under the main altar of the monastery church in 1936 (Gut 1999:105–110). These burials cannot be understood from the Habsburg perspective. During the Habsburg reign only one person chose to be buried in Carinthia—Maria Anna (died 1789), daughter of Maria Theresa, who had joined a convent there (Leitner 1989:102). It is primarily through the intentions and fate of the monks rather than through the identity of the bones that we can understand their present location.

Violence

The most radical and destructive postdepositional process in European history, both in scale and quantity, was exhumation of emperors, kings, queens, and their family members during the French revolution. "Let all the coffins of these divinized monsters be broken open! Let their memory be condemned!" wrote journalist Lebrun in a poem that was published February 6, 1793, in Paris (E. Brown 1985:252). By the end of the year any archaeological testimony of the royal funeral ceremony (Giesey 1960) had disappeared. The bodies from Saint-Denis were thrown into two pits on the north side of the abbey (one called the Valois pit, holding the remains from Merovingian, Carolingian, Capetian, and Valois dynasties; the other, the Bourbon pit). During exhumation people took teeth, hair, bones, and other relics. But in 1817, three years after the accession of Louis XVIII, the desecrated royal bones were exhumed once again. Since it was impossible to single out individual bodies, the bones were put in five coffins (four for the Valois pit and one large one for the Bourbons) and reburied within the abbey in a ceremony. Eventually funerary monuments were also returned to the abbey (E. Brown 1985:255–256).

During domestic conflicts violence was often directed against royal corpses. King Wenceslas IV of Bohemia was desecrated only a year after his death when the monastery of Zbraslaw (Königsaal, south of Prague) was plundered and set on fire by raiding Taborites in 1420. According to one account, men put the cadaver on the altar, adorned it with a crown made from hay, and poured beer over it (Millauer 1830:59–60; Bláhová 1997:102). The remains were collected by a loyal man and buried but were exhumed and reburied at Prague Cathedral in 1424 in a huge public funerary ceremony (Meyer 2000:140). At Notre-Dame-de-Cléry, Huguenotts played ball with the head of Louis XI in 1562 (E. Brown 1985:250), and at Saint-Denis the cadaver of Henry IV was struck by a woman during the exhumation in 1793 (E. Brown 1985:253).

During wars, tombs were also frequently desecrated; grave goods were stolen, and the bones were disturbed or thrown out. The grave of Duke Frederick II (Grave IX) at Heiligenkreuz (see figure 12.2) was probably opened and plundered by the Turks (Niemetz 1974:22).

Ritual Deposition of Bones

While the relics of Christian martyrs were exhumed from the early Middle Ages on and distributed through Europe, in the later Middle Ages some royal corpses achieved saintly status. Once canonized, the bodies were exhumed in the ritual of translation and the relics were moved to a more honorable position and distributed (Finucane 1981:52–53). French King Louis IX was canonized 27 years after his death in 1297. When his grandson Philip IV "the Fair" wanted to move the remains from Saint-Denis to Paris, the monks first refused to give up the bones but finally gave in. In 1306 Philip was able to translate the upper part of the king's head to Saint-Chapelle. One rib was awarded to Notre-Dame; Louis' chin, teeth, and mandible, which were considered the inferior part of the head, were left at Saint-Denis. In 1304 Philip had already presented one of Louis' finger joints to the king of Norway (Brown 1980).

Discussion

Variability in mortuary treatment has been interpreted as the result of age, gender, wealth, social position and affiliation, prestige, occupation, kinship ties, ideology, level of grief, and circumstances and cause of death (Binford 1971; E. Brown 1981; Goldstein 1995:116; Häusler 1968; Hodder 1982b; MacDonald 2001; Pader 1982; Saxe 1970; Shay 1985; Steuer 1968; Tainter 1978). Hence the evidence from Medieval and post-Medieval Europe shows that no factor alone can be held responsible for variability.

Unfortunately for the archaeologists, high-status individuals are not always buried where they lived or died. Although exceptions exist (Murphy and Mallory 2000), there has been very little discussion of people's mobility and its meaning for the mortuary record. In Europe, transport of the corpse was a status marker, and if a corpse had to be transported it was treated. How the corpse was treated depended on the place of death, the distance from the burial place, the climate, and the prospective time before burial of a body. But a simple correlation between status and treatment does not explain variability, since not everybody was transported. Additionally, societal change and individual decisions have played a role (Daniell 1997:87–92). Though evisceration became slowly detached from its original function and a sign for distinct status, some people rejected it. Others did not receive such treatment because they had died (or at least were believed to have died) from a communicable disease. But most important is the point that evisceration and excarnation can be understood only in the context of a belief system that abhorred destruction of the bones through fire.

Another serious methodological problem is that dead people are mobile not only before or during, but also after the funeral. In Medieval and post-Medieval Europe, bones were frequently exhumed (see, for example, Daniell 1997:93; Weiss-Krejci 2001). Whatever the reason for exhumation, in dynastic contexts bones were usually reburied. Though the majority of dynastic reburials indeed took place in a ritual, the new mortuary context may be entirely different from the earlier one. None of these ceremonies can be considered funeral rites, despite the ritual mortuary context of the remains. The postfuneral ceremony can also completely mask the reasons for exhumation. Such exhumation acts can sometimes be explained within the framework of ancestor veneration but often result from a range of nonritualistic activities.

Härke (1994, 1997) has argued that burials can reveal past reality through functional data. These data, which mainly consist of information that physical anthropologists gain from skeletal remains, would form undistorted and unbiased evidence that could be contrasted with a second data type, the intentional data. Intentional data (such as burial type, grave construction, and grave goods) do not reflect past reality but the thinking of the ritual community. Härke has applied this methodology to analyze Anglo-Saxon burials and has shown that the contrast between the two data types may reveal ancient ideology behind the burial ritual (Härke 1994:35–37). Nevertheless, the evidence from dynastic Europe shows that this approach can work only when bodies show signs of burial in the flesh. The analysis of disarticulated bones that may be older than their context or come from somewhere else will surely bias any analysis. Such skeletal data are also intentional and will reflect only the ideology of the community that performed the reburial.

Tombs that hold primary and secondary remains are frequently interpreted as evidence for human sacrifice (Parker Pearson 1999:18), even when "victims" lack signs of violent death. In historic European dynastic mortuary contexts, evidence for human sacrifice and "non-persons" (Arnold and Wicker 2001:xii) does not exist. The frequent combinations of double or multiple, same-sex or mixed-sex burials and combinations of articulated and disarticulated bones result from a behavior in which excarnation, body storage, collective burial practices, multiple burial practices, and postfuneral relocation played an equally important part. As Ucko has already argued in discussing the Merina, an interpretation of such burials as sacrifices "would be quite out of place" (Ucko 1969:269).[4]

While one may argue that such observations may be restricted to historic Europe, a specific burial ideology should not a priori be ascribed to any ancient society without careful consideration. If we want to uncover past realities all possibilities have to be considered. A first step would be to develop methodologies to distinguish which burials are the result of funeral rites from those that are not. This would imply the application of a wider variety of examination techniques for disarticulated bones and an increased utilization of skeletal biological data. A close collaboration between archaeologists and bioarchaeologists may further help to understand the nature of such evidence.

In European dynastic contexts the older the bones, the rarer the chance that they still reflect funerals. But if funeral redefines a person's status, so do exhumation and reburial. The evidence from burial deposits with disarticulated remains may neither hold any information on the status of a person at the time of death nor reflect the intentions of the community that participated in the funeral. But the analysis of jumbled, incomplete, and disarticulated bones may display ideological change and social process and therefore open a different window to understanding ancient human behavior.

Acknowledgments

This research was funded by the Austrian Science Foundation (FWF–Project H140–SPR). The paper was completed under a grant by the Portuguese Science Foundation (FCT–Project SFRH/BPD/8608/2002). I would like to thank the following people for contributing information and supplying literature: Jeffrey Bada, Norman Hammond, Heinrich Härke, Lois Lane, Gerhard Trnka, and Jean Wilson. My special thanks go to the editors for inviting me to participate in their book.

Notes

1. According to historical sources from later times, Klosterneuburg was the primary burial place of Henry "the Cruel." Historians debate when the transfer of corpses from Klosterneuburg to Heiligenkreuz took place (Koch 1976). If Klosterneuburg was indeed the primary burial place, the articulated bones in Coffin X would point to transfer not too long after primary burial, when the flesh had not yet decayed.

2. Dauphin Francis (who died in 1538) was stored in Tournon; Charles Duke of Orléans (who died in 1545) was stored in the abbey of St. Lucien near Beauvais.

3. In England and France, the use of effigies permitted long time periods between death and funeral (Giesey 1960:112; Metcalf and Huntington 1991:171).

4. Ucko (1969:269) also said that a costly tomb may not necessarily imply a ruling family. This is also true for Europe. In Vienna, for example, several burial crypts hold elaborate metal coffins, but only a few crypts served as burial places for the Habsburgs. As J. Brown (1981:29) has argued, it is not necessarily wealth distinction in graves that marks social variables but the right to a special burial location.

13

Death and Remembrance in Medieval France

A Case Study from the Augustinian Monastery of Saint-Jean-des-Vignes, Soissons

Stephan Naji

The Abbey of Saint-Jean-des-Vignes was established circa 1076 on a hill over-looking the Medieval town of Soissons, France (figure 13.1). Abbey construction was in three main phases: Romanesque, Gothic, and a large-scale restoration in the Baroque style (figure 13.2). The present-day Gothic church was started in 1220 and finished around 1521. "The establishment of the abbey was part of the religious reform movement that swept over Europe after the millennium. Communal life at Saint-Jean-des-Vignes was organized around a rule for ordained clerics based on a letter written by Saint Augustine in the fourth century. Members of the community were thus not monks but regular canons, commonly called Augustinians" (Bonde et al. 1990).

The abbey rapidly grew, and the canons of Saint-Jean reached their optimal number of 90 at the end of the twelfth century (Bonde and Maines 1994). Even though the size of monasteries varied considerably, ranging from half a dozen individuals to more than 300 as in Cluny, France (Lawrence 1984), Saint-Jean was an important congregation, especially when its land and possessions—including 40 parishes, farms, and mills—are considered (Bonde et al. 1990).

For this study, 24 burials (figure 13.3) excavated and analyzed at Saint-Jean-des-Vignes are considered. This sample comes from two locations: the chapter room and the cloister. Evidence of postdepositional disturbance is present in 14 of the burials (table 13.1). We have, for example, reuse of a sarcophagus, "shovel marks" on various bones, and construction of a built-tomb on top of an individual.

This preliminary research attempts to explain the various burial practices analyzed thus far at Saint-Jean. This study offers an explanation regarding the seemingly peculiar treatment of certain burials. I will first explore how Medieval people viewed the bodies of the dead, especially in regards to older skeletal re-

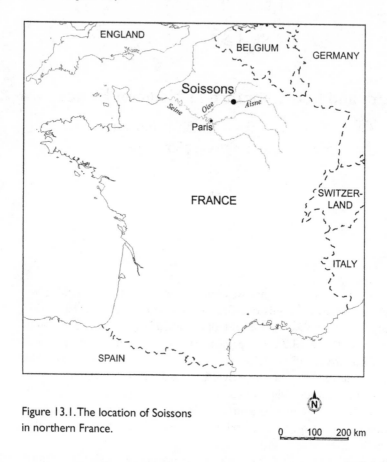

Figure 13.1. The location of Soissons in northern France.

mains, and how remembrance of the dead was manifested, particularly through prayers. Then I will describe various burial practices seen in Saint-Jean-des-Vignes, as well as other contemporary or similar Medieval sites.

The Treatment of the Body and Perceptions of It in the Middle Ages

Historical Perspectives

In *L'homme devant la mort,* Philippe Ariès proposes an explanation for the evolution of the attitude toward the dead body (Ariès 1977). Ariès illustrates a clear change in the view of death as natural and ineluctable, which started in the fifth century and continued until the eighteenth century. For Ariès, this evolution has three essential phases.

The first phase emphasized the fear of the dead body. The dead were believed to be tainted and thus able to contaminate the living (Leviticus 21:1–4, 22:4; Numbers 19:11–16). Therefore, the Roman legislation that prescribed "that a

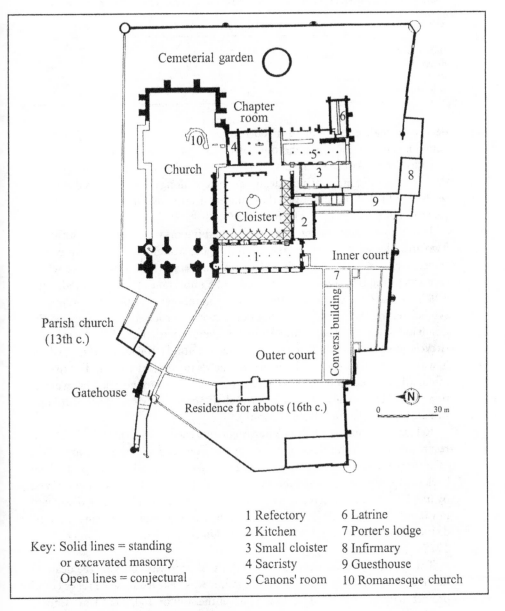

Figure 13.2. The Abbey of Saint-Jean-des-Vignes.

Key: Solid lines = standing or excavated masonry
Open lines = conjectural

1 Refectory
2 Kitchen
3 Small cloister
4 Sacristy
5 Canons' room
6 Latrine
7 Porter's lodge
8 Infirmary
9 Guesthouse
10 Romanesque church

Table 13.1. Frequencies of Anomalies in the Burials of the Cloister and the Chapter Room

Anomaly	Frequency
Shovel marks	16.5%
Reuse of sarcophagus	29.0%
Redistribution of bones	37.5%
Disturbance	41.7%

dead man shall not be buried or burned in the city"[1] (Rush 1941:123) was a common interdiction since the time of the Roman Twelve Tables of law and Theodos' code (Ariès 1977; Rush 1941). Thus, Christians followed the example drawn from antiquity, when the dead were placed along the roads outside the city walls. The first Christians reused these ancient necropolises until official cemeteries were built next to them (Treffort 1996).

In addition to fear of the body is a second important issue: burial location. Two attitudes seem to have coexisted in the early Middle Ages. The first can be traced back to the first monastic and eremitic movements in the Near East, where location of the burial was not believed to be important (Meslin and Palanque 1967). In the Christian community, however, another tradition was followed; symbolized by the fear of *not* being buried with a proper grave, it became the dominant ideology. This attitude directly stemmed from the New Testament (Revelation 11:9) and the Code of Canon Law (Catholic University 1967), where it was said that to ensure the peace of the dead, funeral rites and above all inhumation were required. This concept was also linked to the belief in resurrection day: "He who lies without a burial shall not be resurrected"[2] (Cabrol and Leclercq 1953, chapter "Résurrection").

Religious authorities such as Saint Augustine tried to explain that God could resurrect anyone, regardless of the fate of his body. As noted by Saint Augustine, "Far from us the fear that the all-mighty Lord, to resurrect bodies and bring them back to life, cannot summon everything that was devoured by beast or consumed by fire, all that was scattered in ashes or in dust, washed out by water, dissipated in vapor"[3] (Augustin 1949:534). Even so, the fear that mortal remains could be disturbed or denied burial rapidly grew within the Christian community (Ariès 1977).

This is where the second phase started; the shift toward burying the dead *ad sanctos* (near the body of the saints) began. It was believed that the relics could protect the body and would help the fate of the soul on Judgment Day (Cabrol and Leclercq 1953, chapter "Ad Sanctos"). It seems that the fate of the body did not matter anymore, so long as it was ad sanctos. This could be one explanation for the behavior of the canons regarding the bones. When the graves had to be disturbed for a new burial, they were not considered desecrated because the remains would still be kept on sacred ground. It was common to exhume old bones to make room for new graves and to gather these bones in specific places

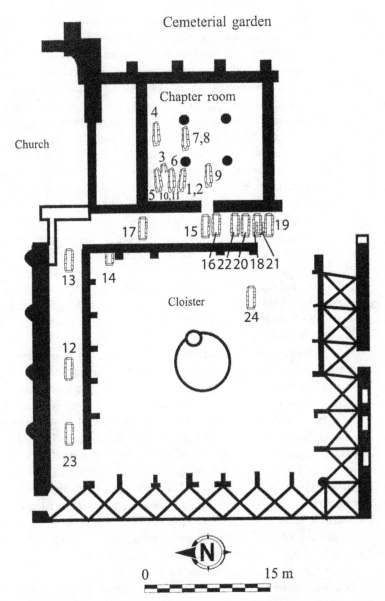

Figure 13.3. Schematic representation of the burials in the cloister and in the chapter room. Some burials contain two or more individuals, as indicated by the paired numbers.

(Breton 1867). This partially accounts for the origin of ossuaries or charnel pits. In this context the constant disturbances observed at Saint-Jean-des-Vignes could be explained. Because sacred space was scarce within the limit of the abbey, and because a great number of people wanted to be buried within this space, the only solution was the reuse of the same space.

In addition, there was also an economic motivation for this shift. The first Christian burials of the fifth and sixth centuries were usually made, for those who could afford it, with offerings. The wealthiest interments, such as royal graves, could contain gold, jewelry, or other precious items. Looters were aware of this fact and would commonly rob rich graves. It is rare to find a grave of that period that has not been at least partially looted (Treffort 1996). This trend changed only in the seventh and especially the eighth century with the reform of Charlemagne, which definitely put an end to grave offerings (Treffort 1996).

The third phase started when the cemeteries moved inside the town walls. Originally outside the town walls, cemeteries had attracted burials of both saints and other members of the population. The external cemeteries expanded with cemeterial churches, as opposed to each town's cathedral church, to receive those who wanted to pray over the relics. This phenomenon, along with the fact that towns were expanding, rendered the boundary between the burial grounds and the town imprecise, and eventually the cemeteries were located inside the towns (Salin 1949).

Ultimately, functional distinction for the cemeterial and the cathedral church converged, and religious authorities relaxed the prohibition of burying the dead within the city wall (Ariès 1977; Durand 1988). The link between churches and cemeteries was established.

After this, cemeteries were recognized not only as containing bodies but also as a sacred ground devoted to the commemoration of the past souls. In the twelfth century, Honorius of Autun, a monk writing in Germany, said that it was more beneficial to be buried ad sanctos because the grave reminds people of the dead and the prayers made by all visitors will profit the dead (Lefevre 1954).

The only official rule that the Church kept repeating for centuries in its synods was the fact that bodies should not be buried within the church itself but should be buried around it. The very fact that this rule had to be repeated over and over again (Synods of Mayence 813, Tribur 895, Nantes 900, and so forth) shows that it was not respected and that churches were indeed used as burial grounds (Durand de Mende 1854 [1284]). These aspects of burial practices can still be seen today in old churches in France where the floor consists entirely of gravestones (Colardelle 1989). Thus, whenever the congregation entered they would literally walk on graves and in turn remember the dead.

This familiarity with death is illustrated in cemeteries, when bones could literally be seen everywhere. A lost glass window of the fourteenth century from the sacristy of the Abbey of Saint-Denis near Paris, France, shows the sainted king Louis IX (1214–1270) in a cemetery picking up bones from the ground and placing them in a bag to commemorate them (Labarge 1968). This glass window, known from drawings, refers to an episode of the king's life in Sidon, where he buried the remains of the dead from the war against the Saracens (Le Nain de Tillemont 1965) when no one else dared to touch the bones.

Treatment of the Body

Inhumation or Cremation?

The treatment of the body has evolved from the beginning of Christianity to the end of the Medieval period. Before Christianity, both inhumation and cremation were practiced. At the beginning of the Christian tradition, however, inhumation became the dominant disposal form. One explanation could be that the early Christians were following the example of Christ, who was buried according to Jewish law (Rush 1941). Inhumation was only officially adopted during the fourth century, however, with the death of the first Christian emperor, Constantine (Riché 1973). Even though cremation was considered an outrageous act (Amos 2:1), Saint Augustine did not condemn it (see note 3). However, the Church remained relatively tolerant of cremation until Charlemagne forbade the practice in the eighth century under penalty of death (Riché 1973). Nevertheless, the Church always reserved the right to dispose of specific bodies, mainly the outlawed, by means of fire. In this case, cremation served as a purification event that cleansed the offense made against God or society (Duby 1967).

Preparation of the Body

Numerous examples from texts, painting, and sculpture show various ways of disposing of the dead. The oldest written examples come directly from the Bible. The dead person's eyes were closed as if in sleep (Genesis 46:4); the corpse was washed (Acts 9:39), anointed with perfumes (John 12:7, 19:40; Mark 16:1), and then wrapped in a shroud (John 19:40; Matthew 27:59), with linen wrappings used to bind the hands and feet together and a facecloth covering the deceased's face (John 11:44, 20:7). The body was afterwards carried on a bier (2 Samuel 3:31; Luke 7:14), and the mourning customs, chiefly lamentation, began (Ecclesiastes 38:16; Jeremiah 9:16–21). However, it seems that during the Middle Ages slight variations occurred. The body was still wrapped in a shroud that was knotted at the head and feet or covered with wrappings, but the face apparently could be left open or covered by the shroud itself (Boase 1972).

The body was usually put in the grave without much delay (Acts 5:5, 10). However, because considerable importance was attached to the place of burial, it was natural to seek a grave in the deceased's own territory or in a sacred place. Therefore, for those dying far from home, special practices were employed to prepare the body for transport (see chapter by Weiss-Krejci, this volume). Dismemberment, with removal of the flesh from the body and boiling of the bones, was practiced to create relics or simply to make transportation easier. When relics were sought, certain parts of the body, such as the heart, would be buried separately (Boase 1972). When Louis IX of France died in 1270 near Tunis, his body was boiled in water and wine to separate the flesh from the bones, and his heart and entrails were removed to be buried in the Benedictine abbey of Monreale near Palermo, Italy (Le Nain de Tillemont 1965). Embalming was also utilized, though this was unusual because it necessitated the use of skilled practitioners. One example is the embalming of Henri I of England, who died near Rouen, France (Boase 1972), and was transported back to England for burial. These practices were reserved for the wealthy and were thus a rare event.

The body was treated formally; even ritually it was not shunned. In the interval between death and burial, bodies were kept in private houses; they were handled, watched, and prayed over, and their presence was accepted with apparent equanimity. Corpse treatment in the interval between death and burial tended, however, to emphasize the dichotomy between personalized and depersonalized bodies. Bodies of the middle and upper classes were treated carefully and with respect; those of the poor received more casual treatment (Harding 2000).

Inhumation of the Body

The deceased were laid to rest in a variety of ways. Most of the variations were a function of wealth, social status, and material circumstances and include interment in the soil, in constructed tombs of various types, and in monolithic sarcophagi. In some cases, tombs were carved directly into a bedrock outcrop. The early Medieval use of stone sarcophagi simply prolonged more ancient traditional practices (Ariès 1977).

At the end of the Carolingian dynasty, wooden or lead coffins began to be substituted for stone sarcophagi. At the same time coffins with cephalic space— a Medieval practice perhaps developed around the ninth or tenth century—were used, diminishing in frequency over the course of the thirteenth century. It seems, however, that between the ninth and the twelfth century wooden coffins were used for body transport alone, and corpses were not buried with the coffins. Instead, the remains were placed directly into the earth or in a constructed tomb or sarcophagus. Only around the thirteenth century did the body come to be regularly buried within the coffin (Durand 1988).

Position and Orientation of the Body

Body position is more problematic, and there seems to be no universal trend that crosscuts cemeteries. The most common positions involved placing the hands over the pelvis, the arms crossed on the chest or lying by the sides of the body (Daniell 1997). Furthermore, according to the tradition of the high and later Middle Ages, the body was to be placed with the feet toward the east in expectation of the last day (Catholic University 1967). However, certain scholars were advocating the reverse position: "One must bury the dead where his head is to be turned to the east and his feet to the west"[4] (Durand de Mende 1854 [1284]). Additionally, another belief was that certain categories of people, such as the priests and bishops, were to be buried with their head to the east so that "in death as in life, he faces his flock" (Ucko 1969:270).

Regardless of the evolution of burial practices throughout the Middle Ages, it would seem that the orientation of the grave was influenced more by the orientation of the associated grave monument than by specific rites (Young 1977). Because burials were placed in churches and since churches had to be oriented east–west, with the façade to the west and the choir to the east, placing the graves in the building's axis could easily be confused with the building's orientation. When G. Durand de Mende wrote about orientation, it simply confirmed the use of an old tradition. However, it does not seem that there are any official Church texts prescribing this specific orientation.

The "Afterlife" of the Body

The presumption of an afterlife and a continuing immaterial entity called the soul is fundamental to mortuary practices. Death, the passage from being-in-existence to being-without-life, was understood not as the separation of the soul from the body but as the loss of every vital sign. The dead person was no longer the living soul, which he had become through creation, because his spirit had left him to return to God. Death was viewed in the context of resurrection, not in that of immortality (Léon-Dufour 1980). The salvatory need of the soul dictated many of the rituals enacted over the body. Belief in the resurrection of the body as an aspect of immortality added significant complications to the treatment of mortal remains. Resurrection implies the restoration of the body—not the earthly body but rather the spiritual body (1 Corinthians 15:44–48): "That is why they are said to be spiritual." Thus, it is possible to consider the dead body as primarily belonging to this world and its treatment as a reflection of priorities and concerns to do with life rather than the afterlife (Harding 2000).

There is an important distinction between attitudes about the corpse that can be identified with a person and attitudes about the depersonalized corpse. Corpses were embodied with both a sense of respect for the social persona and a sense of fear, depending on whether the person looking at the body was a relative or a stranger (Harding 2000). However, once the individuality of the body was dissolved, either with time or for other reasons, the remains (usually the bones) were considered as material objects and thus were treated pragmatically. Despite the continual recycling of burial location mentioned earlier, the Christian burial sites served as a reminder of mortality and conferred some sanctity on the place where the dead were stored (Levefre 1954).

Evidence for Augustinian Funerary Rituals

The eleventh-century rediscovery of the Rule of Saint Augustine was one of the great events in the Western monastic tradition. The Augustinian Rule was elaborated from a letter (CCXI) that Saint Augustine wrote to his sister around A.D. 423. "In this letter Saint Augustine rebukes the nuns of the monastery in which his sister had been prioress, for certain turbulent manifestations of dissatisfaction with her successor and lays down general rules for their guidance" (Schaff 1956). The Augustinian Rule influenced all subsequent thinking about monastic life and even provided the formal basis for three major institutions: the canons regular, the Order of Prémontré, and the Dominicans (Lawrence 1984).

Unfortunately, the rule was not specific about day-to-day life. The Augustianian Rule mostly focuses on the spirituality of monasticism rather than practical guidance on how to organize a community. It does not address everyday activity or the care of the dead (Augustin 1984). For a typical Augustinian community, the most useful written information about monastic life and burial had to come from custumals, or customaries. These latter treatises recorded the narrative practices of specific monasteries. They were compiled to supplement the general instruction of the rule and contained detailed regulations for the celebration of the divine office as well as for every activity that filled the monastic day. They also often drew on various traditional monastic sources, such as the Benedictine Rule and the Synod of Aachen (Lawrence 1984). One discussion of specific mortuary practices relates the actions intended to commemorate the dead in the chapter room by reading from the *libero capituli* or on special anniversaries to "provide four burning [lights] for the chapter room"[5] (Bonde et al. 1990:197).

Further relevant information can be found within various other documents. For instance, Saint Augustine also wrote a letter in A.D. 420–421 (*De Cura Gerenda pro Mortuis*) to his friend Paul of Nola regarding the care of the dead (Augustin 1948). Paul had asked Saint Augustine about the significance of burial ad sanctos. Saint Augustine replied, referring to one of his previous writings, *De Civitate Dei* (Augustin 1949), that the burial is not necessary for the salvation of the soul of the dead because the body itself became insensible: "Do not fear those who kill the body but are powerless to kill the soul" (Matthew 10:28). Only the living worry about burying the bodies of the dead; the dead do not care. Nonetheless, Saint Augustine understood the significance of caring for the dead body in the context of our love for the flesh as an expression of life. In this context he advocated that the body should not be despised: "The bodies of the dead are not on this account to be despised and cast aside; least of all the bodies of the just and faithful, which the spirit has holily employed as organs and instruments for all good works"[6] (Augustin 1949:532). The actual justification for a burial is then better understood within *humanitas,* the mercifulness of the act of burying the dead in consideration for who the person was in life. In addition, the usefulness of the grave is more obviously understood as the living showing their faith in the resurrection. Again, Saint Augustine, speaking about the charity of Tobias in caring the dead, said that "these instances do not show that corpses have any life, but they indicate that God's providence extends over the bodies of the dead, and that such pious works are pleasing to Him, as cherishing faith in the resurrection"[7] (Augustin 1949:532).

Furthermore, burials helped perpetuate the memory of the dead via visual markers, which were useful to stimulate prayers to relieve their souls. Saint Augustine insisted that the honor the dead deserved was useful only to comfort the living (Augustin 1948:chapter III). Finally, burying the dead ad sanctos helped the soul in the afterlife, because saints were the only ones assured of going directly to Heaven (Treffort 1996); if in life the deceased was worthy, then in death he might benefit from this proximity (Augustin 1948:chapter IV).

From these clues, it seems that the treatment of the dead is important in the fact that it reflects our perception of the individual in life. There are two aspects to this idea. The first is that to the Christian the concept of burials ad sanctos is helpful for the soul because of the proximity of the saints. The other is that, in general, burying someone is an act of mercy that every Christian should respect, even though it mainly serves the living.

The Role of Prayers

Historical Perspectives

Historians have for some time reflected on the fact that Catholicism was "a cult of the living in the service of the dead" (Gordon and Marshall 2000:2). Prayers for the dead seem to have always been part of Christian rituals. One of the earlier references is in the Old Testament (2 Maccabees 12:39–45), where Judas Machabee prays for the salvation of his dead men who sinned in battle. In the New Testament, Paul prays and begs God's mercy for Onesiphorous, who had just died (2 Timothy 1:18). In addition, several tombstones at the beginning of the Christian era carried inscriptions regarding prayer for the dead (Cabrol and Leclercq 1953, chapter "Prière des Morts"). Similarly, there are several mentions of anniversaries of death. Saint Augustine cites the testimony of 2 Maccabees 12:43 in favor of prayers for the dead (Augustin 1948:459), but he especially stresses the fact that prayers for the dead will benefit only those who have so lived as to be able to receive benefit from them (Augustin 1869; 1949:650).

In these references, we can see two trends. The first one is the commemoration of the dead and the celebration of their memory (McLaughlin 1994). The second one is the intercession for the dead, where the living try to help the soul of the dead.

> The prominence of the dead in late medieval Latin Christianity was preeminently the result of the conjunction of two compelling ideas. The first was the gradual evolution and eventual formalization of the belief that the majority of the faithful dead did not proceed immediately to the beatific vision, but underwent a painful purgation of the debt due for their sins in the intermediary state (and place) of Purgatory. The second was the conviction, predicated upon the theory that all faithful Christians in this world and in the next were incorporated in a single communion of saints, that the living had the ability (and the duty) to ease the deads' suffering in Purgatory. (Gordon and Marshall 2000:3)

This second notion became the object of a solemn magisterial pronouncement in an ecumenical council, Lyons II (1274) (Catholic University 1967). There it was declared that souls undergoing purification after death could be assisted by the intercessory prayers of the living, by masses, almsgiving, prayer in general, and other devout practices according to the custom of the Church (Denziger 1963:856). Following this event, Pope Sixtus IV in his 1476 papal bull "Salvator noster" (Denziger 1963:1398) granted the "first plenary indulgences applicable to the souls in purgatory."

One link between these two notions can be illustrated by the evolution of the Mass. Before Charlemagne, the Mass reflected the universality of humanity, dead or alive. After Charlemagne, the Mass was only for the dead and for certain living people. Charlemagne basically replaced the Gallic canon with the Roman one. The important change is that the names of the dead, traditionally said in prayers along with the living, were to be mentioned separately. The commemoration of the dead became an intercession for the dead (Treffort 1996).

The celebration of masses for the dead also underwent some changes, from a single mass per day up to the twelfth century (Ariès 1977) to the desire of an almost continuous celebration, especially in monastic context. In addition, the development of private masses after the thirteenth century, especially among the monastic orders, multiplied the celebrations of masses for the dead. These masses were celebrated in exchange for money, allowing churches and monasteries to extend the power of intercession to many more souls, while at the same time benefiting financially. This phenomenon became so popular that hundreds of masses had to be celebrated each day. Thus, the number of priests, ordained monks, and canons increased, as well as the number of commemorative chapels. This trend culminated in the seventeenth century, at which time in the church of Saint Benoit in Paris, for example, 10,000 masses were supposed to be said for Simon Colbert. Not surprisingly, the priests quickly fell behind in their celebrations (Ariès 1977).

The last fact that needs to be considered in relation to prayer and remembrance is the development of anonymous tombs. The actual location of the body seems to have slowly become dissociated from the tomb itself. Prior to the ninth or tenth century, the first trend of burying ad sanctos illustrates this phenomenon. Grave identity did not matter as long as one knew that one's grave was ad sanctos. However, a second trend started in the eleventh century whereby monumental tombs placed in the church (and for the less wealthy, plaques fixed to the wall of the church or the cloister buildings with posthumous inscriptions) physically symbolized the grave (Lebeuf 1954).

The evolution of the treatment of the dead throughout the Middle Ages clearly indicates that interceding prayers for the salvation of the soul were a main concern dominating the actual fate of the material remains. Furthermore, the development of anonymous graves only reinforced the concept of sacred ground over sacred body and could thus explain, in part, how the living viewed skeletal remains.

Burial Practices at Saint-Jean-des-Vignes

Description

During excavations that have taken place at Saint-Jean-des-Vignes since 1982, various human remains have been recovered (Bonde and Maines 1999, 2000, 2001; Wallace 1985). These remains were found in three main structures: graves, ossuaries, and backfill.

Four main burial locations were used in the abbey (see figure 13.2). In order of significance, starting with the most important, these were the church, the chapter room, the cloister, and a cemetery area lying to the east of the church and cloister ranges (Bonde and Maines 1994). Excavations confirmed the presence of burials in each of these locations. In addition, the abbey obituary reveals that at least one abbot and the founder of the abbey, Hugues de Chateau Thierry, were buried within the church (Bonde et al. 1990). Textual evidence shows that the chapter room was used as a privileged burial ground for important patrons, such as Bishop Haymard of Provins, who became a canon in the abbey in 1218 just before he died. Texts also reveal the presence of at least one patroness, Adelaid, who died in the 1140s and was buried in the Romanesque chapter room (Bonde et al. 1990). This paper will focus on the cloister and the chapter room; the church has not yet revealed sufficient remains to be studied.

One striking aspect of the repartition of burials at Saint-Jean is the incredible density of burials. For example, in the eastern cloister gallery alone, burials are almost always adjacent to each other, if not overlapping. Space between two burials is very rare and never larger than a few centimeters.

Several burial practices were followed at the abbey. Primary burials included built tombs, partially built tombs, pit graves, anthropomorphic tombs, and sarcophagi. Secondary burials such as ossuaries and redeposited whole or partial individuals within a primary burial have also been recovered. The only feature common to most of the graves is that all the individuals seemed to have been buried in some type of shroud. Several types of shrouds were used during the Middle Ages. We have evidence for at least two single-piece shrouds and wrappings, as evidenced by inferred body positions (Duday 1985; Duday et al. 1990; Duday and Sellier 1990) and the bronze pins recovered from one burial. Additionally, the bronze staining present on two skeletons attests to the former presence of pins (Bonde and Maines 2000).

Peculiarities

Several aspects of a number of these burials are noteworthy and require comment. These include, first, the presence of cuts on some bones. These cuts are straight depressions of about 2 to 3 millimeters in width and 2 millimeters deep that cross the length of the bones with no remodeling and one border slightly beveled inward. The cuts from both the ossuaries and burials have been interpreted as postmortem shovel marks. Second, we also find bones of several individuals "piled up" within the same sarcophagus, illustrating a redeposit of major skeletal elements, such as the cranium from an older burial together with an articulated individual, and the constant disturbance of old burials for newer ones. Finally, at the end of the 2000 season, the author excavated another peculiar skeleton. The upper right part of a skeleton (CL-21)—vertebrae, ribs, humerus, and hand—was found underneath a wall of a built-tomb (CL-18). These remains corresponded to the left side of a skeleton unearthed in 1999 within CL-18, which contained a fully articulated individual. Subsequently, the author managed to identify the cranium of the crushed skeleton among other bones in an adjacent ossuary. The mandible was found lying just west of the body beneath another stone. Most of the long bones other than the humeri were missing but might also be present in the ossuary, waiting to be identified (Bonde and Maines 2000). Altogether, 58 percent of the burials had been tampered with in one form or another.

These findings strike one as being rather rude on the part of the gravedigger. While we cannot know who the gravediggers were at any given moment of the abbey's history, the most likely candidates would come from among the community's lay brothers resident at the site. Granted, an outsider may have been employed to do the task, but one would nevertheless think that within the monastery a certain care would have been taken when dealing with the community's dead.

These findings invited a consideration of the relative importance of older bones in the eyes of the canons and more generally of the Church. Were the bones not sacred per se, as opposed to the fleshed body or the actual location of the bones, and thus little care was required for their manipulation? In this case, the remains found in Saint-Jean would not be extraordinary. Alternatively, perhaps the bones were to have been venerated as prescribed by present-day Catholicism, so that "the body was considered as a temple of the soul, a temple of the Holy Ghost" (Rush 1941) and thus was worthy of respect in life and death (1 Corinthians 3:16, 6:19). Here, evidence at Saint-Jean would indicate an example of negligence within the abbey.

Archaeological Evidence for Similar Burial Practices

Marc Durand has written extensively about Medieval cemeteries in the region of Saint-Jean-des-Vignes (Durand 1988). His review reveals several similar patterns of burial disturbances. The cemetery of Saint-Pierre in Senlis contained numerous burials from the late Middle Ages undercutting one another. At the contemporary necropolis of Montataire is clear reuse of stone sarcophagi with various combinations of primary and secondary inhumations as well as the presence of bones in the backfill of the grave cuts. The cluniac priory of Saint-Nicolas d'Acy (eleventh–seventeenth centuries) reveals the same pattern of grave disorder (Durand 1991).

The same situation is found in other regions of France—for example, east of Saint-Jean, in Savoie, in the eleventh-century church of Sainte-Croix, Drome

(Colardelle 1981), or in Champagne, in the thirteenth–fourteenth-century church of Saint-Symphorien de Thibie (Billoin and Gape 1997). These examples can be found throughout France from the Merovingian period (Colardelle 1981, 1989; Treffort 1996) to the end of the Middle Ages. Although no case was found that matched the "crushed individual," it would seem that disregard for the bones of previously interred individuals was widespread, whether in monasteries, churches, or rural cemeteries.

Interpretation

In light of the numerous examples of burial disturbances in Medieval cemeteries, it would seem that the peculiarities found in Saint-Jean are not unusual after all. In a monastic context where burial space is limited, the canons seem to have adopted the only solution possible for the great number of individuals who wished to be buried within the sacred enclosure of the abbey. This solution was to reuse sacred spaces as often as necessary to respond to the living population concerned with the fate of their bodies. Priority was for the living, or rather the recent dead, over previous generations. Older bones were reorganized in ossuaries or backfilled into the latest burials. Commemorative plaques and stones were probably used in some cases, as illustrated by some gravestones reused in the sixteenth-century abbot's residence of Saint-Jean-des-Vignes as a step in the staircase.

Another explanation could be invoked for the disturbances of skeletons, especially when parts of a skeleton seem to be missing. Because burying ad sanctos implies having saint's relics, one could argue that some bones may have been stolen to create relics or to diminish the prestige of Saint-Jean. Stealing relics was a common phenomenon throughout the Middle Ages. The very well-documented twelfth-century theft of the relic of Saint Petroc, an early Medieval Cornish saint from the Abbey of Bodmin, England, to the Abbey of Saint-Meén in Brittany, is a good example of such political acts (Jankulak 2000). Similarly, the theft of Saint Mark's relics from Alexandria in 828 by the Venetians (Dale 2000) illustrates the political importance of such bones and creates alternative scenarios for potential disturbances in sacred burial places. A prominent monastery such as Saint-Jean could have enticed individuals to do just that.

Excavations of the burials revealed that some care had been taken to minimize the damage in some instances. In 2001 the author excavated a burial (CL-22) with a clear cut from another grave that followed the vertebral column of the skeleton. The gravedigger did go through one arm and one leg, but the rest was perfectly preserved and left undisturbed (Bonde and Maines 2001).

Another element to consider is the reuse of stone sarcophagi in the chapter room for burial. Even with the argument of saving time, space, and money by using an existing sarcophagus, we also have to consider that this place was the second most important burial location. In addition, the density of burials in this part of the abbey is much less pronounced than in the cloister. The argument of space cannot be used appropriately in reference to the chapter room. I would also discard time and money as valid arguments. Saint-Jean was a wealthy abbey and would have no need to save money on important individuals. There is also no evidence of sudden mass deaths that would have pressured the canons into burying their dead in haste. It seems they had the manpower and the money to deal with their dead in the timeframe they wanted. A more hypothetical explanation such as the association of relatives or proximity to socially or politically important figures seems more likely and would have facilitated the commemoration of the deceased.

One consequence of these observations is the demonstration that secondary burials in a monastic context could carry more interpretations than has been previously accepted. Even though manipulation of bones in Medieval burials seems to be rather common, the reason why such manipulations were originally made is still hypothetical. The explanations sought in this paper for the secondary treatment of bones are only a preliminary approach to a much vaster issue—namely, the treatment of nonsaints' remains in monastic contexts. These explanations, however, allow us to widen the scope of interpretations for such remains in other cemeteries and hopefully will motivate others to question similar practices in different contexts. Studies from other sites and religious orders are needed to understand the complete picture of monastic burial practices, to explain not only how the remains were handled, but also why they were handled in such a way.

Conclusions

The perception of mortal remains has evolved considerably between the fifth century and the eighteenth century, having changed from fear and reverence of the dead body to day-to-day familiarity with bones. Thus, the archaeological record should reflect such an evolution and complexity. Of course, "evolution" and "complexity" are two of the most difficult aspects of history to reach through the material record. However, sometimes we can get a glimpse of at least one of these aspects.

Saint-Jean-des-Vignes has revealed that old bones and personalized burials were not the main concern of Medieval canons or their early modern successors, at least for the burials studied. Shovel marks, the reuse of sarcophagi in the chapter room, and the skeleton crushed under a built-tomb in the cloister all reflect a common fact of the Medieval period: sacred space was precious and limited. Thus, it is not surprising to find in a Medieval monastery evidence of what seems to be signs of disrespect for the dead, since Medieval people were concerned less with the expression of respect and remembrance of the body and more with that of the soul.

Acknowledgments

I would like to thank Jane Buikstra for providing me with the opportunity to write and publish this article, the motivation to tackle such vast issues, and the means to approach the field of mortuary practices. I could not have started this enterprise without the help of Sheila Bonde and Clark Maines, with whom I have enthusiastically worked on the wonderful site of Saint-Jean-des-Vignes, France. I also thank them for their valuable comments on a previous draft of this chapter that allowed me to stay on track the entire time. Finally, I would like to thank Henry Duday, who made me a strong believer of his "anthropologie de terrain" and who motivated me to explore the amazing world of the dead. My thanks also go to Valerie Prilop, who patiently proofread my text.

Notes

1. Cicero, *De Legibus*, vol. 2, pages 23 and 58. "Hominem morum inuit lex in XII, in urbe ne sepelito neve urito." Translation by Rush.

2. "Insepultus javeat, non ressurgat." Translation by author.

3. Saint Augustine, *De Civitate Dei*, book 22, chapter 20: "Absit autem, ut ad resuscitanda corpora vitaeque reddenda non possit omnipotentia Creatoris omnia revocare, quae vel bestiae vel ignis absumpsit, vel in pulverem cineremve conlapsum vel in umorem solutum vel in auras est exhalatum." Translation by Combes.

4. "On doit ensevelir le mort de telle sorte que sa tête soit tournée à l'occident et ses pieds à l'ouest." Translation by C. Barthelemy.

5. Lectio 31: "ad anniversaria duplicia mortuorum quator ardentes in capitulo provideat." Translation by Maines.

6. Saint Augustine, *De Civitate Dei*, book 1, chapter 13, page 11: "Non ideo contemnenda et abiecienda sunt corpora defunctorum maximeque iustorum atque fidelium, quibus tamquam organis et vasis ad omina bona opera sancte usus est spiritus." Translation by Combes.

7. Saint Augustine, *De Civitate Dei*, book 1, chapter 13, page 11: "Verum istae auctoritates non hoc admonet, quod inest ullus cadaveribus sensus, sed as Dei poividentiam, cui placent etiam talia pietatis officia, corpora mortuorum pertinere significant propter fidem ressurrectionis astruendam." Translation by Combes.

14

Mortuary Practices and Ritual Use of Human Bone in Tibet

Nancy J. Malville

Tibetan Buddhist mortuary practices are strongly influenced by the doctrine of rebirth, which regards death as "an experience that is repeated at certain intervals" (Maraini 2000:171 [1951]). "The life we live is not the gift of a god, but merely an episode in a sequence of different lives, an installment in an endless serial" (Migot 1955:100). The most important considerations when someone dies are to say prayers to guide the soul of the deceased into a new rebirth and to dispose of the cast-off old body as quickly and completely as possible. "A funeral is not a particularly sad occasion though relatives may well be crying. The death is over and done with, and all that remains is the practical matter of the disposal of the body" (Norbu and Turnbull 1970:109).

Sometimes certain skeletal elements are retained for rituals in which the use of human skulls and femurs reinforces the central theme in Buddhism of impermanence and nonattachment. Human bones not only serve as reminders of the inevitability of death but are also perceived by some as powerful ritual objects for making contact with the various gods and demons of the rich pantheon of Tibetan deities and dangerous spirits.

The earliest forms of burial in Tibet were probably cremation and exposure of the dead to be eaten by birds and animals (Hummel 1961; Laufer 1923; Loseries 1993). Special treatment was given to certain high-status individuals such as Tibetan royalty, whose burial tombs may still be seen at Chunggye in the Yarlung Valley (Ngapo et al. 1981). A traveler in Tibet from 1316 to 1330, Friar Odoric of Pordonene, was told that the inhabitants had once practiced a form of ancestral worship in which they showed respect for their deceased fathers by preserving the skulls and drinking from these skulls on certain occasions (Eliade 1974 [1951]; Laufer 1923). Eliade (1974 [1951]) suggests that this custom may have been influenced by such Asian shamanic practices as, for example, that of the Yukagir of Siberia, who preserved the skulls, bones, and dried flesh of their deceased shamans and distributed these relics to their relatives for religious purposes and for use in divination (Jochelson 1926). Even today, Tibetans sometimes preserve the skulls of respected *rinpoches* for use in making religious offerings (Tamdin Wangdu, personal communication).

Disposal of the Body

The *Tibetan Book of the Dead* (Tib. *bar-do'i-thos-grol*) teaches that the five inner elements of the body (earth, water, fire, air, and space) gradually dissolve into one another at the time of a natural death (Freemantle and Trungpa 1975).[1] Tibetans employ five methods of disposing of the dead, four of which are symbolically associated with the first four of these elements. Preservation of the body with salt is a fifth method, appropriate only for certain high-status individuals. Usually an astrologer-lama is consulted to make certain that the right way of dealing with the body is chosen (Norbu and Turnbull 1970). The choice of method depends also on the age and status of the deceased individual, the circumstances of death, and practical considerations such as stony ground, frozen rivers, or the availability of firewood.

Cremation is the preferred method of corpse disposal in Tibet, as in India and Nepal, but the scarcity of firewood in many barren parts of Tibet makes cremation very expensive or even impossible for the common people (David-Neel 1986 [1927]). For this reason, it was customary in the past to cremate only high lamas (Loseries 1993), who were sometimes "incinerated in a big cauldron filled with butter" (David-Neel 1986:135 [1927]). The cremation site is often located close to the sky on a high ridge, "that area on earth closest to space, the mountain top, where symbolically emptiness and the manifest meet" (Downs 1980:196).

Sky or celestial burial, a practice of ancient origin in which the body is cut up and fed to vultures, is a common alternative to cremation in Tibet (Loseries 1993; Ngapo et al. 1981; Shen and Liu 1953) and in arid regions of Nepal such as Mustang. The vultures that dispose of human remains are regarded as sacred birds because of their important role in the celestial burial and also because of the belief that they do not harm any small creatures (Ngapo et al. 1981). Among the mountain nomads and at some of the more remote sky burial sites in Tibet such as Kongpo and Tsang, the corpses are simply taken into the mountains (Norbu and Turnbull 1970) or to a charnel ground (Loseries 1993) for exposure to wild beasts and dogs. Dogs that feed on the exposed corpses are considered to be guides for the dead. Exposure of the dead to animals is an ancient burial custom dating back to prehistoric times in Eurasia (Hummel 1961; Loseries 1993). In the Anatolian settlement of Çatal Huyuk (dating from about 5800 B.C.) in what is now southern Turkey, researchers have uncovered wall murals at three so-called vulture shrines that depict scenes of vultures pecking at headless corpses. One possible interpretation is that such scenes reflected part of the burial process, in which dead bodies were exposed for defleshing (Palmqvist 1993).

At the sacred mountain of Mt. Kailash in western Tibet, the charnel ground of the 84 Mahasiddhas (Drachom Ngagye Durtrö) provides an example of a sky burial site where bodies are offered to animals because vultures are lacking. Reserved for deceased monks and lamas according to one source (Chan 1994), the site is located on a high rocky shelf at an elevation of about 16,000 feet at the beginning of the circumambulation route (*kora*) around Mt. Kailash (figure 14.1). It is a desolate setting with hundreds of small stone cairns and a few scattered human body parts lying about. On the occasion of the annual Saka Dawa festival at the nearby Tarboche flagpole,[2] sorrowful Tibetan pilgrims wander among the cairns, often leaving hair, fingernails, and clothing as symbolic deaths at this site and also at a second site farther along the kora route at an elevation of nearly 18,000 feet (author's personal observations 1999).

Not all deceased individuals qualify for cremation or sky burial, because these methods are regarded as honorable methods of corpse disposal. The alternative methods, burial in the earth or disposal of the corpse in a river, are considered dishonorable and are used only for victims of dreaded diseases such as smallpox or leprosy, people who have died violent deaths, and poor people who have nobody to look after them (Loseries 1993; Ngapo et al. 1981; Norbu and Turnbull 1970). According to one source, undesirable individuals such as murderers and criminals are denied celestial burial and even water burial but are placed under the earth because "if their souls are trapped underground, they will not be reincarnated and their kind will become extinct" (Ngapo et al. 1981:91). Certain ethnic minorities, such as the Lopas in Tibet (Ngapo et al. 1981) and the Lepcha, Mun, and Bonthing in Sikkim (Loseries 1993), bury their dead in the ground.

Small children are often treated differently from adults because, according to some interpretations, they are considered to be spiritually undeveloped. For example, children younger than the age of eight are denied burial at the ancient charnel ground of Drigunthil (Loseries 1993). Sometimes the bodies of deceased children are disposed of in a river (Norbu and Turnbull 1970) or left in a mountain cave to be consumed by wild animals (Ngapo et al. 1981). "When infants die, their bodies are put in porcelain jars covered with lids and thrown into the river, though sometimes these jars are kept for a long time in the families' storerooms" (Ngapo et al. 1981:90–91). It is customary for Sherpas in Nepal to bury the body of a deceased child in the ground, often near a stream (Jangbu Sherpa, personal communication).

The fifth way of dealing with the dead, drying and preserving the body with salt, is reserved primarily for a few high-ranking lamas (Shen and Liu 1953; Valli and Summers 1994). Even the salt water that drips from the lama's corpse is mixed with clay and formed into tiny images of Buddha to which miraculous powers are attributed (Shen and Liu 1953). Following the death in 1989 of the Tenth Panchen Lama, his body was preserved in a glass case in Tashilhumpo

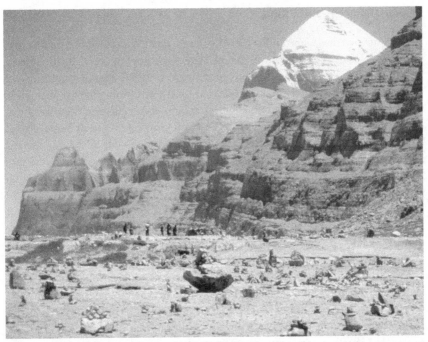

Figure 14.1. The charnel ground of the 84 Mahasiddhas, located at an elevation of about 16,000 feet, below the sacred Mt. Kailash in western Tibet. Photograph by John Mckim Malville.

Monastery in Shigatse (Batchelor 1998). When the Shey Tulku died in 1991 in Dolpo, Nepal, his body was packed in salt in the meditative posture. Pilgrims gathered in front of the body to light lamps and pray, taking home with them "a bit of the salt that had escaped from the bamboo mat containing the body" because "these precious crystals are said to have the power to heal" (Valli and Summers 1994:137). The ashes or preserved bodies of high-ranking lamas are sometimes placed in stupas or *chörtens* (Tucci 1973), as in the case of Dalai Lamas, whose bodies are enshrined in reliquary stupas within the Potala (Batchelor 1998; Chan 1994).

In exceptional cases even a layman's body may be preserved with salt (Norbu and Turnbull 1970). For example, when the youngest brother of the present Dalai Lama died at about two years of age, the astrologer-lama consulted for the death horoscope instructed the family to preserve the dead boy's body with salt and to keep it in the cellar so that he could be reborn in the same house (Jetsun Pema 1997). His reincarnation, Tenzin Choegyal, was recognized by special butter markings placed on the body of the dead boy. He was later recognized also as the reincarnation of Ngari Rinpoche, a close friend of the thirteenth Dalai Lama.

Tibetan Buddhist Death Rites

When someone dies, Tibetan Buddhists call in a lama to perform the death rites. The body of the deceased is covered with sheets and kept in the home for at least 24 hours while relatives and friends participate in ritual chanting and prayers designed to send the spirit of the deceased on its way. Sometimes a shaman is summoned in addition to a lama, and both religious specialists may cooperate in the rituals. Downs (1980) documented a cremation ceremony in Nepal in the Sherpa village of Gompa Zhung (Junbesi) in which the Buddhist shaman danced and drummed, traveling in his trance to the world of the dead. The shaman was seeking the spirit of the newly deceased man to bring him back so that the lama could instruct him about the after-death experience.

The main purpose of the death rites is to make certain that the soul does not remain behind with the body but sets off on the proper pathway toward a new rebirth (Mumford 1989; Norbu and Turnbull 1970).[3] The rites may continue for several days, depending on the ability of the family to pay for the services of a lama (Mumford 1989; Jangbu Sherpa, personal communication), and most Tibetans continue to light lamps and pray for the deceased every 7 days until the 49th day after death (Tamdin Wangdu, personal communication).

The actual details of the death rites may differ from one region to another. Mumford (1989) documented the ceremonies associated with the cremation of a young Tibetan Buddhist woman in Manang District, northern Nepal. The officiating lama first calculated the death horoscope (*rtsis*) to determine the timeliness of the death, the immediate cause of death, and the prognosis for future rebirth. The horoscope reading determined even the timing of the removal of the corpse from the house and the direction in which it was to be carried to the cremation site.

The evening following the cremation of the corpse, the lama performed a ceremony (*za 'dre kha sgyur*) to exorcise the death demon (*gshed-ma*) and prevent it from harming other family members. During the 49-day period following death, burnt offerings were made each day to feed the deceased's spirit and those of wandering ghosts, especially those demanding repayment for debts incurred during the deceased's past lives. The family of the deceased woman distributed rice cakes (*tshogs*) to members of surrounding villages to "pay all debts and accumulate merit" for the deceased (Mumford 1989:205).

The lama performed the "severance" rite (*gcod* or *chöd*), in which he called upon the deceased to visualize a fierce manifestation of the goddess Ma-cig lab-dron cutting up her body as food for a great banquet for gods and demons. The lama instructed the deceased woman to renounce her body and, as an act of generosity, to give it as food to all beings in the three realms (that is, the earth, the underworld, and the heavens). The gcod ritual "achieves what the lamas call the union of two truth levels: the severance 'cuts away' [the corpse's] ignorance, while at the same time the 'cut pieces' of her corpse are identified with the rice cakes [tshogs] that are distributed to the other villages" (Mumford 1989:206). The fearsome imagery of the severance rite text calls to mind the Bon shamanic traditions that preceded Buddhism in Tibet:

> Since I must die anyway, I give my body to all the guests [both invited and uninvited, who come to feed on the flesh that is visualized as the food of a banquet]. All come, I'll feed you! Those who like meat, take my flesh. Those who like blood, take my blood. Those who like bones, take my bones. Those who like skin to wear, take my skin. Take it all, I don't need it. . . . Break the bones and suck the marrow. Have enough, be pleased in the night and in the day, sing songs of happiness! (Mumford 1989:206–207)

The lama then called the spirit of the dead into a paper effigy (sbyang-bu) and read from the Tibetan Book of the Dead to guide the consciousness of the deceased on the proper path to rebirth (Freemantle and Trungpa 1975; Tucci 1980 [1970]). "Like a Baedeker of the world beyond, [the book] gives astonishingly detailed descriptions of the visions that appear in the mind of the dead, from the first until the forty-ninth day after it has left the body; that is to say, until the moment when it is on the point of entering a new bodily envelope. . . . The crucial phase in the cosmic history of the individual occurs in the first days after death" (Maraini 2000:171–172 [1951]). It is common for the Bardo ritual of instruction to be performed once a week during the next 49 days (Mumford 1989; Norbu and Turnbull 1970).

Sky burial sites (durtro, dur-khrod) may be set apart by a stone circle, as at Tsurphu in Tibet (Loseries 1993), or located on a high rock platform, as at Sera (Ngapo et al. 1981; Loseries 1993). One of the most auspicious sites for sky burial is the great cemetery of Drikungthil, which is said to be "identical with the most famous of the eight Indian charnel grounds, Silbatshal . . . to which it is connected by a rainbow" (Loseries 1993:180).

Although the whole family attends the funeral, usually only a few family members or their representatives witness the sky burial (Ngapo et al. 1981; Tamdin Wangdu, personal communication). They watch from a distance, because the actual work is done by specialists, the stobs-ldan, who burn pine and juniper wood to attract the vultures and sprinkle tsampa (roasted barley flour) on the fire. "The cutting of the flesh has to be done in a certain way, and as soon as it starts the birds gather, sometimes hundreds of them. The bones have to be taken and broken, pounded to a powder, and mixed with a little barley flour, or tsampa. This too is eaten by the birds. If they take everything, it is a good sign" (Norbu and Turnbull 1970:110).

In the 1960s and 1970s, the Chinese officials, who appeared to regard sky burial as "a bizarre ritual of a primitive people," banned sky burials in Tibet along with other religious practices (Faison 1999:A4). Tibetans later regained limited rights to practice their traditional form of burial. At the sky burial site of Sera, the ancient ritual of corpse disposal is now regulated by the city of Lhasa

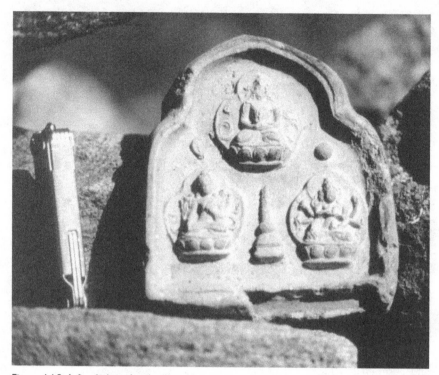

Figure 14.2. A fired clay *ts'a-ts'a* placed by relatives of the deceased inside the sacred cave of Sengge Phuk (Lion's Cave) in upper Solu, Nepal. A pocket knife provides scale. Photograph by John Mckim Malville.

and the corpse cutters are paid government employees. Loseries (1993:187) comments that "[w]ith its total suppression of religious activity the unpopular communist regime in Tibet unwittingly caused a complete reorientation towards the essential significance of charnel ground traditions." She notes also that "[a]s wood for cremation is very costly in Lhasa, and transport back to China is also rather expensive, most Chinese now settled in Lhasa have to resort to sky burial—ironically, considering that the Chinese invaders exterminated nearly all the vultures for sheer amusement. Nowadays, every effort is made to increase their number again" (Loseries 1993:184).

Disposal of Bone Fragments Remaining from Cremation or Exposure

After the body has been fed to the birds, it is considered to be a bad sign if anything is left behind because "only the bodies of the condemned, it is believed, are shunned by the birds" (Shen and Liu 1953:151). It is important for the deceased person to give away everything as an act of generosity. "If any of the bone is left, it must be burned to ashes and scattered far and wide. Every morsel of the corpse must be disposed of, so that the soul is free to leave it" (Ngapo et al. 1981:90).

Sometimes the family may build a small stone cairn (*chaitya*) over the ash and bone fragments remaining from cremation or exposure of the corpse to animals. In the Khumbu region of Nepal, the bodies of Sherpas killed on mountaineering expeditions to Mt. Everest and other neighboring peaks are carried down the mountain, if at all possible, to a cremation site on a ridge near Lobouche. Firewood is transported to the site, and relatives of the deceased come to participate in funeral ceremonies and to mark the site of the cremation with a stone cairn (Ortner 1999).

Another common treatment of cremation remains in Tibet and Nepal is to mold them into miniature chörtens or into medallions known as *ts'a-ts'a* or *sa-tsch'a* (David-Neel 1986 [1927]; Shen and Liu 1953; Tucci 1973; Waddell 1972 [1895]). The family of the deceased takes the cremated remains to the lamas, who then pulverize the fragments in a mortar, mix them with clay, and mold them into small clay tablets (often totaling 108) using stamps bearing the images of chörtens or buddhas. The lamas perform this service free of charge for poor people but expect generous donations from wealthy families (Jangbu Sherpa, personal communication). The relatives will later place the ts'a-ts'a near monasteries or in sacred caves and other remote locations. One such example is the sacred cave of Sengge Phuk (Lion's Cave), a remote pilgrimage destination in upper Solu, Nepal, near the Tibetan refugee monastery of Thubten Choling. Numerous ts'a-ts'a made of fired clay have been placed on ledges inside the cave and on the ledge above its mouth (figure 14.2).

Use of Human Bones in Tantric Ritual

Thubten Jigme Norbu, elder brother of the Dalai Lama, warns that everyone must stay at the sky burial site until all remains have been consumed by vultures because "certain tantric sects call for the use of certain parts of the body, such as the skull or the thighbone, for secret rituals. No family would want the bones of a relative used in this way, unless he himself so wished it, or the astrologer recommended it" (Norbu and Turnbull 1970:110).

The tantric method, which seeks to achieve swift enlightenment through the union of opposites, offers techniques "for utilizing all things good and evil to that end" (Blofeld 1970:31). Tantric practitioners believe that "the vital force" of the bone's "previous owner" remains within the bone, giving the bone power in tantric rituals (Beer 1999:264). The skeletal elements most commonly used are the skull and the femur, the skull for making cups and hand-drums and the femur for thighbone trumpets and bone ornaments. Sometimes skull-cups and thighbone trumpets are fashioned from copper instead of human bone.

Skull-Cup

The skull-cup (Skt. *kapala*; Tib. *thod phur*) is made from the oval upper section of a human cranium. Many skull-cups are elaborately decorated and lined with brass or silver. The skull-cup serves as a libation vessel for many wrathful and protective Buddhist deities and is often depicted in tantric iconography as being filled with warm blood or the heart of an enemy (Beer 1999). Many levels of complex symbolic meaning are associated with the iconographic depiction and use of the human skull-cup in Tibetan Buddhism. When used by an ascetic or hermit as a begging bowl or food vessel, the skull serves as a "constant reminder of death and impermanence, the ephemeral transitoriness of life that engenders renunciation" (Beer 1999:264). One explanation given by lamas for the use of a skull in making sacred offerings is that it is a "natural vessel" not made by human hands that provides an image of the "natural, unelaborated state of pure aware-ness" (Kohn 2001:136). Instructions for selecting the proper skulls for making offerings to deities such as Amitabha, the Buddha of Endless Light, are outlined in a Tibetan text that transmits teachings from medieval India (Laufer 1923). The text specifies that a skull used for making an offering to the gods should be that of a person "known to have been profoundly religious, or to have possessed other high qualifications, such as rank, nobility, wisdom, or learning. . . . Skulls of women and children born out of wedlock are unsuitable for sacred purposes" (Laufer 1923:15).

Different criteria are used in selecting skulls for other types of ritual. Because of the occult power that certain skulls are believed to possess, the skull of a murder or execution victim is thought to have the greatest tantric power, the skull of someone who has died from a violent or accidental death has medium power, whereas the skull of a person who died peacefully in old age has virtually no power. "The skull of a child who died during the onset of puberty also has great potency, as do the skulls of a miscegenated or misbegotten child of unknown paternity, born from the forbidden union of castes, out of wedlock, from sexual misdemeanor, or particularly from incest" (Beer 1999:263).

Hand Drum

The double-sided hand drum (Skt. *damaru*; Tib. *da ma ru, rnga chung*) is a ritual implement associated with Shiva that has roots extending back to the ancient Harappan civilization of the Indus Valley (Beer 1999). The damaru of Shiva, which symbolizes Shiva and his consort Shakti joined in conjugal union, is de-picted iconographically as the joined skull-caps of two human crania, preferably those of an adolescent boy and girl. Although some damaru used today in Ti-betan Buddhist ritual are made from human skulls obtained from charnel grounds or sky burial sites, the drums are more commonly made from wood or fashioned from skulls salvaged from sources such as "unclaimed Indian accident

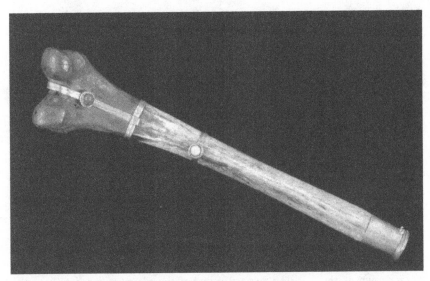

Figure 14.3. A Tibetan shaman's trumpet (*kang-ling*) made from a human femur studded with coral and turquoise stones and fitted with a mouthpiece at the proximal end. The sound of the kang-ling, said to resemble the neighing of a horse, is believed to call in ghosts and to assist in communication with souls of the dead. Photograph by John Mckim Malville.

victims, cremation ground debris, or 'water-burials' washed ashore on the mouth of the River Ganges" (Beer 1999:258). Damaru from unknown sources such as these would possess little occult power for tantric ritual but would still be of symbolic value.

Thighbone Trumpet

The thighbone trumpet (Tib. *rkang gling, rkang dung*; figure 14.3) is used by Tibetan shamans of both the Bon and the Buddhist tradition in many rituals of exorcism and weather control (Beer 1999). The sound of the *kang-ling* is believed to call in ghosts and to assist in communication with souls of the dead (Jangbu Sherpa, personal communication) and is said to be "pleasing to the wrathful deities, but terrifying to evil spirits" (Beer 1999:259). According to the tantric tradition, "the left femur of a sixteen-year-old brahmin girl" is most effective against evil spirits, followed by "the femur of a 'twice-born' brahmin . . . followed by the thighbone of a murder victim, then a person who died from a sudden accidental death, then one who died from a virulent or contagious disease" (Beer 1999:259).[4] Other sources state that femurs from criminals or those who have died a violent death are the preferred sources (Laufer 1923; Waddell 1972 [1895]). It is said that during the elaborate ceremony consecrating the trumpets, the officiating lama "bites off a portion of the bone-skin; otherwise the blast of the trumpet would not be sufficiently powerful to summon, or to terrify the demons" (Laufer 1923:10).

Bone Ornaments

Intricately carved bone ornaments are worn as part of the elaborate costumes used in Tibetan sacred dances (Beer 1999), particularly in certain ritual shamanistic dances intended to propitiate evil spirits and exorcise demons (Laufer 1923). Although bone ornaments and rosary beads are usually carved from yak bone in Tibet (Tamdin Wangdu, personal communication), several sources specify that human bone is sometimes used in ornaments intended for ceremonial purposes. Laufer (1923:10) describes a bone apron collected in Tibet for the Blackstone Expedition of 1908–1910 as being composed of "forty-one large plaques exquisitely carved from supposedly human femora and connected by double chains of round or square bone beads." Waddell, writing in 1895 about the Tibetan sorcerer known as the *nag-pa* ("expert in incantations") provided details of the sorcerer's costume such as his tall conical hat and his "sash of human bones (*rus-rgyan*) carved with fiends and mystic symbols" (Waddell 1972:483 [1895]). Migot (1955:198) observed dancers at Tangu gompa in Jyekundo, northeastern Tibet, who wore over their whirling skirts "a sort of apron of human bones hung in long loops like necklaces" and carried in their right hands "a little drum, made of the cranial cavities of two children with a covering of human skin." In recalling her childhood in Lhasa, a younger sister of the Dalai Lama tells of the Tibetan New Year ceremonies known as Torgya in which the masked skeleton dancers wore over their black costumes "chains made of human bones . . . [which] made sinister, almost supernatural noises at the slightest movement" (Jetsun Pema 1997:27 [1996]).

Ritual Use of Human Bone in Public Ceremony

The 3 public days of the 18-day Buddhist festival of Mani Rimdu in northeastern Nepal demonstrate the ritual use of human bone in ancient ceremonies and dances dating back to the ninth century in Tibet (Kite et al. 1988; Kohn 2001). The Mani Rimdu festival, which celebrates the triumph of the Buddhist tantric master Padmasambhava over the Bon shamans, originated in Tibet at Mindroling and Rombuk monasteries and was transmitted to Nepal by the Zatrul Rinpoche. Although these Tibetan monasteries have been essentially destroyed by the Chinese, Mani Rimdu is now celebrated annually at the Sherpa monasteries of Tengboche, Thami, and Chiwong and, in a somewhat different form, at the Tibetan refugee monastery of Tubten Choling (Kohn 2001). The most important public event of the Mani Rimdu festival is the public empowerment ceremony in which the Rinpoche distributes small blood-red *mani* ("long-life") pills to all

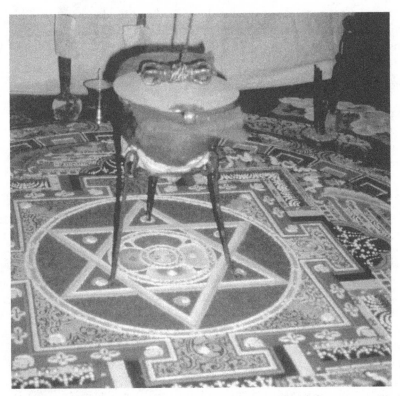

Figure 14.4. Empowerment of the *mani* ("long-life") pills distributed to all participants at the Mani Rimdu festival at Chiwong monastery, Solukhumbu, Nepal. The blood-red pills are empowered by being placed for 10 days in a human skull set on a tripod over an elaborate sand painting, during which time the monks chant prayers over the pills. Photograph by John Mckim Malville.

participants to confer spiritual blessings on them. Prior to the public ceremony, the pills have been empowered through being placed for 10 days in a human skull covered with a magic bronze mirror and other ritual objects and set on a tripod over an elaborate sand painting, or *mandala* (figure 14.4). During this time the monks have chanted prayers of empowerment over the pills (Kite et al. 1988; Kohn 2001). The particular skull currently used at Chiwong is said to have belonged to a soldier who died in battle (Kohn 2001).

The second public day of Mani Rimdu is the day of masked dances. A pair of thighbone trumpets announces the entrance of each dance group. In the seventh dance, the dance of the Four Great Protectors, the dancer representing Mahakala carries a skull-cup in one hand and a curved chopper in another (Kite et al. 1988; Kohn 2001). Damaru drums are carried in the ninth dance by the Sky Walker dancers, and in the tenth dance, the Buddhist yogi known as the Seer carries a thighbone trumpet and a damaru as he clowns and amuses the crowd with his own comic version of the tantric gcod rite of offering his body to all flesh-eating demons (Kohn 2001).

Charnel Ground at Sermathang, Nepal

A Sherpa charnel ground at Sermathang in Helambu, the region of Nepal just north of the Kathmandu Valley, provides examples of some of the mortuary practices discussed here (Jangbu Sherpa, personal communication). Sometime prior to 1960 the victims of a smallpox epidemic were hastily buried in the ground at this site without the benefit of religious ceremonies or prayers. The main concern at the time was to prevent the further spread of disease by disposing of the corpses as quickly as possible. About 20 years ago, Kancha Lama exhumed and cremated the remains, conducting the rituals and prayers necessary for proper guidance of the souls of the deceased. Before cremating the bones, the lama selected and saved several femurs and skulls for ritual use. Because there were no relatives to object, it was considered acceptable for him to take these bones (Jangbu Sherpa, personal communication). Kancha Lama then built at the site a small monastery, which is now supervised by Chantal Rinpoche, a lama from Kathmandu. In both the Hindu and Buddhist tantric traditions, charnel grounds were believed to be places of great and dangerous power where "tantrics and yogins gathered . . . [and] highly esoteric initiations and rituals were performed" (Beer 1999:251). In the mid 1990s, Nawang Sherap Lama, a tantric lama from Boudhanath, Nepal, built a small house at the charnel ground in which he lived for three years, three months, and three days. During this time he received nightly visits from the spirits of departed Tibetan teachers such as Padmasambhava and Milarepa, who communicated their teachings to him in dreams. The lama, who is recognized by some as a tantric *geshe* (one who has acquired his knowledge through communication with spirits and ghosts rather than through texts), says that he was able to protect himself from dangerous spirits because he was prepared with strong *mantras* (incantations) to repeat, whereas some monks who had not been sufficiently prepared had gone mad or died in the charnel grounds (Nawang Sherap Lama, personal communication).[5]

Summary

In accordance with the Tibetan Buddhist doctrines of rebirth and impermanence, the most important considerations at the time of death are to say prayers for guiding the soul toward a new rebirth and to dispose of the corpse as quickly and completely as possible.

Tibetan Buddhists have five ways of dealing with the dead: cremation, sky burial or exposure, water burial, earth burial, and preservation with salt. The choice of method depends on (1) the advice of the lama-astrologer consulted for the death horoscope; (2) the age and social status of the deceased; (3) the conditions of death; and (4) practical considerations such as availability of firewood or vultures.

Cremation is the preferred disposal form, but where firewood is scarce, the common method is sky burial or exposure. Water burial and earth burial are regarded as dishonorable and are reserved mainly for young children, the very poor, victims of contagious disease, murderers, and criminals.

Complete disposal of the body in a sky burial is considered important for several reasons. It is said to be a good sign if the vultures take everything because this frees the soul to leave the old body and proceed toward a new rebirth. It also ensures that the deceased leaves behind no skeletal elements that could be used by tantric practitioners. Ash and bone fragments remaining after cremation or exposure to animals may be disposed of by building small cairns over the remains or by incorporating them into small clay tablets.

Skulls and femurs are the skeletal elements most commonly retained for use in occult ritual. According to the mystical tantric beliefs of ancient India and Tibet, human bone has power in ritual because the bone retains the vital force of the person from whom the bone is taken. Skulls are made into cups and drums; femurs, into thighbone trumpets and bone ornaments. The most powerful sources of bone for tantric ritual are held to be "twice-born" Brahmins (because of their high caste and purity), adolescents (because of their awakening sexual powers), victims of violent death or contagious disease, and criminals. Because bones from these sources are difficult to obtain, tantric practitioners often must make do with bones of unknown persons salvaged from any available source (Beer 1999).

Acknowledgments

I am most grateful for the assistance of Jangbu Sherpa, Nawang Sherap Lama, Loyang Choedon, and Adam Kay in providing information for this study and to Tamdin Wangdu, J. McKim Malville, and Sallie Greenwood for their helpful comments on early drafts of the manuscript.

Notes

1. Chogyam Trungpa writes in his commentary to the *Tibetan Book of the Dead*, "Physically you feel heavy when the earth element dissolves into water; and when water dissolves into fire you find that the circulation begins to cease functioning. When fire dissolves into air, any feeling of warmth or growth begins to dissolve; and when air dissolves into space you lose the last feeling of contact with the physical world" (Freemantle and Trungpa 1975:4).

2. Saka Dawa, the most important festival of Mt. Kailash, is held annually at the great flagpole of Tarboche on the full moon of May–June. The celebration commemorates the birth, enlightenment, and death of Buddha.

3. Included among the Tibetan pantheon of demons are *"gShin-'dre,* wandering evil spirits of the dead (Skt. *pretas*) who have failed to find rebirth" (Mumford 1989:142). Chan (1994:279) notes that at the charnel ground of the 84 Mahasiddhas near Mt. Kailash, the epithet *shendri* is used in reference to the "horrendous" stench due to "countless 'sky-burials' over the centuries."

4. In an interview with Nawang Sherap Lama conducted in June 2001 by Adam Kay (Jangbu Sherpa, translator), Nawang Sherap indicated that the bones themselves have no special power but are ritual symbols. It is the mantras chanted over the bones that put power into them. He explained that monks who have studied bones examine details such as skull sutures and lines in femurs to determine which bones are best to collect for ritual purposes. It is unclear whether in speaking of "lines" Nawang Sherap was referring to the epiphyseal disks or to muscle attachment lines such as the linea aspera. The epiphyses (growth plates) of the femur provide good indicators of age at death because they unite during puberty, at which time growth stops. Union of the epiphyses occurs two to three years earlier in females than in males (Bass 1971).

5. "And as the world is apt to trouble one's mind with its sensuous appeals and the renunciations one has to force on oneself, those lamas have recourse to a practice meant to give them a direct, concrete experience of the vanity of whatever belongs to the world of change and appearance. In the dark fortnight, when night's mystery and terrors are deeper, they retire to the fields where human corpses are exposed, beat a drum made of a human skull, play a flute made of the shin bone of a sixteen-year-old girl, put on a robe plaited with human bones . . . and shout at the top of their voice evoking those monstrous deities and rousing deep, long echoes in the lonely darkness. . . . No wonder if the power of suggestion in that dark, silent desert is such that the images of the gods actually appear before the hallucinated eyes of the lamas made of less stern stuff, and if quite a few cannot bear the sight of those ghosts and are driven mad with fright or die in a fit of terror" (Tucci 1973:80).

III

Sacrifice, Violence, and Veneration

Gordon F. M. Rakita and Jane E. Buikstra

The final section, much like the preceding one, deals with how corpses are treated. However, of special interest are contexts in which the living and the dead are objects to be sacrificed, venerated, consumed, or even subject to unusual acts of violence. In the first chapter in this section, the ancient Maya are the setting for Duncan's study of the possible violation of the human body as part of a complex ritual sequence. Duncan utilizes a model of ritual violence to examine and interpret a collection of interments from the Petén region of the Postclassic Maya. Expanding upon Bloch's (1992) model that links violence and veneration within the same ritual structure, Duncan explains the patterns he observes in terms of an indigenous population being subordinated by foreign invaders. Grave location, body treatment, and grave goods are key variables in interpreting this record. Duncan concludes that violence expressed in mortuary rituals may be related to ethnic groups' striving to reproduce their social identity vis-à-vis other groups.

Further emphasizing the need for carefully collected and analyzed data, and contrasting with the examples of rapid change in mortuary behavior noted in the chapters in Section 1 by Charles, Chapman, and Cannon, Stodder provides a case study of possible cannibalism among the New Guinea Aitape. Using treatment and taphonomic condition of animal bone to broaden contextual perspective, she examines several alternative ritual and nonceremonial scenarios to define depositional processes. In doing so, she emphasizes the value of integrating osteological, archaeological, and ethnographic data. Stodder concludes that there are several viable alternatives to cannibalism in the case, particularly when the possibility of secondary mortuary treatments is considered.

Examining ancient Andean ritual practices, Verano details the excavation of the remains of over 90 sacrificial victims from the Pyramid of the Moon of the prehistoric Moche region of Peru. Osteological examination of the skeletal remains suggests that symbolic preparation and displays of defleshed individuals rather than cannibalism provides a more parsimonious explanation of the unusual treatments accorded these individuals. Verano cogently discusses the role such displays may have played within Moche society.

The chapter by Forgey and Williams continues the focus on ancient Andean contexts with an examination of the Nazca trophy heads. The authors explore the question of whether the heads represent actual trophies taken from vanquished enemies or are relics of revered ancestors. Detailed examinations of archaeological contexts and formal variability in these curated human remains are used to assess both current and historical theories. Forgey and Williams' analysis of variation in imagery, disposal method, preparation, and demography of trophy heads suggests that that variation may be caused by temporal differences in ritual use of the trophies. This study is a further example of how skeletal biological data can enhance interpretations of mortuary practices.

Returning to Mayan society, Beck and Sievert's chapter explores bones recovered from the "Sacred Cenote" at Chichén Itzá. The Cenote has been described as a location where rituals of human sacrifice took place. Beck and Sievert use remains from collections at Harvard's Peabody Museum to explore alternative routes by which male and female adults and children entered the Cenote. Their careful concern for perimortem and postmortem alteration, coupled with ethnohistoric information, leads to a rich interpretation of Maya social and cosmological attitudes about death and rebirth.

Finally, McNeill's contribution concentrates on the Chamorro people of Micronesia, whose reverence for the ancestors was documented by early Spanish accounts of continued contact with ancestors' remains. McNeill presents an example of postmortem procurement and use of human skeletal material. The Chamorro practiced a variety of mortuary treatments, including curating skulls of two generations of individuals in houses and interments within house compounds. A third form of postmortem treatment, the manufacture of ancestors' remains into projectile points, is the subject of this study. McNeill looks at bones removed from interments, their age and sex profiles, and evidence for manufacture and use of spear points manufactured from human bone. Depositional contexts for bone points is also considered. This study presents an excellent example of the use of osteological data in the interpretation of unusual mortuary practices. It also presents a valuable cautionary tale, illustrating how some secondary processing of human remains may be unrelated to ancestor veneration.

15

Understanding Veneration and Violation in the Archaeological Record

William N. Duncan

"Upon the death of nobles and high-ranking dignitaries . . . their bodies were cruelly disemboweled and monstrously severed into pieces, which were cast into boiling water. Then, when the bones were loosened from the flesh, they were sent or carried to the place reserved for interment."

E. Brown 1981:221

"Traitors were also subjected to evisceration. The rebel William Wallace got the full treatment in 1305. He was drawn through London's streets at the tail of a horse to the place of his execution where he was hanged, but taken down still living. His innards were cut out and burned. The body was then quartered and decapitated, the limbs sent into Scotland, the head mounted at London Bridge. As he had committed many crimes, so he suffered in many ways."

Finucane 1981:50–51

Whether the surviving members of society wish to venerate or violate the deceased is one concern that impacts postmortem treatment of the body (Shay 1985). Veneration includes aiding the soul to a final resting place and/or honoring the memory of the deceased. Kings, saints, and individuals who are joining the ancestors are among those who receive such honors. Violation includes denying the deceased a resting place or destroying the soul of the deceased. Such treatment is generally reserved for individuals who behaved in culturally inappropriate ways (for example, violated taboos, were witches, committed crimes, or were aliens) or died under culturally undesirable circumstances (such as violence, diseases, suicide, and death in battle; what Bloch and Parry [1982:15] call "bad death"). Violation has been shown historically and ethnographically to result in idiosyncratic mortuary practices in Europe (Finucane 1981:41; Foucault 1995 [1977]), Africa (Goody 1962:142), the Southwest United States (Darling 1998; Walker 1998), the Northwest Coast of North America (Kan 1989:132), Mesoamerica (López Austin 1988:231–236), and worldwide surveys (Shay 1985). As the above quotes from Brown and Finucane suggest, though, processes of violation and veneration may involve similar acts, producing deposits in the material record that are, for the archaeologist, dishearteningly similar. Consequently it is frequently difficult to discern processes of violation and veneration among mortuary deposits in the archaeological record.

Past attempts to investigate such deposits have often avoided differentiating veneration from violation. Examples include research addressing the presence of cannibalism in the Southwest United States (for example, Turner and Turner 1999; White 1992) and in Europe (for example, Russell 1987; Villa 1992). These authors analyzed the deposits using formal criteria, comparing the treatment and context of human remains in question with animal remains that were butchered and with local human deposits clearly not attributable to cannibalism. However, as Parker Pearson (1999) and Conklin (1995) have acknowledged, this formal approach fails to discern whether the deposits reflect attempts to venerate or violate because cannibalism is used for either purpose.

Responding to these formal analyses, researchers have emphasized a contextual approach for understanding violence in the material record. Parker Pearson (1999), Walker (1998), and others (for example, Darling 1998; Ogilvie and Hilton 2000) note that what constitutes violation differs within and between cultures. Thus, we need to understand violence within the context of the culture under consideration. One notable attempt to operationalize this was made by Walker (1998). Walker suggested that we consider the life history of artifacts and features in the archaeological record to identify patterns reflecting ritual violence. Using this approach, he suggested that some of the deposits originally thought to reflect cannibalism in the Southwest United States were actually the product of witch executions (Walker 1998). Whether or not the deposits in question in the American Southwest are the products of cannibalism or witch executions, Walker's approach improves on formal attempts (for example, Turner and Turner 1999; White 1992) by utilizing the historical record to understand processes of violation specific to Pueblo society. The question remains, though: how might we understand violation and veneration in cultures further removed from direct historical records?

One option for exploring processes of violence and veneration in the past is to consider mortuary practices in light of ethnographic models of ritual. Maurice Bloch (1992) proposes one such model, suggesting that veneration and violation are variants on the same ritual structure. Bloch's model is useful on two levels: it can help us understand why veneration and violation produce deposits that look alike; and it may serve as a guide for constructing scenarios about veneration and violation in the past that may be evaluated in light of other data. This chapter, then, has three goals: (1) to outline Bloch's model (1992) and consider ethnographic and historic examples of mortuary practices in light of it; (2) to consider the scope of applicability of Bloch's model; and (3) to interpret a series of interments from the Maya Postclassic (A.D. 950–1524) (Duncan 1999) in terms of Bloch's model. The Maya example suggests that Bloch's ritual model provides

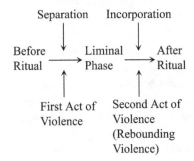

Figure 15.1. Bloch's model (1992) of ritual violence.

fruitful avenues for teasing apart some, if not all, processes of veneration and violation in the material record.

Bloch's Model

Bloch (1992) argues that cross-cultural similarities between ritual structures stem from the fact that most cultures view human life as occurring within a transcendental framework. For Bloch, ritual is what connects everyday life to that which is transcendental, and ritual involves two things: a three-stage process and violence as a mechanism to move the ritual process between stages (Bloch 1992). As a concept, ritual violence still remains somewhat ill defined in the literature. However, researchers such as Hubert and Mauss (1964 [1899]), Eliade (1959), in particular Bloch (1992) in cultural anthropology, and Walker (1998) in archaeology have noted that ritual often involves some darker, or "kratophanous," aspects (Eliade 1959). As shown in figure 15.1, the three-stage process that Bloch uses is similar to that of van Gennep (1960 [1908]), comprising separation, liminality, and incorporation. The first act of violence moves the ritual participants into a liminal phase by destroying that which is antithetical to the transcendental aspects of society (Bloch 1992). Bloch (1992) argues that this act detaches the participants from the everyday and affirms the place of the sacred/transcendental aspects in the worldview. However, most people cannot remain detached from the everyday forever; they have to reenter everyday life. The second act of violence is what is novel about Bloch's model (1992). He argues that the second act of violence is a rebounding event, in which the individual exits the liminal phase in a fashion that subordinates the everyday to the transcendental (Bloch 1992). The point is that participants do not want to exit the ritual process in the same condition they entered. By subordinating the everyday to the transcendental aspects of the worldview, the participants reproduce the worldview of society and simultaneously undergo a fundamental change themselves.

Bloch's model is relevant for the current discussion because it considers veneration and violation in mortuary practices to be forms of this same ritual structure. For Bloch, biological birth and death imply change, which are threatening to societies that have worldviews incorporating transcendental ideals that go beyond the historical present. Thus funerals are an attempt "to negate the individual life and death, and replace it by a notion of continual life," thereby affirming a victory over biological birth and death (Bloch 1982:228). In Bloch's model, helping the deceased achieve such victory over death and commemorating it constitutes veneration. Violation denies such victory. Ethnographic and historic examples of mortuary practices suggest that veneration and violation may produce similar deposits because (1) they both utilize violence as a mechanism; (2) what constitutes violation and veneration may be contested and negotiated within a given society and thus may change over time; and (3) some acts of violation may create symbols from the deceased's body parts that are treated reverentially in later rituals.

Veneration

Bloch derived his model from work among the Merina of Madagascar (Bloch 1971, 1982). The Merina are divided into what Bloch calls demes—local kin groups that have clearly defined, discrete territories. Demes are ideally endogamous, and the relationship between the people of the deme (both living people and ancestors) and the land is thought to be unchanging and permanent. Each deme has a number of tombs that collectively house the ancestors, and these tombs are seen as "the medium of the merging of the ancestors, deme, and land" (Bloch 1982:213). The importance of the deme in Merina society cannot be overstated. Reaffirming the unity and permanence of the deme is "the most sacred, most imperative duty of the living and it alone ensures the continuing strength of the blessing passed on within the deme, because the power of life in blessing depends on the non-dispersal of the land/ancestor substance of the deme" (Bloch 1982:213). Reaffirming the unity of the deme, though, consists of the destruction of images of change and division, which are antithetical to the continued existence of the deme. Several symbols of change and division exist in Merina society, but the individual lineages that exist within the demes (with which women are associated) and biological birth and death are particularly relevant to funerals (Bloch 1982).

The first part of the funeral consists of burying the deceased in a single grave outside the collective tomb (Bloch 1982); in this event, pollution and mourning are emphasized. Women relatives mourn (sit on piles of trash while mourning and weep) and are polluted, while others isolate themselves from the corpse and grave. The secondary funeral ritual, called the *famadihana*, involves placing the bones of the individuals in the collective tomb. The famadihana emphasizes blessing, fertility, and unity in a joyous return of the bones to the ancestral tomb. The women exhume the bones and carry them from the grave to the tomb. However, rather than simply taking the corpses to the famadihana, the women are actively harassed by the men en route to the tomb (Bloch 1982). Upon arriving at the tomb, the men enter and take out the ancestors' remains, placing them with the newly deceased on the women's shoulders. After the men request blessings, the corpses are rewrapped in shrouds and the women throw the bones in the air (which over time contributes to the destruction of the individuals' remains). The ceremony ends with the men replacing the collective remains in the tomb.

The first portion of the funeral sees the creation of the association between women and putrefaction and sorrow (Bloch 1982:217). This is an "ideal image of . . . the world of women, pollution, sorrow, and individuality," all of which are antithetical to the unity of the deme (Bloch 1982:218). The first act of violence is the destruction of this ideal, manifest in the harassment of the women and the throwing of the bones. This represents an assault on individuality and biological birth and death. The rebounding violence occurs when the men place the collective group of remains in the tomb, symbolizing the incorporation of the individuals by the collective. To Bloch, this is a violent act because the entry into the tomb subordinates the violated image (the individual) to the transcendent symbol of Merina life—the collective tomb of the deme (Bloch 1992:48). The famadihana symbolizes the victory of the permanence of the tomb and deme over biological birth, death, and individuality. In this case, the violence is directed toward that which is threatening to society: the concept of individuality and the death of the individual. The recently deceased are honored by becoming part of the collective group of ancestors and being incorporated into the ideal symbol of the Merina deme.

Violation

Preventing enemies from having the appropriate funerary rituals denies the potential for their victory over death (Bloch 1982:228–229). Bloch (1982) calls this kind of violence "predation," and it may be negative or positive. Negative predation occurs when individuals simply prohibit enemies or criminals from receiving the appropriate rituals, and this is often accompanied by defacement of the individual. As an example Bloch (1982:228–229) considers the fighting over the corpse of Hector in the *Iliad*. The ideal that is affirmed in Greek life is "the perfect youthful body" (Bloch 1982:228), and the perfect death is "to die young, in the prime of life, and then . . . be cremated so that disfiguration and decay do not occur" (Bloch 1982:228). The Trojans wanted to ensure that the ideal would not be corrupted. The Greeks, though, wanted the body for the opposite reason. By disfiguring Hector's corpse, the Greeks denied the Trojans an important symbol.

Similarly, the statement by Finucane (1981:50–51) quoted at the beginning of the chapter demonstrates that in the later Middle Ages in Europe, traitors and murderers were often hanged, drawn, quartered, or otherwise, and they could be denied burial in a Christian graveyard if they refused to admit their crime and ask for forgiveness. This denial of burial in sacred ground was a punishment in addition to the physical suffering they would endure while dying, because they would be denied passage into heaven and were either destined for hell or "refused any kind of posthumous existence whatsoever" (Finucane 1981:58). In the European case, the heretic or criminal refusing to admit his or her crimes was more threatening to society than the common criminal (Finucane 1981:57). Since authority was derived from God, failure to repent and show fear of damnation struck at the heart of social authority. Both veneration and negative predation utilize violence, but they differ with respect to their object. The object of violence in veneration is the symbol of biological birth and death (for example, the complex of symbols representing individualism among the Merina) that needs to be subordinated to the transcendental ideal. However, the object of violence in negative predation is the deviant or outsider who threatens society (Finucane 1981:56–58).

Juxtaposed with the treatment of heretics in Late Medieval Europe is the practice of dismembering and boiling the bones of some nobles and high-ranking dignitaries. Dignitaries who died far away from home were dismembered and boiled to prepare the remains for transport to their chosen burial place (E. Brown 1981; see also Weiss-Krejci this volume). In 1299 Boniface VIII challenged this practice by papal bull, claiming that the dismemberment and boiling of the deceased was "not only abominable in the sight of God but also abhorrent to the human mind" (E. Brown 1981:221). Anyone found continuing the practice after the bull in 1299 was excommunicated and the body in question was to be denied Christian burial (E. Brown 1981:222). Thus Boniface attempted to turn the treatment previously symbolizing veneration into an act of violation! The effect of the bull, though, was to make such dismemberment and boiling more desirable than ever. As E. Brown (1981:264) notes, "After 1300 separate burial of the body's parts was a privilege which only the most favored could obtain and it thus became a sure sign of status and distinction." Within the same society we see that what constitutes veneration and violation may change over time (and indeed may be interchangeable over a very short period of time), and the ability to practice acts of veneration and violation may reflect social status.

Unfortunately for archaeologists, the situation gets worse. As Bloch points out, there are multiple kinds of violation. Positive predation is "not a matter of depriving your enemies of their substance by denying them . . . a funeral. It is rather a matter of taking over their corpses and allocating to yourself the vitality which they hold" (Bloch 1982:229). Scalping among North American Plains cultures is one such example (Owsley 1994:337). Owsley (1994:337) notes that taking scalps was a symbol of bravery and prowess in battle. However, the scalps had religious significance as well. Among Puebloans, scalps were used in ceremonies to bring rain and were often referred to as seeds (Owsley 1994:337). Among the Hopi, scalps were sometimes used as a kind of sympathetic magic, seen in cases where young boys were fed scalps to increase bravery. Bloch (1982:229) also suggests that headhunting among the Jivaro and Iban had similar motivations. Positive predation involves "establishing apparently immortal human structures . . . by creating an image of an inverted reproduction which ultimately requires the symbolic or actual presence of outsiders, who are there to have their vitality conquered, but who, unlike the main participants, do not then go on to conquer" (Bloch 1992:44).

Unlike negative predation, the vitality of the victims is incorporated into or utilized by the main participants as a way of reproducing society (Bloch 1982). This fits into Bloch's model because violence is directed at outsiders, who are seen as antithetical to society. The rebounding action is the incorporation of the symbol of the destruction of the outsider into various purposes associated with affirming the transcendence of society. The problem for archaeologists is that these symbols of the violated enemy (often a body part of the enemy) may be treated with reverence. For example, in East Sumba, Indonesia, upon warriors' return from a successful headhunting raid, "the head was cleaned of its flesh and 'beautified' before being brought to the village, so that it appeared 'pure' and 'noble'" (Hoskins 1996a:228). Thus we understand at least three reasons why violation and veneration appear similar in the archaeological record: (1) they operate using the same ritual structure and employ violence as a mechanism; (2) what constitutes and who deserves veneration and violation may change over time within the same society; and (3) violation may produce material symbols that are treated reverentially in later rituals.

The Model's Applicability

Bloch (1992:1) advertises his model as identifying the "irreducible core of the ritual process." Before turning to an archaeological example, it is worth identifying the scope of applicability of Bloch's model; by that I mean where it is appropriate to apply Bloch's model and what aspects of mortuary practices his model might ignore. Bloch acknowledges that the model describes ritual in cultures that recognize a distinction between everyday life and some other time/space that is divorced from historical context. Clearly not all cultures recognize such a clear distinction in their worldview (Read 1998). That said, even where such divisions exist, as Parker Pearson notes, rarely in any culture is human experience so easily "compartmentalized between the ritualized and the everyday" (Parker Pearson 1999:33). Thus it is worth considering how the sacred and the profane fit into a given culture's worldview when applying Bloch's model. Focusing on ideal relationships ignores more subtle aspects of negotiation that are important parts of mortuary practices (Parker Pearson 1999). For example, David Graeber (1995) has demonstrated among the Merina of Madagascar that Bloch's model does not account for different attitudes toward the ancestors. Men generally will not talk about the ancestors as hostile, while women do. This likely stems from the fact that men want to be remembered when they are ancestors. The men want to overshadow earlier ancestors and their children. Thus, they must make people respect the ancestors but not respect the ancestors too much. Women, though, are not likely to become revered ancestors, and they focus more on the cruelty of angry ancestors. Therefore, there is a more complex relationship between ambition and remembering and forgetting than Bloch's model suggests.

Bloch's model also ignores a considerable amount of historical variability with respect to specific practices (Hoskins 1996b). For example, Bloch's concept of positive predation essentializes the role violence plays in societies that practice headhunting (Hoskins 1996b). Needham (1976) notes that while it is a common theme, there is no a priori connection between head taking and procuring the vitality of enemies. Hoskins (1996b) echoes this sentiment, noting that while certain themes run through headhunting rituals in southeastern Asia, it is an inappropriate oversimplification (and perhaps an inappropriate projection) to boil down the variation of headhunting practices to Bloch's "irreducible core." Finally, as Hoskins (1996b) points out, Bloch's model fails to capture and explore important distinctions between real and imagined violence.

The Postclassic Maya Case

There are several reasons to think Bloch's model is applicable to the Postclassic Maya. First, the sacred in Mesoamerican worldview is not manifest exactly like the unchanging ahistorical time and space that Bloch suggests exists for the Merina. However, change and particular processes of termination and regeneration permeate the Mesoamerican landscape. Second, violence, particularly in the Postclassic (Soustelle 1984), appears to have been systemic in Maya culture. Evidence for this is seen in iconography (Demarest 1984), in the use of defensive walls and moats (Rice et al. 1997), and in ethnohistoric documents (Jones 1998). Ethnographic and ethnohistoric lines of evidence (Gossen 1986) indicate that for the Maya, like most Mesoamerican cultures, violence was a generative concept used for social reproduction.

Third, numerous ethnographic (for example, Boremanse 1998) and ethnohistoric (Tozzer 1941) accounts indicate that the Maya had a concept of a soul that transcended the biological body or was reborn after biological death. For example, among the highland Tzotzil (Freidel et al. 1993:245) and Zinacanteco Maya (Vogt 1976:18), a vital force (ch'ulel) was considered to be present in humans as well as in inanimate objects. Like many Mesoamerican cultures (Furst 1995), Maya groups have multiple concepts that fall under the category of soul. Similarly, the northern Lacandon Maya in Chiapas, Mexico, distinguish between the pixan (the soul), the kisnin (a ghost), and the sol (the corporeal aspect of the individual) (Boremanse 1998:96–98). After death the pixan continues to an afterlife, the kisnin remains in a solitary existence on the earth, and the sol resides in the remains of the individual. Under some circumstances the portion of the soul that continues cannot be destroyed and reborn in a weaker state or suspended in its journey. Among the Lacandon, people who violate supernatural sanctions (such as those who commit incest or murder) have their souls tormented in an

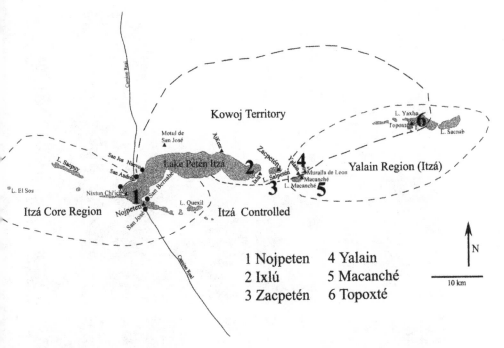

Figure 15.2. Seventeeth-century political geography around the Petén lakes, Guatemala (adapted from Jones 1998:6, Map 3).

underworld. In the case of murderers, the soul is burned and "becomes smaller and smaller until it is ultimately annihilated" (Boremanse 1998:71).

There also appears to be the potential for positive predation among the Maya. For example, Tzotzil Maya speakers of Chiapas report that when a pole symbolizing the World Tree is ceremonially raised in village plazas, a living chicken is crushed under it, thereby transferring a life force to the World Tree (Stross 1998:32). Stross (1998:32) also notes "that similar sacrifices with human victims have taken place in historical times as a final phase of bridge construction in Chiapas, in order to provide the bridge with a soul, giving it the strength to withstand the forces of nature."

During the Postclassic (A.D. 950–1524), three ethnic groups lived around the Petén lakes in northern Guatemala (figure 15.2). The Itzá and the Kowoj dominated the political landscape around the lakes to the south and north, respectively. A third ethnic group, the Yalain, appear to have lived on the southeastern portion of the lakes region (Jones 1998). Excavations under Proyecto Maya Colonial have identified three recurrent types of interments around the lakes during the Postclassic: skull pairs; skull rows resembling Mexica *tzompantli* (figure 15.3); and mass graves (Duncan 1999).

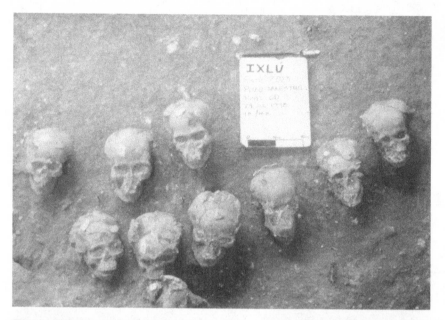

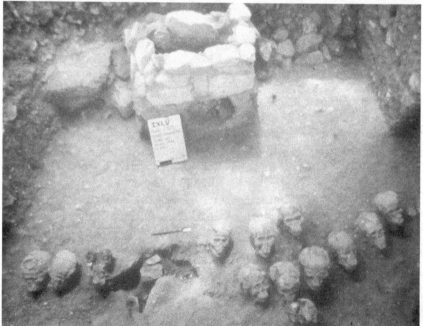

Figure 15.3. Close-up (above) of skull rows (below) from Ixlú, Structure 2023. Photographs by Don Rice.

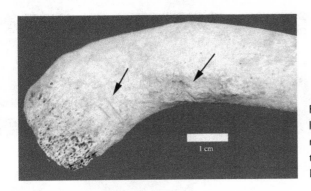

Figure 15.4. Cut marks on lateral anterior aspect of right clavicle, Ixlú, Structure 2023. Photograph by Don Rice.

1 cm

Skull pairs have been reported at Ixlú (Duncan 1999) and on Nojpeten (Cowgill 1963). At Ixlú, excavations by Proyecto Maya Colonial produced three pairs of skulls on an east–west line (Duncan 1999), on opposite sides of a small shrine (as defined by Proskouriakoff [1962]). Two of the skulls in pairs were interred in the same construction episode as the skull rows (see discussion below). All six skulls faced east, with five having articulated cervical vertebrae (Duncan 1999). All are young adults, and those for which sex could be determined are male (three of six). On the west side of the building, perpendicular to the crania were four postcrania in a north–south line (Duncan 1999). All four are young adult males (Duncan 1999). These individuals lacked crania, hands, and feet (Duncan 1999). While the axial skeletons (minus the skulls) were articulated, the limb bones and scapulae were placed in bundles on top (Duncan 1999). Cut marks were found on the clavicles (as shown in figure 15.4), on the distal humeri, on the lateral border of the scapulae, and on a femoral neck. The color of the cut marks was similar to that of the surrounding bone, indicating perimortem dismemberment (Duncan 1999). The only associated grave goods were isolated sherds and some animal bone fragments (Duncan 1999). The skulls and postcrania were placed on top of a plaster floor at the base of the shrine, suggesting that their placement was relevant to the construction of the structure. Cowgill (1963) reports finding a single skull pair from Nojpeten. These faced one another; however, since they were found in a test pit, no other information (such as architectural context) was available.

Skull rows, resembling Mexica tzompantli, have been recovered from Ixlú (Duncan 1999) and Macanché (Mark Aldenderfer, field notes). The skulls at Ixlú were placed in two rows, containing a total of 15 skulls. These were found in the middle of the same building as the skull pairs but on a higher level and are considered to be related to the construction of the building. Prior to the placement of the skulls in the ground, the floor under them appears to have been burned. Two semicomplete vases, as well as a small cache of deer bones, were found on the same level as the skull rows. All of the skulls in the rows were facing east, and at least some have articulated cervical vertebrae. The skulls in the rows

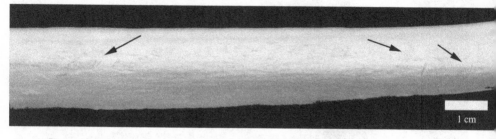

Figure 15.5. Cut marks on right tibia, Zacpetén, Operation 1000. Note that cut marks are present on various places along the shaft. Photograph by Don Rice.

are from adolescent to young adult individuals (15–30 years), and those for which sex could be estimated (8 of 15) were male. A similar skull row was found on the Macanché mainland. Twelve west-facing crania were found in two rows in the fill of a "non-descript mound" (P. Rice 1986:264). Field notes suggest that all were probably adult males (Mark Aldenderfer, field notes); however, attempts to locate these skulls have proven fruitless so far. No associated grave goods were reported.

Mass graves have been reported from Topoxté (Bullard 1970) and Zacpetén (Pugh 2001). Pugh's (2001) test excavations (consisting of three test pits) at Zacpetén produced the remains of 9 adults and children (including an infant) in a mass grave (Op. 1000). Cut marks were identified from this context on rib fragments and on the shaft of one tibia. The individuals appear to have been dismembered, placed in the pit in one episode (all remains were found in the same stratum), and covered with limestone rocks. However, unlike the postcrania at Ixlú, the tibia exhibited cut marks in various places along the shaft (figure 15.5), suggesting something other than just dismemberment. A radiocarbon date taken from immediately below the mass grave was from A.D. 1415± 20 (Pugh 2001). Bullard (1970) described a similar mass grave from Topoxté. He found human bones in the western portion of the Mayapán-style temple assemblage at Topoxté that were mixed with rocks and earth. These individuals also included the remains of adults and children. No grave goods were recovered from either mass grave.

Previous work suggests that these types of interments were ethnically group-specific (Duncan 1999) and that the mass grave reflects an attempt to hinder the journey of the souls or terminate the individuals and have them reborn in a weaker state, while the skull rows and pairs do not (Duncan 2000). When compared to seventeenth-century social-group boundaries suggested by ethnohistoric data (Duncan 1999), the cases of the skull rows and mass graves do not appear to reflect ethnic divisions (see figure 15.2). The Kowoj controlled the northern edge of Lake Petén Itzá, with the Yalain to the east and the Itzá to the south (although the relationship between the Yalain and the Itzá is unclear; Jones

1998). While Flores, Macanché, and Topoxté fall within the Itzá-Yalain boundaries, Ixlú and Zacpetén fall within the Kowoj territory.

However, when the mortuary practices are considered in terms of ethnically specific architecture and ceramics, the fact that the interment types reflect ethnic divisions becomes clear (Duncan 1999). The mass graves, at both Zacpetén and Topoxté, are found in conjunction with Mayapán-style temple assemblages (Pugh 2001). These assemblages were constructed by the Kowoj and have several components (figure 15.6). First is a temple with terraces, and a medial altar against the back wall. Second, to the left of the temple (facing the temple) is an oratorio. Third, a raised shrine is located in front of the temple. Fourth, a statue shrine is located between the temple and the raised shrine. Finally, a colonnaded hall is found at a right angle to the temple. A variation of these assemblages is found at Mayapán, from which, ethnohistoric sources suggest, at least some portion of the Kowoj migrated (Jones 1998). The skull pairs and rows are not known to be associated with any one type of civic architecture. However, Ixlú, Yalain, and El Fango (a site in the savannah region south of Lake Petén Itzá) share similar architectural assemblages that are not found in conjunction with the Mayapán-style temple assemblages (Don Rice, personal communication 2001). This shared architectural pattern involves a south-facing open hall facing two or

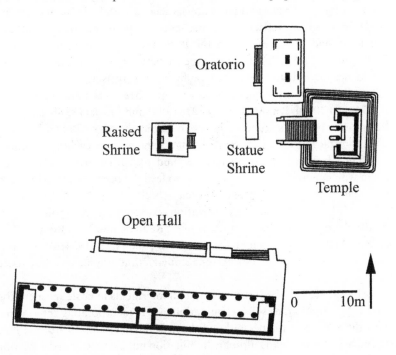

Figure 15.6. Mayapán-style temple assemblage (reproduced with permission from Pugh 2001:18, Figure 1–4).

more north-facing smaller open halls (Don Rice, personal communication 2001). This may be an Itzá/Yalain architectural assemblage. Minimally, though, the architectural assemblages appear to break down into Kowoj and non-Kowoj (Don Rice, personal communication 2001).

Leslie Cecil (2001) identified ceramic types that are ethnic identifiers. She argues that Clemencia Cream ware and red-and-black decorated pottery reflect Kowoj occupation. Itzá specific ceramics are somewhat more difficult to identify, owing in part to more emphasis on excavating Kowoj sites; however, she suggests that Vitzil Orange-Red ware pottery and the presence of reptilian motifs reflects Itzá occupation (Cecil 2001).

Thus we have identified, minimally, architectural assemblages and ceramic groups that reflect Kowoj and non-Kowoj occupation. The mass graves are found associated with Mayapán-style temple assemblages, Clemencia Cream wares, and red-and-black decoration at Zacpetén and Topoxté and thus are Kowoj-specific (Cecil 2001:529; Duncan 1999). The correlation between the skull rows and skull pairs at the same sites with the non-Kowoj architectural assemblages as well as the presence of non-Kowoj (Itzá?) ceramics suggest that the skull burials in Petén reflect non-Kowoj occupation. If the architectural and ceramic evidence are in fact indicative of ethnic group differences around the lakes, then the skull rows and pairs are associated with Itzá/Yalain occupation, while the mass graves reflect Kowoj occupation. Interethnic-group conflict was systemic around the lakes during the Postclassic, and boundaries frequently shifted (Jones 1998). Thus the incongruence between ethnohistorical and material evidence regarding political geography is not surprising.

These interments represent different attempts to terminate or to regenerate the soul (Duncan 2000). Becker (1988, 1992, 1993) and Mock (1998b) suggest that different interments may reflect these goals among the Maya. Becker has demonstrated that burials (the disposal of human remains) and caches (intentionally interred goods) may have been subsumed under what he terms an "earth offering," in which individuals were presented to feed the earth god or to impregnate the earth in a "death-planting-rebirth cycle" (Becker 1993:49). As Becker (1992: 190) notes, "impregnation (or fertilization) created by excavation for a grave provides the basis for rebirth and new life." Redfield and Villa Rojas (1934; in Yucatán), McGee (1990; among the Lacandon), and Nash (1985; among Tzeltal speakers in Chiapas, Mexico) present similar ethnographic cases of regeneration.

Mock (1998a, 1998b) argues that not all interments indicate regeneration of the soul. She argues that some termination events incorporating interments involve "the erasure of the personhood through flaying/mutilation of the human face and head, not only the ultimate humiliation but also the final destruction of an individual's identity" (Mock 1998b:119). In the Popol Vuh, when the gods destroyed their third attempt to make humans, they did so through "humiliation, destruction, and demolition" (Tedlock 1996:71). The Books of Chilam Balam also indicate that the outgoing Jaguar priest was said to have had his face "flattened" at the end of a *k'atun* (a 20-year cycle; Edmonson 1984:97). Archaeologically, Mock (1998b) argues that the skull pit at Colha (Op. 2011) is the product of a similar termination event. Cut marks consistent with flaying were found on the faces of 20 of the 30 skulls from the pit (Massey 1989; Mock 1998b). Mock (1998b:120) interprets the skulls as the product of an event terminating individual identity, with "their communication to the Otherworld closed forever." I suggest, though, that rather than representing total destruction of the individuals (as Mock implies), this violation for the Maya was used to create an enduring symbol of the objects' weakness. To continue the example from the *Popol Vuh,* after their violation, the manikins (the third attempt by the gods to make humans) variously seek refuge in houses, trees, and caves but are denied passage every time. The monkeys in the forest are left as a symbol of the manikins' destruction. The monkeys were reborn as a kind of enduring symbol of the manikins' "incompetence" and subhuman state: "And it used to be said that the monkeys in the forests today are a sign of this. They were left as a sign because wood alone was used for [the manikins'] flesh by the builder and sculptor. So this is why monkeys look like people: they are a sign" (Tedlock 1996:73). Creating the monkeys as an enduring symbol of weakness may have also involved removing them from the birth-death-replanting cycle that Becker (see above) describes. Removing them from the natural progression of transformation highlights their weakness, turning them into a lasting symbol of subhuman incompetence, which is the ultimate violation.

How though, might we distinguish between attempts to influence the soul using the material record? Carr (1995) provides the most comprehensive Human Relations Area Files study on mortuary practices completed to date in terms of numbers of practices and variables considered, analyzing 29 cultural determinants and 46 variables of practice from 31 nonstate societies. In his study, he found that archaeologically manifest correlates exist that reflect the journey of the soul and the nature of the soul after death.

The cultural determinants (Carr 1995:134 [determinants 81a, 81b, 82, 83, 84, 86]) under consideration are (1) beliefs about the afterlife; (2) beliefs about the nature of the soul (other than its journey) and its effect on the living; (3) beliefs about the nature of the journey of the soul into the afterlife; (4) beliefs about a soul's existence; (5) beliefs about reincarnation of the soul; and (6) beliefs about universal orders and their symbols. While almost all of Carr's variables of mortuary practice reflected multiple determinants (social, religious, and psychological), the variables included here (see below) reflected these determinants most frequently (Carr 1995:137, Table 5). These variables are body preparation and treatment, form of disposal, grave location, and kinds of grave goods. Some variables are modified because of problems of category definition and relevant aspects of the Maya culture. Distinguishing attempts to terminate the soul's journey versus allowing it to continue hinges on finding the four correlates reflecting termination co-occurring archaeologically as a suite. As shown below, individual variables may be ambiguous, and it is certainly possible to find an archaeological deposit in which some variables reflect termination and others reflect regeneration. Finding a deposit in which each variable reflects an attempt either to suspend the soul's journey or to cause the soul to be reborn in a weaker state would provide a preponderance of evidence suggesting that the deposit represents an act of violation.

Variable: Body Preparation and Treatment

Carr (1995) separates body preparation and treatment. Preparation relates to ornamentation (such as covering with pigment), and treatment (such as mutilation, embalming, cremation) relates to processing. However, the present study collapses these categories, as they may overlap. As mentioned above, Mock (1998b) suggests that for the Maya, individuals for whom the journey of the soul was terminated were humiliated and destroyed. Mock (1998b:117) specifically argues that this humiliation could take the form of cut marks and burning, in particular on the face. Evidence for this includes destruction of monumental masks at Cerros (Mock 1998b:117) and the burning of the faces of the gods' third attempt to make the human race in the *Popol Vuh*. Cut marks and burning alone, though, are insufficient evidence for identifying termination. For example, elite burials of the Cocom lineage at Mayapán involved cutting an individual's head in half on the coronal plane and rebuilding the face, cremating the body, and placing the ashes in the skull (Tozzer 1941:130). Defacement in a general sense is the destruction or violation of whatever is the essence of the object (*sensu* Taussig 1999). Thus archaeologically one would expect body treatment, whether in the form of cut marks or smashing remains or burning to be done in a manner that reflects destruction, not simply dismemberment or preparation for later use. Cut marks congruent with flaying, such as on the face or on the diaphyses of long bones, suggest an attempt to terminate the soul's journey.

Among the Maya, spoken language and the mouth are symbolically meaningful as the seat of the soul and the source of power (Gossen 1986:7). Stuart (1995:190–191) has suggested that the word *ajaw* means "the shouter," in addition to "lord." Nash (1985) notes that the soul leaves through the tongue after death. Finding a cache of mandibles that had been removed from the skull of various individuals and buried under a shrine would suggest not an attempt to terminate the souls' journey but an attempt to appropriate the individuals' power or essence in some fashion. Finding an individual's mandible with cut marks covering the mandible, crushed, or having teeth extracted outside of some dedicatory context would be congruent with an attempt to deface the individual by destroying a source of power.

The face is an important locus for such activities. As mentioned above, Mock provides various examples from ethnohistory and indigenous texts of how the face is targeted among the Maya when one attempts to violate or insult an individual. Taussig (1999) argues that this is common cross-culturally. Thus, body preparation that reflects an attempt to destroy or deflesh human remains—in particular, that which targets the face in some fashion—is congruent with an attempt to terminate an individual's soul or suspend its journey.

Variable: Form of Disposal

Carr (1995) found that form of disposal (such as a mass grave) reflects philosophical and religious beliefs. If Mock (1998b) is correct that forgetting the individual is part of a termination event, then this forgetting should be manifest in forms of disposal that obscure individual identity. Cross-culturally, mass burials commonly have the purpose of obscuring individuals' identities (Cannon 1995). Sometimes, individuals' souls may be obscured as they move into a collective group of ancestors, and this is reflected by placement into an ossuary (Graeber 1995). However, among the Maya it appears that individual souls are remembered when veneration occurs. Evidence for this can be found in the tombs of Rio Azul. As Hall (1989) notes, the increase in kingly power in the Early Classic appears to have been accompanied by an increasing emphasis on identifying the individual kings in royal lineages in iconography on tomb walls. If souls are regenerated, then individuals should be recognizable archaeologically. Termination or suspension of the soul's journey should be manifest in a form of disposal that does not maintain individual identity in the grave.

Variable: Grave Location

The current use of grave location as a variable deviates slightly from Carr's (1995). Carr (1995) found that grave orientation relative to real and mythical landscapes and to cardinal directions infrequently reflects the determinants in question cross-culturally. When grave orientation did reflect a cross-cultural pattern, the most common determinants to influence these variables were the determinants considered here. However, grave location relative to architecture is considered here since all of the interments in question are in public areas and the cardinal directions were relevant to Maya cosmology (Ashmore 1991; Ashmore and Geller this volume). For the Maya, east was associated with rebirth; west, by contrast, was associated with death. Similarly, organization along north and south lines may reflect an attempt to link cosmic layers along an *axis mundi,* with placement to the north evoking the heavens and the south associated with the underworld (Ashmore and Geller this volume).

As with body treatment and preparation, though, grave location is a potentially ambiguous variable. The significance of the cardinal directions (and spatial organization in general) is not in question (Gossen 1986). How this is manifest archaeologically and the degree to which we may decipher the meaning of direction archaeologically are less obvious. For example, among the Lacandon an important ritual object is the god pot: a ceramic incense burner with a face on one side. These pots are ensouled through being painted, being sung to, and other acts. These pots face east while they are in use and are turned to face west when they are ceremonially killed (Tozzer 1907; McGee 1990). However, they are located on the west side of the god house (Tozzer 1907). Benches for the participants in rituals with the god pots are placed on the east side of the god pots so that the participants may face the pots. The significance of an eastern orientation thus does not always translate into placement and orientation of significant things on and toward the east. Similarly, archaeological studies have found tremendous variation in orientation across the Maya lowlands on regional and intrasite levels through time (Ashmore and Geller this volume; Welsh 1988). Should we use grave location relative to architecture in an effort to understand the meaning of interments in the Maya area? Although the variable is potentially ambiguous, I think the answer is a guarded yes. Ashmore and Geller (this volume) note that at Tikal and Copán "superimposition of royal burials and their shrines may define a particular spot [in the respective acropoli] . . . as a specific *axis mundi*." Placement of royal burials in northern acropoli associates the royalty with their place in the heavens. Similarly, Welsh (1988) found that eastern shrine groups on the edges of plazas are an important locus for burials in the Classic period. Thus, in conjunction with other lines of data, we may utilize orientation relative to architecture to gain insight into the meanings of burials. For this study, then, interments east or north of architecture should reflect regeneration of the soul or some association with the heavens. Finding interments to the west or south of architecture, though, would suggest that the burials reflect an attempt to hinder the soul's progress or association with the underworld.

Variable: Kinds of Grave Goods

Carr (1995) found that kinds of grave goods varied with the determinants in question here in terms of functional types, local versus nonlocal goods, and items that were broken or unbroken. Ethnographic (Vogt 1998), ethnohistoric (Tozzer 1941), and archaeological evidence (Welsh 1988) indicates that goods were placed in graves to provision the individual's soul in the afterlife among numerous Maya groups. Ethnographic (Vogt 1998) and ethnohistoric (Tozzer 1941) sources also demonstrate that smashing vessels and censers and razing buildings were part of termination rituals. Smashed grave goods or an absence of grave goods suggests that the interment represents an attempt to hinder the soul or have it reborn in a weakened state, while unbroken vessels or nonlocal goods indicate regeneration of the soul.

Because of the potential ambiguity of any single variable, finding any one of the correlates reflecting soul termination does not provide sufficient basis for concluding that the interments reflect an attempt to terminate the soul. Of the 30 skulls at Colha, 20 exhibit cut marks on the face. However, cut marks are insufficient evidence to conclude that the individuals had their souls harmed. As mentioned above, some elite burials at Mayapán involved cutting off and rebuilding individuals' faces, cremating their body, and placing the ashes in the skull (Tozzer 1941:130). Clearly, the manifestation of a single variable, such as cut marks, can be part of either violation or veneration. To make a convincing case, each of the correlates reflecting termination must co-occur archaeologically. In addition to the cut marks on the skulls at Colha, ceramics in the deposit were intentionally broken (as suggested by the absence of matching sherds) and were placed in the pit (Mock 1998b). The skulls were placed on the west side of a staircase, and there "was no obvious pattern in the placement of the skulls except age: the skulls of older adults were found in the top layer of skulls" (Mock 1998b:114). Following the interment of the skulls, the structure was burned (Mock 1998b). Thus, the Colha skull pit conforms to each of the archaeological correlates for termination of the soul's journey, and I suggest that the most parsimonious interpretation of the Colha skull pit is that it was created through an act of violation.

Interpretations

A consideration of the three types of Postclassic interments in light of Bloch's model suggests that the mass graves represent an act of violation in the form of negative predation. The form of disposal reflects loss of individual identity, and the body treatment suggests dismemberment as well as some kind of defleshing, evident in the transverse cut marks found along the shaft of a tibia. The mass graves are located on the west side of the Mayapán-style temple assemblages, on the opposite side of the plaza from the temple on the east, and there is a dearth of grave goods. As with the skulls in the Colha skull pit, the variables are congruent with predicted behaviors reflecting the hindering of the souls' journey. Endocannibalism (generally not an act of violence; see Conklin 1995; Poole 1982) can produce similar kinds of interments (Buikstra 2001). However, the absence of pot polish and absence of evidence of burning suggests that the mass graves were not the product of endocannibalism. Thus, the individuals in the mass grave appear to have had their souls' journeys disrupted like the manikins in the *Popol Vuh,* creating an enduring symbol of their destruction.

The skull pairs and skull rows around the Petén lakes do not appear to reflect an attempt to terminate or hinder the soul's journey, though. Neither the rows nor the pairs were associated with a single kind of architecture. Further, the skull rows were facing opposite directions. While there was a dearth of grave goods, there were no signs of defacement, as seen at Colha (Mock 1998b). I suggest that the skull rows and skull pairs reflect either (1) the symbolic destruction of the body and the continuation of the soul that Bloch (1982) discusses or (2) positive predation. In either case the soul continues, but we cannot know in what form.

Both scenarios are possible for the Maya. As shown above, Landa (Tozzer 1941:111–130) demonstrates that the use of skulls may be part of veneration. However, as Miller (1999) notes, the iconography and epigraphy in the Maya area associated with the sacrifice of captured enemy rulers suggests that decapitation of enemies was a part of violation. This interpretation is bolstered by research on the iconography and timing associated with the use of skulls and skull racks in Mesoamerica (Bill et al. 2000). Read (1998) argues that, like most Mesoamerican cultures, Mexica calendrical ceremonies were designed to signify the end of a period and the beginning of a new one. Moser (1973) notes that seven of the 20-day Mexica month ceremonies involve adding to tzompantli. Further, as Miller (1999) notes, the relationship between skulls and rebirth is seen in the *Popol Vuh*. When the severed head of One Hunahpu, the father of the story's hero twins, is placed in a calabash tree, it spits in the hand of Blood Moon, the daughter of an underworld lord, making her pregnant with the hero twins (Tedlock 1996:36). Finally, among the Tzutujil Maya in the highlands of Guatemala, maize seeds are referred to as "interred ones" or "little skulls" (Carlsen and Prechtel 1991:28). Thus, there is a connection between skulls and rebirth in Maya literature. Ultimately we cannot know whether the skulls reflect veneration and the soul continued as a victory over death or whether positive predation occurred and the soul continued after it had been appropriated from an enemy. However, evidence from the codices suggests that individuals used to make tzompantli were most likely enemies, and thus their skulls reflect positive predation. As noted above, Moser (1973) has shown that enemies were typically used to add to tzompantli. Also, the Codex Mendoza shows captors holding their captives by the hair.

By itself, the above scenario makes a nice story. However, it becomes increasingly persuasive when considered within the context of Late Postclassic social history and political geography. The Itzá appear to have roots in Petén reaching back to the Early Classic (Boot 1995), and they likely maintained contact with other Itzá groups at the major centers of the North (Chichén Itzá and Mayapán) throughout the Postclassic (Rockmore 1998). The earliest records of the Kowoj, though, are from Mayapán in Yucatán (Roys 1962). Ethnohistoric evidence suggests that the Kowoj migrated to the Petén lakes region after the fall of Mayapán around A.D. 1450 (Jones 1998). The single ^{14}C date that was taken from immediately below the bone layer was A.D. 1415± 20, or 35 years before the fall of Mayapán (Pugh 2001; although as Cecil [2001:549] notes, Kowoj occupation may stem from A.D. 1000). Further, settlement in defendable locations (D. Rice 1986), the use of defensive walls and moats (D. Rice and P. Rice 1981), and ethnohistoric documents (Jones 1998) indicate that the Itzá and Kowoj were clearly enemies, warfare was systemic, and territorial boundaries shifted frequently. Thus the political environment of the Late Postclassic is consistent with one in which we might expect to find a new group, the Kowoj, attempting to reproduce their collective identity through the destruction and subordination of outsiders.

Acknowledgments

Funding for this project was provided in part by the National Science Foundation, by Southern Illinois University–Carbondale, and by Prudence and Don Rice. I would like to thank the editors for inviting my participation in this volume. Don Rice kindly made his photographs available for use. Don Rice, Leslie Cecil, and Tim Pugh provided assistance and clarification regarding architectural and ceramic data from Petén. Jason González provided much-needed assistance with the figures. Andy Hofling, Erica Hill, Kay Read, Carmen Arendt, and the students of Proyecto Maya Colonial and SIUC provided invaluable comments throughout the writing process, no doubt improving this chapter's substance and style. All remaining errors are my own.

16

The Bioarchaeology and Taphonomy of Mortuary Ritual on the Sepik Coast, Papua New Guinea

Ann L. W. Stodder

The analysis of human and animal bone fragments from a site on the north coast of New Guinea suggests that preconceived notions of what constitutes a burial or a ritual deposit can influence the trajectory and outcome of field investigations and can color our interpretation of archaeological remains. Our conception of the activities that constitute mortuary behavior and how these might be visible in the archaeological record need to be flexible and our methods of inquiry fine grained.

Site 23 is a small cultural deposit on a hilltop just inland from the quiet coastal town of Aitape, about 50 kilometers east of the border of Papua New Guinea and Irian Jaya. In 1996 members of the Field Museum's New Guinea Research Program (NGRP) conducted archaeological testing at this site and several others. The excavation of four 1 x 2 meter and one 1 x 1 meter units yielded an assemblage of shell, sherds, a few items of ground stone, 1,060 fragments of human bone, and 2,306 fragments of animal bone deposited in a natural limestone crevice. Site 23 is dated to circa A.D. 700 (Terrell and Welsch 1997). No architectural structures or features of any kind were recorded in the field. This small deposit was interpreted as a domestic midden. The shell is from marine and mangrove environments and appears to represent food remains rather than exotic shell for ornament manufacture or trade (Gerber and Schecter 2002). The mixture of animal and human bone fragments suggested that the human remains had been cannibalized and then buried with other food debris.

The bioarchaeological analysis was presented as an exercise in collecting taphonomy data to answer the "was it or wasn't it cannibalism?" question. In contrast to the American Southwest, where debate has focused on the validity of bioarchaeologically based identifications of cannibalism (Billman et al. 2000; Dongoske et al. 2000; Turner and Turner 1999), "the case of past cannibalism in parts of Papua New Guinea is no longer an issue for the majority of Melanesian scholars" (Goldman 1999:19). There are "burgeoning ethnographic confirmations of precolonial cannibalism" among Highland people including the Bimin-Kukusimin, Gimi, Hua, Foi, Daribi, and peoples of the Strickland-Bosavi region of inland southern Papua New Guinea such as the Kalui, Etoro, Bedamini, Same, Gebusi, Kubor, and Onabasulu (Goldman 1999:19; see also Brown and Tuzin 1983; Lindenbaum 1979). However, there is no ethnographic evidence that people in the Aitape area ever practiced cannibalism, and the ethnohistoric records of mortuary behavior suggested that the Site 23 data should be examined in a broader interpretive context.

The Vertebrate Faunal Assemblage

The faunal assemblage from Site 23 is predominately pig and human, and as indicated in table 16.1, one-fourth of the bone is so fragmented that it could only be designated as either pig or human. Dog teeth and fish remains constitute only 2 percent of the assemblage. This contrasts with the faunal remains from two other sites tested: Site 16, where the assemblage is almost exclusively human bone; and Site 46, for which the assemblage is almost half pig bone and only 6 percent human bone and also includes a range of food species (turtle, fish, and phalanger—a squirrel-like marsupial). The anatomical distribution of both the pig and human bone from Site 23 is also striking (table 16.2). The human bone is 78 percent postcranial. The assemblage of pig remains, which represents a minimum of 11 individuals, is almost exclusively (96 percent) mandible fragments and teeth. There are 20 or so pig maxilla fragments and 4 skull vault fragments. Less than 4 percent of the pig bone is from postcranial elements, and these are primarily a single set of caudal vertebrae. In sum, the assemblage is basically human postcranial remains and pig mandibles: not what one expects in a domestic midden.

Table 16.1. Vertebrate Faunal Components from Three New Guinea Research Program Sites

Species	Site 23 (NISP = 3,366) %	Site 46 (NISP = 132) %	Site 16 (NISP = 554) %
Human	34	6	96
Pig	31	42	1
Pig/human	25	8	0
Dog	1	4	0
Fish	1	10	1
Turtle	0	6	0
Indeterminate	8	20	1
Other	0	4	1

Note: NISP = number of individual specimens.

Table 16.2. Anatomical Distribution of Pig and Human Bone, Site 23

Segment	Human (NISP = 1,060) %	Pig (NISP = 1,011) %
Cranial	14.2	69.0
Dental	7.5	27.2
Cranial and dental total	*21.7*	*96.2*
Axial	18.9	2.2
Upper limb	6.4	0.0
Lower limb	27.5	0.5
Hand/foot	10.9	0.3
Indeterminate postcranial	14.6	0.8
Postcranial total	*78.3*	*3.8*

Note: NISP = number of individual specimens.

The human remains were determined to represent a minimum of seven individuals—four adults and three subadults—based on analysis of tibiae and dentition (table 16.3). A 4–6-year-old and a 2-year-old are represented by dentition and cranial fragments, and an individual estimated at about 6 months in utero is represented by a petrous portion of the temporal. The adults include two males, one female, and one individual of unknown sex. The adult bone assemblage includes fragments from hands and feet (11 percent of 1,060 fragments) and axial elements (19 percent). Leg and foot bones account for 28 percent of the fragments. Arm and hand bones account for only 6 percent of the assemblage, and the radius is particularly underrepresented.

There is a nearly complete human mandible, as well as cranial fragments from at least two adults, but cranial remains are underrepresented. The upper region of the cranial vault is not represented at all, and most of the bone is from the temporals and occipital (figure 16.1). The more complete remains of an adult male (figure 16.2) were found in the northwest corner of the site.

With the exception of this spatially distinct subassemblage, the infracranial and cranial remains could not be associated or reconstructed into individuals. There were long bones found next to each other, and in one area a stack of long bone shafts was found, but the bones were not in anatomical position. Some of the same elements from clearly different individuals were found in close proximity, including two anterior fragments of first cervical vertebrae and tibia fragments with differential robusticity (indicating that they were from both male and female individuals). In sum, the human remains were not articulated, and they were not consistently distributed in coherent anatomical groups, but neither were they randomly distributed across the site.

Comparison of the vertical distribution of the shell, pig, and human bone (figure 16.3) suggests that the human bone may have been predominant at the bottom of the deposit, with pig bone and shell predominating above. The scale of

Table 16.3. Identifiable Human Bone, Site 23

Element	NISP	MNE	MNI
Occipital	11	1	1A
Frontal	9	2	1A, 1SA
Malar	1	1	1A
Mandible	47	2	1A, 1SA
Maxilla	6	1	1A
Parietal	16	2	1A, 1SA
Temporal	29	3	2A, 1SA
Zygomatic	3	2	1A, 1SA?
Dentition	79		3A, 2SA
Clavicle	2	1	1A
Scapula	7	2	2A
Rib	83	?	1A
Vertebra, cervical	6	3	2A
Vertebra, thoracic	67	7	2A
Vertebra, lumbar	2	1	1A
Sacrum	2	1	1A
Innominate	22	2	2A
Humerus	51	3	2A (2L, 1R)
Radius	3	2	2A (1L, 1S?)
Ulna	8	2	1A (1L, 1R)
Hand phalanges, proximal	7	1	1A
Hand phalanges, medial	11	11?	2A?
Hand phalanges, distal	2	2	1A
Femur	41	2	2A
Tibia	205	6	4A
Fibula	39	4	2A (2R, 2L)
Patella	6	1	1A (1L)
Talus	3	2	2A (2L)
Calcaneus	12	2	1A (1L, 1R)
Navicular	3	3	2A (2L, 1R)
Foot phalanges, proximal	5	5?	1A
Foot phalanges, medial	6	6	1A

Note: NISP = number of individual specimens; MNE = minimum number of elements; MNI = minimum number of individuals represented; A = adult, SA = subadult, L = left, R = right, S? = side unknown.

vertical provenience varies slightly in different excavation units, so the interpretation of these data is limited. But this presents the possibility that human bone was deposited first, followed by the pig mandibles, and then more shell and bone fragments.

Taphonomy

Taphonomic analysis was performed with the goal of reconstructing the cultural and natural processes that contributed to the extremely fragmentary condition of

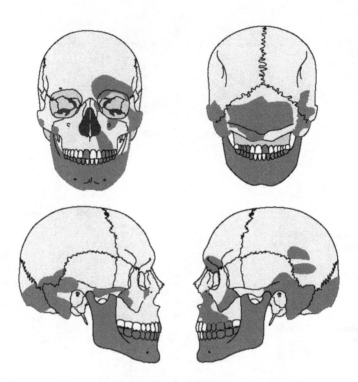

Figure 16.1. Composite reconstruction of identifiable cranial fragments.

these remains. After preliminary sorting in the field, the bone fragments were cleaned, inventoried, and analyzed in the A. B. Lewis Laboratory in the Department of Anthropology at the Field Museum. Modern breaks due to excavation and transport were noted before the bone was cleaned, and these were repaired prior to analysis. After cleaning, inventory, and anatomical identification, refitting was attempted for bone fragments within provenience units, and then within anatomical groups from all units. Refit sets of bone fragments were assigned a conjoin set number. Each of the conjoined sets—reconstructed portions of skeletal elements—was analyzed as a single entity, that is, taphonomy data was collected for the entire set, not for each individual fragment.

The taphonomy data collection protocol closely follows the methods described by White (1992). As listed in table 16.4, the observations can be conceptually grouped into five categories: (1) preservation and condition of the bone, (2) tool marks, (3) animal-inflicted damage, (4) fractures, and (5) fracture products. The categories are not mutually exclusive, since a chop mark or animal chewing can both be related to bone fracture. With such a fragmentary assem-

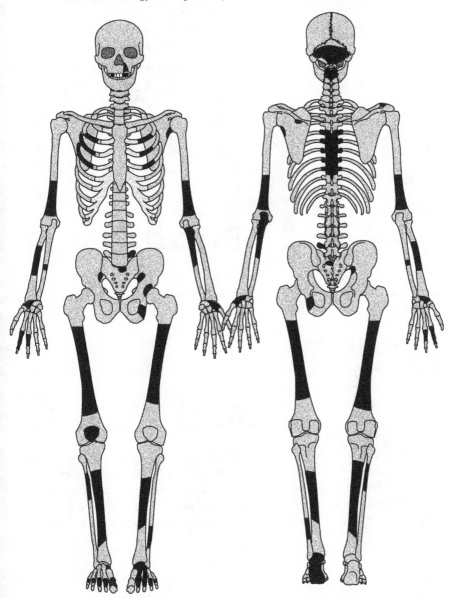

Figure 16.2. Elements present (dark shading) from Individual 2E-2, Site 23.

blage, it was important to try to distinguish animal-induced damage from naturally occurring and from human-induced damage. This is difficult to do without overestimating the degree of our understanding of these processes and without underestimating the degree of overlap, mimic, and similarity between the marks left on bone by cultural, animal, and environmental agents.

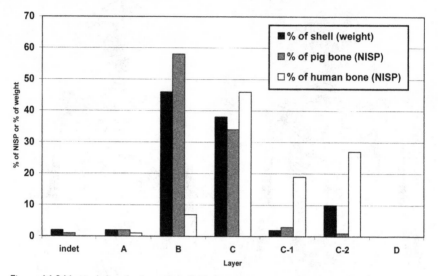

Figure 16.3. Vertical distribution of shell, pig bone, and human bone from Site 23.

Preservation and Condition

The average size of the human bone fragments is 2.3 centimeters, and 1.8 centimeters is the average size of pig bone fragments. The largest human bone fragment is 16.5 centimeters long, and one pig mandible fragment is 12.8 centimeters long. As indicated in table 16.4, about half of the bone fragments exhibit rolling or rounding from abrasion.

There is very little end polish, beveling, or weathering, but the pig bone is on average slightly more weathered than the human bone. Less than 1 percent of the human bone exhibits thermal alteration (two fragments). Thirteen percent of the pig bone fragments show discoloration due to thermal alteration. One fragment is blackened; the others are red or red and partly gray. None is cracked or calcined.

Tool Marks

Tool marks (including cut marks, scrape marks, chop marks, and a broader shallower mark referred to here as a U-shaped groove) are present on 21 human bone fragments, 6 pig bone fragments, and 3 fragments in the pig-or-human category. The cut marks do not resemble those made with stone tools—narrow and V-shaped. Instead they are somewhat shallower and more closely resemble marks made by bamboo tools in replicative studies conducted by Spenneman (1990) in his investigations of Fijian cannibalism. Expedient and extremely sharp, bamboo knives are routinely made and used in a range of activities in gardening and

Table 16.4. Taphonomy Summary, Human and Pig Bone, Site 23

Category	Human		Pig		Pig or Human	
	Nw/Nobs	%w	Nw/Nobs	%w	Nw/Nobs	%w
Preservation and Condition						
Weathering	Mean = 0.74		Mean = 1.47		Mean = 1.10	
(0–6 scale)[a]	N = 452		N = 313		N = 123	
	SD = 0.98		SD = 1.02		SD = 1.03	
Rolling/rounding	238/448	53	147/312	47	104/208	50
End polish	2/439	<1	0/310	0	4/206	2
Beveled fracture	1/436	<1	0/310	0	1/206	1
Thermal alteration	2/446	<1	41/311	13	7/209	3
Tool marks						
Tool marks: any	21/505	4	6/438	1	3/124	2
Chop marks	5/446	1	3/313	1	3/208	1
Scrape marks	3/444	1	0/313	0	0/207	0
Cut marks	7/443	2	1/313	<1	2/207	1
U-shaped groove	7/443	2	2/313	<1	0	0
Animal damage						
Chew marks: any	177/505	35	57/425	13	44/124	35
Ovoid pits	56/446	13	10/312	3	16/208	8
Rodent gnaw	0/466	0	0/313	0	1/208	<1
Tooth puncture	7/446	2	0/313	0	2/208	1
Trampling/random striae	67/447	15	61/312	20	41/208	20
Cranial fracture						
Internal cranial fracture	4/35	11	0/4	0	0/3	0
External cranial fracture	4/7	57	0/1	0	0/0	0
Cross-sutural fracture	7/47	15	0/1	0	0/0	0
Postcranial fracture						
Perimortem	115/268	43	7/12	58	13/18	72
Postmortem	153/268	57	5/12	42	5/18	28
Fracture products						
Inner conchoidal scar	1/105	1	0/10	0	0/21	0
Outer conchoidal scar	0/31	0	0/12	0	0/0	0
Incipient fracture crack	5/33	15	0/12	0	0/0	0
Peeling	30/360	9	21/293	7	10/190	5
Percussion pits	10/446	2	1/313	<1	1/208	<1
Crushing	3/444	<1	0/312	0	0/209	0
Adhering flake	1/382	<1	0/295	0	0/195	0

Notes: Nw = number of fragments evidencing category of wear or mark; Nobs = number of observable fragments; %w = percentage of sample with wear or mark.

[a] Behrensmeyer 1978.

hunting (Loving 1976; Steensberg 1980). They also have ritual uses in head-hunting ceremonies, as observed by Haddon among the Kiwai and Mawatta peoples of Borneo (1901:115) and documented for the Asmat (Zegwaard 1959) and the Mianmin (Gardner 1999) of New Guinea. Shell tools might also have been used. These make shorter cut marks with interior striations, somewhat

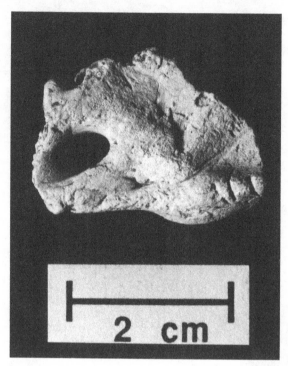

Figure 16.4. Petrous fragment with cut mark (NGRP 23/ 4514). Copyright by the Field Museum, neg. #A113871_12, photographer John Weinstein.

shallower cut marks than those made by stone tools (DeGusta 1999; Toth and Woods 1989).

The U-shaped grooves are relatively shallow, elongated grooves or notches with a U-shaped cross section. They are distinguished from rodent gnawing and chewing damage by their orientation, patterning, and co-occurrence with other alterations like ovoid pits made by tooth cusps. The U-shaped grooves vary in length and width, and in the number and the orientation of the grooves relative to each other and the bone element. The products of several different taphonomic agents are probably represented in this category, given the variability in mark morphology and location. Some might be tooth-furrows such as described by Milner and Smith (1989:44). But the likelihood of this possibility is challenged by the occurrence of the grooves in what would appear to be extremely difficult areas to chew on and by the lack of other chewing marks on more "accessible" portions of the same fragments. The U-shaped grooves do not match the morphology of experimentally generated marks made in clay with pig incisors, which exhibit more distinct edges and near-grooves formed by the lateral curvature of the incisor crowns. The U-shaped grooves seem more likely to have been made by a wood, bamboo, shell, sea urchin spine, or bone tool. They occur almost exclusively on nontubular elements from the cranial and axial regions.

The cut marks and U-shaped grooves are in locations indicating decapitation and disarticulation: the petrous and mastoids (figure 16.4), the first cervical vertebra (figure 16.5) of two individuals, the anterior superior iliac spine, and the greater sciatic notch in two individuals. This consistency suggests deliberate patterned processing. Other cut marks are located on the frontal bone just above the orbit, on phalanges, and on mandible fragments. Scrape marks are present on a temporal fragment, a metacarpal, and a patella fragment. Chop marks are present on three long bone shaft splinters, a parietal fragment, and an ilium fragment.

In the pig bone assemblage, cut marks are present on a mandibular ramus fragment; chop marks are present on the proximal surface of a mandibular condyle and on two caudal vertebrae; U-shaped grooves are present on a maxilla fragment and an unidentifiable bone fragment.

Animal Damage

Trampling and chewing damage are abundant on both human and nonhuman bone. Rodent gnawing is present on only one fragment, but at least one type of chew mark appears on 35 percent of all human bone fragments (177 of 505), on 13 percent of pig bone (57 of 425), and on 27 percent of the entire assemblage (307 of 1,143).

One of the most common alterations to the surface of the bone fragments is referred to as "ovoid pits" (figure 16.6). These are present on 13 percent of human bone fragments (56 of 446)—including some tooth roots—and on 3 percent of the pig bone (10 of 312).

Where multiple pits appear on a single fragment, they may overlap or have linear alignment. Half-pits are sometimes present adjacent to a fracture edge. On some refit specimens, the pits cross fracture edges, indicating a role in the bone failure. The pits average 4.75 millimeters and range from 1.5 millimeters to as large as 9.7 millimeters in diameter. The interior of some pits have multiple punctations, and others exhibit parallel curved striations. The working hypothesis for this study is that the pits are the result of pig masticatory activity, since they resemble impressions of pig molar crowns made in modeling clay. The sideways grinding masticatory motion of pigs (Herring 1976) seems likely to have produced the parallel striations within the ovoid pits.

Pig scavenging has been observed to create scoring, tooth punctures, and furrows in bone (Berryman 2002; Gladikas 1978; Greenfield 1988). Pigs and dogs are both active scavengers of bone in Pacific communities (Spenneman 1990, 1994), but the size of the larger ovoid pits suggests that they were made by adult pig molars.

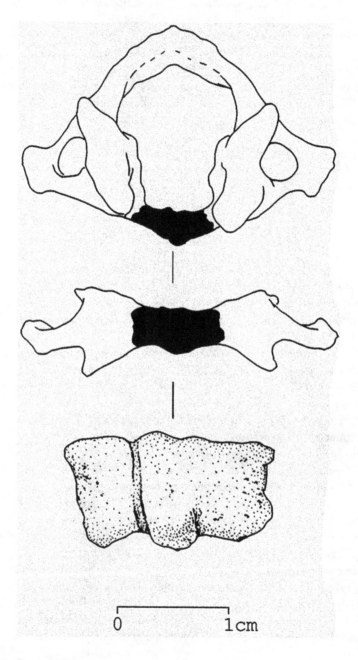

Figure 16.5. Location of cut marks on first cervical vertebra.

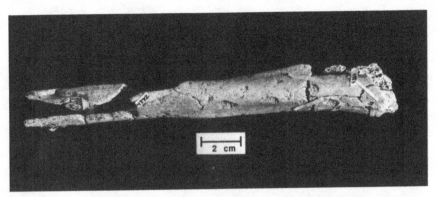

Figure 16.6. Partially reconstructed humerus with ovoid pits (NGRP 23/4880). Copyright by the Field Museum, neg. #A113870_13, photographer John Weinstein.

Fractures

Fractures on tubular elements (long bones, phalanges, metacarpals, metatarsals, and ribs) were categorized as perimortem or postmortem according to their shape, using Marshall's guidelines (1989). Spiral, V-shaped, saw-toothed, and flaking fractures were grouped as perimortem—fractures to bone in the vital state. Stepped, longitudinal, perpendicular, and irregular-perpendicular were counted as postmortem fractures that affected the bone in its nonvital state. Of the 268 fracture edges on human tubular bone fragments, 45 percent of the fractures affected the bone perimortem (115 of 268) and 57 percent of the fractures were inflicted postmortem. In the assemblage of human remains, 21 long bones are represented, but none has an intact end. The fracture patterns in the reconstructed diaphyses suggest that the midportions of the bones were broken in their nonvital state: they exhibit step and longitudinal fractures. The long bones appear to have been buried with at least their shafts intact, rather than having been broken up for marrow extraction. The articular ends and the proximal and distal portions of the long bone shafts may have been broken during disarticulation, or they may have been eaten by animals, or both. The extremely small assemblage of 12 observable pig bone tubular fragments exhibits 58 percent perimortem fractures and 42 percent postmortem fractures.

Fracture Products

Incipient fracture cracks (White 1992:137) are the most abundant fracture product observed in the human bone, present in four long bone fragments and a mandibular condyle. These cracks are incomplete fractures that radiate from the location of a loading point on the bone, and they are associated with perimortem damage. None was observed on the pig bone, but as with much of the taphonomy

data, this may be at least in part an artifact of the paucity of tubular bone fragments in the pig assemblage. All of the incipient fracture cracks observed are
associated with animal chewing damage; none resulted from tool use—at least as
visible on the bone fragments.

Peeling is present in 9 percent and 7 percent of the human and pig bone fragments, respectively. Peeling occurs as a result of the fracturing and pulling apart
of a green bone (White 1992:140). One instance of peeling in the human assemblage is associated with a tool mark, and 12 are associated with animal chewing
marks. Percussion pits are present on 2 percent of human bone fragments and less
than 1 percent of the pig and pig/human fragments. Two of the 10 percussion pits
on human bone are associated with tool marks, but none is associated with chew
marks. The pattern of co-occurrence or lack of fracture products with tool marks
and with animal chew marks supports the evidence above that a great deal of the
damage to the assemblage was inflicted by animals, some of which may have
obliterated evidence of human agency in the creation of the assemblage.

The Taphonomic Signatures of Cannibalism

The predominant rationale for systematic taphonomy studies in the assessment
of cannibalism centers on the question of whether human bone shows evidence of
having been treated similarly to nonhuman bone that is accepted as representing
food remains (White 1992:339). Villa and coworkers (1986:431) outlined four
types of evidence on which a hypothesis of dietary cannibalism must be based: (1)
similar butchering techniques in the animal and human remains, allowing for
anatomical differences; (2) similar patterns of long bone breakage; (3) identical
patterns of postprocessing discard of human and animal remains; and (4) evidence of cooking (if present), indicating comparable treatment of human and
animal remains.

Perimortem damage attributable to human and animal agents is present in
human and nonhuman bone from Site 23. The same types of tool marks, presumably made by the same toolkit, are present on the pig and human bone. Cut marks
on human cervical vertebra and the tool marks on the temporal bones suggest
that decapitation involved cutting the muscles below the chin and at the lower
lateral aspects of the skull. Cut marks on both species suggest that mandibles and
digits from both pigs and humans may have been disarticulated in the same
manner. There is slightly more weathering and more thermal alteration on the pig
bone, and more incipient fracture cracks in the human bone. But the extent to
which we can compare the condition of the pig and human remains is limited. We
cannot compare patterns of long bone breakage or the patterning in other
taphonomic features seen on tubular bones. The bone is so fragmentary and the
animal assemblage so anatomically skewed (mandibles, dentition, cranial fragments, and one tail) that butchering or processing cannot be readily reconstructed for either pigs or people.

However, as with the question of "cannibalism or not," the issue of similar processing of humans and animals is not so difficult to answer in New Guinea. In fact, several ethnographies indicate that human bodies were quite conscientiously and deliberately dismembered and disarticulated in precisely the same manner as pigs. In his treatise on Asmat headhunting, Zegwaard (1959:1026) wrote that "the first ceremony was the butchering. The method described is also applied when a cassowary, pig, crocodile or big lizard is slaughtered. Throughout New Guinea we find regional instructions on the slaughtering of animals and these regional methods are faithfully executed on both animals and human beings."

Goodale's (1995:236) description of Kualong mortuary ritual, which does not involve cannibalism, includes an intriguing observation on preparation of the body: "The skull and jaw bones are certainly removed and sometimes also the long bones of the arm, scapula and collarbones, and their breastbones. (I believe it to be significant that these bones are the same as those in the butchered head portion of a pig.)" Ernst notes that the only major difference in the preparation and consumption of pigs and people among the Onobasulu is the discard of human intestines, for reasons pertaining to the status of the victim as a sorcerer (Ernst 1999:151).

We know cannibalism was practiced in some parts of New Guinea at some times and that in some Melanesian cultures human bodies were processed as part of cannibalism or headhunting activities with the same tools and in the same anatomical sequence as pigs. Both of these cultural practices may have been part of creating the Site 23 bone assemblage and its taphonomic profile.

The Turners propose six characteristics as the minimal taphonomic signature of cannibalism. These include perimortem breakage, cut marks, anvil abrasions or percussion striae, burning, many missing vertebrae, and end polish (Turner and Turner 1995, 1999:24). These criteria are based on the Turners' (1995) extensive study of bone from the American Southwest, although they have been proposed as criteria for the "standardized world definition" of cannibalism (Turner and Turner 1995:1) The Site 23 bone exhibits abundant perimortem breakage, but this is the result of animal chewing in addition to tool-induced damage. Two percent of the bone fragments exhibit cut marks. There are two percussion striae associated with percussion pits in the assemblage. Less than 1 percent of the human bone fragments are burned. There are many missing vertebrae, but 75 fragments are present from cervical thoracic and lumbar areas, and these are from at least two individuals. End polish is present on less than 1 percent of human bone fragments. While the Site 23 assemblage could be seen as meeting these criteria for cannibalism—the frequency of burning is not zero—it does so at a marginal level.

DeGusta's (2000:90) characterization of cannibalized bone from Fiji includes six features: (1) remains found in a midden context, (2) intensive fragmentation, (3) skeletal element distribution that differs from that expected for complete skeletons, (4) lack of evidence for major nonhuman modification, (5) burning on more than 10 percent of human bone, and (6) cut marks on more than 5 percent of human bone. The human bone from Site 23 seems to share the first three characteristics with the Fiji remains, although it seems unlikely that the nonhuman bone assemblage dominated by pig mandibles represents domestic midden refuse. The Site 23 bone has less burning and fewer cut marks than the Fijian material, which may be in part an artifact of the abundant nonhuman modification—for example, rounding, trampling, and animal chewing damage on the Site 23 bone assemblage.

Ethnographic and historical accounts of cannibalism in New Guinea and other parts of Melanesia vary widely in detail and include the killing and consumption of enemies captured in raids (exocannibalism), as well as highly ritualized consumption of all or a few very specific body parts of deceased loved ones or powerful relations (endocannibalism) (Lindenbaum 1979; Brown and Tuzin 1983; Chowning 1991). Each of these variations could leave different archaeological signatures (if any). As DeGusta observes about historical descriptions of cannibalism and noncannibalistic mortuary ritual in Fiji, "these accounts describe such a wide variety of different butchery and consumption practices that virtually any osteological patterning could be accommodated" (1999:240).

Contextualizing Perimortem Mutilation in the Aitape Remains

The taphonomic profile for Site 23 falls within the range of variability in human bone assemblages believed to be cannibalized. But as Kantner (1999) and others (Darling 1998; Dongoske et al. 2000) have written, there are behaviors other than cannibalism that produce perimortem mutilation, including mortuary ritual, warfare, and social control. Consumption of human body parts does not take place in a cultural or ceremonial vacuum. As Ernst remarks about cannibalism in the Onobasulu, "its defining feature is not fundamentally anchored to the beliefs that surround it. The *physical* act of ingesting human flesh is inadequate for defining in any general way a category of sociocultural meaning and practice. Rather, in each instance the question of what it [cannibalism] means for those who practiced it must be asked anew" (Ernst 1999:156). In Melanesia, it was part of the religious and political realms, a factor in the negotiation of relationships between the dead and the living, enemies and allies, family and outsiders, humans and nonhumans. And while the taphonomy data could be used to support an argument for cannibalism in Aitape prehistory, the nonhuman assemblage and the ethnohistoric record of mortuary behavior in New Guinea suggest some alternative scenarios in the creation of this deposit, some of which are listed in table 16.5. With or without cannibalism, other dimensions of mortuary behavior seem to be represented here.

The faunal assemblage from Site 23 is remarkable not only for the fragmentary human remains, but also because it contains the dental remains of at least 11

Table 16.5. Possible Explanations for Contents, Condition, Location of Site 23

Midden contents	Condition of human bone	Disposition of human bone
Cultural		
• Debris from cannibal feast of pigs and humans	• Processed there	• Postcannibalism debris
• Primary or secondary inhumations intruded into domestic food debris deposit	• Processed elsewhere	• Secondary interments
	• Cannibalized	• Primary interments
	• Not cannibalized	• Single event
• Shell and domestic debris used as cover for burials	• Violent death	• Multiple events
	• Natural death	
• Pig feast at burial site		
• Pig mandibles as trophies/personal effects placed at burial site		
Natural		
• Remnant of larger deposit	• Sand, water abrasion	• Washed into crevice from larger deposit uphill or from collapse of structure formerly on site
	• Animal scavenging and bone consumption	• Bone deposited by pigs, dogs

pigs. These include 445 mandible fragments, 22 maxilla fragments, 85 maxilla or mandible fragments, and 275 loose teeth or root fragments (in addition to those in situ in the maxillae and mandibles). At least one juvenile and three confirmed young adults are included. The nearly complete absence of elements from the consumable, fleshy portions of the pig diverges from what we expect to find in a kitchen midden filled with food remains. And as illustrated in figure 16.3, the vertical distribution of pig remains above the bulk of the human remains suggests that these nonhuman remains may have been deposited on top of, or after, the human bone. The concentration of pig mandibles is suggestive of the often-observed practice in parts of New Guinea and Southeast Asia of keeping pig mandibles as hunting trophies (White 1972; Gorecki and Pernetta 1989; Griffin 1998; Hyndman 1991). This is thought to be one factor in the disproportionate number of pig mandibles in some Highland sites (White 1972; Bulmer 1976). Because of the importance of pigs in the Melanesian economy (see, for example, Rappaport 1968) and the integration of the killing and/or trading of pigs in Melanesian mortuary ritual (Jolly 1984; Macintyre 1984; Goodale 1985; Foster 1990), the pig bone strongly suggests a ritual component to the deposit. The pig mandibles could have been buried with the human remains as personal possessions of the deceased or as offerings of wealth and sustenance for the afterlife.

Analysis of the contents of the deposit thus indicates that Site 23 could have been an extant midden in which human remains were interred. People may have been interred in the natural limestone crevice at the top of this small hill and then covered with shell and other material, which served as fill for the grave. The deposit could represent the remains of a feast at which people were consumed and pigs were killed, their edible portions distributed, and their bones disposed of elsewhere.

As described above, the condition of the human bone clearly indicates considerable natural damage to the bone as well as both human- and animal-induced damage. Patterned decapitation and disarticulation is suggested by tool marks at similar locations on the remains of more than one individual (first cervical vertebra, greater sciatic notch). The possibility that at least one skull was processed at this site is suggested by the recovery of a fragment of the anterior rim of the foramen magnum (figure 16.7). Enlargement of the foramen magnum to facilitate the removal of brain tissue, and also for mounting the skull on a pole, is evident in several historic-period skulls from this area of New Guinea (Rieth 1998). However, removal of the brain is a common part of mortuary procedure, in which the skeleton is cleaned after initial decomposition in a temporary grave or on an exposure platform (Stodder and Rieth 2003). This need not be interpreted as a prelude to cannibalism.

Noncultural processes may also be relevant. Could this simply be a peculiar remnant of a larger, now destroyed, deposit? The bone could have washed into a natural limestone crevice, or it could have been deposited there by scavenging animals. Future excavation in the area may reveal a more extensive use area or convincing evidence of habitation structures that would facilitate our understanding of the function of this site. But missing deposits and uncollected data do not answer the question of whether this is a mortuary deposit.

Archaeological Context

The archaeological record for Aitape is virtually nonexistent. The only other human bone found in Aitape is a fossilized 5,000-year-old skull fragment discovered by geologists in 1929 (Chiles 1997; Fenner 1941; Hossfeld 1964, 1965). Other archaeologists have worked in the Sepik-Ramu basin to the east (Swadling et al. 1989, 1991), in the Highlands and foothills (Gorecki 1979; Gorecki and Gillieson 1989), and along the coast between Vanimo and Irian Jaya (Gorecki et al. 1991; Green 1990). But the NGRP excavations were the first archaeological projects conducted in the Aitape area.

Inland, the Ailegun rockshelter in the Jimi-Yuat valley on the fringes of the central Highlands yielded human remains in a niche at the back of the shelter. "Most, if not all of these skeletons were in a secondary burial context. Numerous offerings were scattered in the niche. Among these were one stone axe blade, betel nut bundles, pig jaws, cassowary bones, and fish, bird, and snake bones" (Gorecki and Gillieson 1989:170). The antiquity of this site is not known.

At the Dongan site, a large midden in the Sepik-Ramu basin east of Aitape,

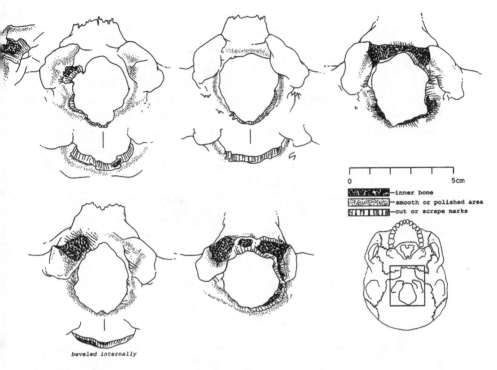

Figure 16.7. Modifications to the foramen magnum on New Guinea crania collected in the early 1900s.

Swadling and coworkers recovered a single human tooth (Swadling et al. 1991), and a small assemblage of human teeth was recovered from the Akari site near Madang (Turner 1993).

To the west of Aitape, small quantities of human bone—several teeth and a few cranial fragments—were found in the midden deposit at Taora Shelter on the coast near the Irian Jaya border (Gorecki et al. 1991). Gorecki also observed caves with multiple individuals along this area of the coast, and Green (1990) visited some of these in the course of in-situ cranial data collection fieldwork. Most of these ossuaries contain only skulls (Gorecki, personal communication, August 18, 1998).

More information directly related to mortuary sites comes from coastal sites in southeastern New Guinea—Flamingo Bay (Egloff 1979), the Milne Bay and Morobe areas (Pietrusewsky 1973), and islands to the east including the D'Entre-casteaux Islands (Egloff 1972), the Trobriands (Austen 1939; Egloff 1972, 1979; Pietrusewsky 1973), and Woodlark Island (Ollier and Pain 1978). Roughly rect-angular structures of upright limestone slabs at Woodlark Island are interpreted as mausoleums or funeral monuments similar to those on the Trobriand Islands (Ollier and Pain 1978; Austen 1939). More commonly human skeletons have been found in funerary pots stored in caves and niches along the coast. Sometimes skulls have been present as well, but as on the north coast, many caves contain only skulls. Egloff also reports some burials in large mounds on Collingwood Bay (1979), and while the antiquity of these burials is uncertain, they do indicate that people were interred in middens. The late Lapita locality on Watom Island (Green and Anson 2000) and a few late prehistoric sites in the Port Moresby–gulf coast area have one or more inhumations associated with villages including Mailu, Motopure, and Nebira 2 (Bulmer 1975).

This brief summary is not exhaustive of New Guinea prehistory, but we believe it is an accurate depiction of the paucity of archaeological activity on the north coast and of the human remains recovered. The archaeological record to date yields few features that fit the classic definition of a primary, undisturbed belowground inhumation (Stodder and Rieth 2003). It is clear that rockshelters and caves were used for the disposal of skeletal remains and for skulls without other bones. In addition to these ossuaries, isolated human remains—teeth and cranial fragments—have also been found in various midden contexts where no mortuary features are evident.

Mortuary Ritual and Human Taphonomy in New Guinea

While the archaeological record is sparse, there is information on mortuary ritual in historical and ethnographic sources on New Guinea. Because this is a place renowned for both linguistic and cultural diversity, overgeneralizing about mortuary behavior on a large scale is unwise, but some consistencies are apparent.

> Death triggers the ceremonies most characteristic of Melanesia, especially of the coastal and lowland regions. Beginning with the funeral, these may culminate years later in great festivals involving dances, masked performances and the dispersing of vast amounts of pork and other food to the participants. . . . Although cremation is practiced in a few places, in many others initial disposal of the body is temporary. It may be exposed on a platform or buried for a few months until decay is complete, but thereafter some or all of the bones may be subject to special treatment. . . . The fate of the bones of the dead varies with the sort of continuing relations desired between their former owners and the living, but often they are deposited in sanctuaries such as caves, or in structures that serve as temples in which the bones will be a focus for future rituals. (Chowning 1986:356–357)

Specifics vary locally and according to gender, age, and social status, but for adults multistage mortuary proceedings were common. For wealthier males in particular it seems that there really is no such thing as an undisturbed primary interment. The use of transit graves and temporary platforms or houses for the several-months-long decomposition stage was followed by exhumation of the

Table 16.6. Interment and Curation of Human Remains in New Guinea

Locality	All	Skull	Mandible	Arm	Leg	Finger	Foot	Rib	Ankle	Any
Central Highlands										
Lake Kutubu						XR				
Lake Kopiago	X	X	X							
Porgera		XR								
Wage/Lai rivers		X	X	X	X					
Mendi				X	X					
Giluwe/Ialibu		X		X	X					
Upper Wahgi	X	X	XR	X	X					
Middle Wahgi		X	X					X		
Chimbu	XR	XR	X	X	X					
Upper Jimi				XR	XR		XR		XR	X
Wonemara	X					X				
Sepik Coast										
Sissano		X		X						
Arop		X		X						

Sources: Highlands: Gorecki 1979:114; Coast: Welsch 1998:146.
Note: X = removed; XR = removed and replaced later.

bones. The bones were cleansed, smoked, and sometimes painted or otherwise decorated.

Which elements were ultimately interred—in a limestone crevice, cave, rock-shelter, or perhaps near a family's garden—varied by locality, as documented in Gorecki's (1979) survey of mortuary behavior information in early patrol reports from the Mount Hagen area of the central Highlands (1950–1965). As shown in table 16.6, skeletons were often interred without the skull and missing one or more other elements. Field Museum curator Albert B. Lewis also recorded information on mortuary behavior. Lewis' diaries from the Joseph N. Field South Pacific Expedition (1909–1914) include these descriptions of mortuary ritual at two villages near Aitape (Sissano and Arop):

> Bodies are buried under the house, being first wrapped in cocoanut leaves, then in *nibung,* and tied with bush rope. For 1 1/2 to 2 days before burial they are placed in a nearly upright position in the house, supported by the house ladder (or similar object). Here the people come to look and mourn. The body is fitted out in best cloths and ornaments. After a certain time, in connection with a sing-sing, the skull and radii are exhumed. The skull is placed in the men's house. The radii are taken by the two nearest relatives (these are definitely determined for all cases) and kept as magical protectors or charms; worn on the breast shield in battle, carried on the canoes to produce wind, etc. (A. B. Lewis, in Welsch 1998:146)

In Arop the dead are not buried, but wrapped up and placed over a small fire in the house. The *nibung* leaf wrapping is arranged so that the fluid from the body is caught in the vessel, and mixed with sago, is eaten by the nearest relatives. They remain there (with the family all around), for at least a year, till completely decayed, when the skeleton is buried, but the skull and radii are kept out. Very thin old men are buried. The radii are used as charms. (A. B. Lewis, in Welsch 1998:146)

The curation of radii in the Highlands and on the coast is intriguing, for these are clearly underrepresented in the Site 23 assemblage. Curation of other skeletal elements seems to have been common as well. Arm and leg bones were given to friends and trade partners to keep or to use as raw material for weapons. The mandible might be kept by a child or parent, perhaps worn in a string bag around the neck. Lewis' collections from the coastal villages include a typical man's bag. Among its contents is a human radius in a magic bundle. A woman's bag contains a polished mandible along with bone hairpins, awls, and betel nut.

While a variety of infracranial elements were kept by friends or relatives and so would not be found with the rest of the skeleton in its final disposition, skulls were subject to an even broader array of processing and curation practices, some of which are listed below. In addition to the literature on mortuary ritual (especially Gorecki 1979; and Lewis as quoted in Welsch 1998), this listing is based on published (Holmes 1897; Dorsey 1897) and original (Rieth 1998) observations of the Field Museum's collection of crania from New Guinea and nearby New Ireland and the Admiralty and Bismarck archipelagos.

Treatments of the skull and possible taphonomic signatures are listed here.

- Decapitation: tool marks at the base of the skull and on the cervical vertebrae (see figure 16.5). However, with sufficient soft-tissue decomposition the skull, mandible, and scalp can be removed without tools; procedures are described at Lake Kutubu in the southern Highlands (Williams 1941), for the Kiwai in the Fly River area (Riley 1925), and others.
- Defleshing: cut and scrape marks at areas of muscle attachment, around the base of the nose and the eyes, and so forth.
- Cleansing: skulls were sometimes smoked as part of cleansing, and this could leave evidence of thermal alteration.
- Removing brains: fractures to occipitals, removal of base of skull, or enlargement of the foramen magnum
- Removing mandible: cut or scrape marks on condyles or rami and at muscle attachment areas on the skull.
- Attaching mandible with fiber: drilled or cut holes in parietals or temporals for attachment of fiber; holes at mandibular notches; grooves or polish at base of nasal cavities, along zygomatic or along inferior surface of mandible, from fiber binding.

- Preparing skull for mounting skull on rack or pole: enlargement of foramen magnum (see figure 16.7) or chopping or breaking out of temporal-parietal junctures for mounting pole laterally through the skull.
- Manufacturing artifacts from skull: tool marks from removal of skull cap for drinking cup; tool marks from removal of central portion of frontal bone (forehead) for amulet; absence of cranial vault or forehead portions.
- Decoration: application of ochre, chalk, or other media for modeling or painting; incised design on parietals and frontal.
- Curation and display: in men's houses, special "skull house," on porch or in entryway of house as pile or bundle; at boundary markers or settlement entrances.
- Ritual travel: in "skull cycle" for several years after death, as described for the Kualong (Goodale 1985).
- Interment: with other skulls in cave or crevice; in family burial area; in bush at place of death; in ancestral shrine.
- Discard: in river or trash heap, of skulls no longer of significance to relatives or owners.

In sum, multistage mortuary ritual is typical for Papua New Guinea, and intact human skeletons in primary interments seem very unlikely to be a common archaeological feature on the north coast or in the Highlands of New Guinea. For those of us accustomed to clearly defined pit features containing extended skeletons with grave goods, the notion of what constitutes a burial and a mortuary feature must be reshaped to accommodate the archaeological record in a place where there is in a sense no such thing as a primary burial. A burial in this area might be one or two bones, or everything except the skull. Bones could be found in primary, secondary, or even tertiary context. They might be encountered in what looks like an earth oven, in a midden, in a natural or constructed limestone crevice, in a rockshelter, or in a cave. The bone(s) might be accompanied by the remains of close relatives, distant ancestors, pigs, cassowaries, or other animals.

Conclusion

Several taphonomic agents contributed to the condition of the bone found at Site 23, and there are several possible explanations for the contents of the deposit. The skewed faunal assemblage could simply be the result of the rest of the deposit disappearing over the last 1,300 years. The bone could be the remains of a cannibal feast complete with 11 pigs. Or it could be the burial of a man with his hunting trophies and his relatives, minus most of their crania and arm bones. It seems reasonable to infer that the bone assemblage from Site 23 is a group of secondary interments. The deposit and the skeletal remains are in a natural limestone crevice: the mortuary location of choice for the nearby central Highland and coastal groups surveyed. The pig mandibles suggest feast remains or a personal trophy array. Skulls were removed with shell or bamboo tools by (in part) severing the longus colli muscle. Mandibles were detached, apparently in a similar manner as they are removed from pig crania. Most of the skull vaults as well as most of the forearm bones are missing. At least one skull seems to have been processed for mounting on a pole by enlargement of the foramen magnum. The long bones especially were damaged by pig, and perhaps also dog, chewing—perhaps when the bones were in a shallow temporary grave or on a platform, prior to their deposition at Site 23.

The taphonomic signature of mortuary ritual on the north coast of New Guinea is complex and presumably variable. Admittedly we know little about it at this early stage in the archaeological exploration of the area. We do not suggest that mortuary practices were the same in A.D. 700 and 1909 or 1952, but the similarities are compelling: just as compelling as the taphonomic suggestion of cannibalism, for which there is no accepted evidence on the north coast. When we go beyond the constraints of the "cannibalism or not" question and examine the Site 23 assemblage in the context of the rich and detailed information on mortuary ritual in Papua New Guinea, these fragments of bone—those that are present and those that are missing—suggest 1,300 years of continuity in several dimensions of mortuary ritual on the Sepik Coast.

Acknowledgments

The author gratefully acknowledges the assistance of John E. Terrell, Timothy Rieth, David Reese, Rob Welsch, Daniel Nolan, Michele T. Douglas, Terry Hunt, and Anne Grauer. The drawings (figures 16.5 and 16.7) are by Eric Wert. The photographs were taken by John Weinstein.

17

Were Nasca Trophy Heads War Trophies or Revered Ancestors?

Insights from the Kroeber Collection

Kathleen Forgey and Sloan R. Williams

Max Uhle coined the term "trophy head" in 1914 to describe the culturally modified human heads he found in the Nazca valley,[1] assuming that they were trophies taken in battle from fallen enemies. Julio Tello (1918) examined several similar heads and concluded that the heads were important symbols of religious and social power, not simply war trophies. Tello argued that the presence of women and children in his sample, in conjunction with the fact that the heads exhibited the "Nasca" cranial deformation, indicated that the heads had not been taken from slain enemies. Thus, these two central figures in Peruvian archaeology first framed the arguments of a controversy that has persisted for nearly a century.

Coelho (1972:79–80) has outlined the following possible uses of Nasca trophy heads: "enemy trophies of warfare, fertility symbols, cult objects, serving a religious purpose, or the cause or result of human sacrifice."[2] Nasca iconography provides support for each of these explanations, leading Coelho to suggest that the heads would be more appropriately termed "ceremonial heads" (1972:45). Silverman (1993:chapter 15), Proulx (1989), and Carmichael (1995) note that the imagery of Paracas and Early Nasca iconography shows a relationship between trophy heads, ancestors, and principles of fertility, regeneration, and rebirth. The frequent depictions of trophy heads in war-related contexts have led many researchers (Roark 1965; Sawyer 1966, 1972; Verano 1995; Zuidema 1972), including Proulx (1971, 1989, 2001), to argue that slain enemies were the source of the artifacts.

Ancestor worship was a key component of Inca and other native religions when the Spanish arrived in 1532. Andean religious, social, and political practices revolved around ancestor worship and are described in great detail by ethnohistorians (Cobo 1990). Knowledge of the concept's importance in later cultures probably led Tello (1918) and Coelho (1972; Neira Avedaño and Coelho

Table 17.1. Chronology of the Nazca Valley

Year	Standard chronology	Phase	Culture name	Kroeber phase	Cultural event
A.D. 1476	Late Horizon				Inca conquest
	Late Intermediate period			Late	Regional cultures re-establis
		4			Societal collapse
	Middle	3			
	Horizon	2	Huaca del Loro	Nasca Y	Wari conquest
A.D. 750		1			
		7	Late Nasca		Reorganization
	Early	6		Nasca B	
	Intermediate	5	Middle Nasca		Transition
	period	4		Nasca A2	
		3	Early Nasca	Nasca A1	Emergence of Nasca culture
A.D. 1		2		Nasca A0	
1000 B.C.	Early Horizon (phases 1–10)		Paracas		Initial permanent occupatio
	Initial period				Unoccupied?
	Preceramic period				Temporary hunter-gatherer occupations

Source: Adapted from Schreiber 1998.

1972) to propose ancestor worship as a potential explanation for the elaborately prepared Nasca trophy heads. In addition to the presence of men, women, and children and the shared "Nasca" cranial deformation pattern, the similar burial treatment received by both the trophy heads and the Nasca dead was used to further support their argument. More recently, Carmichael (1988, 1995) has argued the case for ancestor worship by focusing on evidence for the postmortem manipulation of Nasca dead. He describes several examples of tombs that appeared to have been reopened to remove human body parts and suggests that the Nasca used these objects for the veneration of the dead. Carmichael (1988:379–381) also presents two iconographic images that depict what he believes are images of ancestor worship. One ceramic vessel shows an individual holding a trophy head next to a huge mummy bundle, and the other vessel shows a number of trophy heads inside a step-sided temple or tomb. The detailed ethnohistoric accounts of ancestor worship in the Andes, when combined with the possible examples of the ritual use of human body parts taken from Nasca dead and iconographic depictions, provide support for ancestor veneration as the source of these trophy heads.

Proulx (1971, 1989, 2001) agrees that the Nasca trophy heads have a larger meaning than one of mere war trophy, but he has forcefully argued that warfare was the source of the heads. He believes that the numerous iconographic images linking trophy heads and headless bodies with battle scenes demonstrate that warfare provided the means by which heads were collected. Proulx (2001:Figure 6.10) is particularly impressed by a ceramic image depicting a warrior holding an enemy warrior by the hair with one hand and armed with a knife in the other. He also uses ethnographic analogy, particularly of headhunting as practiced by the Jívaro of Ecuador, to infer Nasca intent (Proulx 1989). Finally, he cites Verano's (1995) osteological analysis, in which 85 percent of the trophy heads he studied were young to middle-aged males, as evidence that the dead were young male warriors.

Although trophy head iconography is common in the Andes, the osteological evidence for trophy heads is relatively rare and is largely confined to late Early Horizon and Early Intermediate periods (table 17.1) in the Río Grande de Nazca drainage system. Approximately 145 trophy heads have been reported from this region. Eighteen of those heads are part of the Kroeber collection housed at the Field Museum in Chicago. The trophy heads from this collection are particularly significant because they, unlike many of the heads, come from archaeologically documented contexts. These heads were recovered from burials and sites excavated in the Nazca valley during two expeditions led by Alfred L. Kroeber in 1925 and 1926 (Kroeber and Collier 1998). This chapter describes our osteological analysis of those remains and discusses the insights that these artifacts provide for the larger issue of the nature and role that trophy heads played in Nasca society and the larger Andean world.

Background

Archaeological Setting

The Nasca culture flourished on the south coast of Peru during the Early Intermediate period (figure 17.1; see table 17.1). The heartland of the Nasca culture is the valley of the Nazca River, one of ten tributaries forming the Río Grande de Nazca drainage. On the basis of ceramic stylistic similarities, Uhle (1914) considered this culture to be a continuation of the Paracas tradition but sufficiently unique to warrant its own style. Its pottery was characterized by pre-fire slip painting depicting complex iconographic themes. The presence of large mounds at the ceremonial site of Cahuachi and large architectural features like the famous Nazca lines initially led archaeologists to assume that the Nasca were a state-level society (Lanning 1967; Lumbreras 1974; Rowe 1963). Recent work (Carmichael 1988, 1995; Schreiber 1998; Silverman 1993; Silverman and Proulx 2002) indicates that these large structures were achieved by a less complex sociopolitical system.

The Early Intermediate period was a time of dynamism in the Nazca valley; settlement patterns changed as people moved from the many small villages scattered over the landscape that they had inhabited in the earlier phases to a small number of much larger towns in the later ones (see Schreiber 1998 and Silverman

2002 for reviews). These settlement changes are explained at least in part by a series of devastating droughts, which forced the Nasca people into large settlements located near a series of underground aqueducts (also called filtration galleries or *pukios*) developed to provide new water sources. The dramatic social and political changes that accompanied these settlement shifts undoubtedly affected all aspects of Nasca social, political, and religious life.

Iconographic Evidence

Depictions of decapitated heads, commonly referred to as trophy heads, appear on ceramic vessels, textiles, and sculpture throughout the pre-Columbian Andes (Blasco Bosqued and Ramos Gomez 1974; Paul 1990; Proulx 1968; Tello 1918; Toussaint-Devine 1984; Uhle 1914). The images are present for over 3,000 years, from their first appearance on sculptures and ceramics in the Initial period (Cordy-Collins 1992) to depictions of Inca trophy head taking and display in the chronicles (Guáman Poma de Ayala 1980:130, 168).

Decapitated heads first appear during the Initial period in the north coast and highlands regions. They are key components of the "decapitator theme" on north coast Cupisnique ceramics (Cordy-Collins 1992). The images continue to hold an important position in the Early Horizon and are found throughout the area of Chavín influence in northern and central Peru (Benson 2001; Burger 1992:Figure 163). Decapitated or trophy head iconography is also common in the altiplano and is seen at Pucará, an Early Horizon and Early Intermediate period site (Chavez 1992; Moseley 1992:Plate 40) and the Middle Horizon site of Tiwanaku (Kolata 1993:Figures 5.23, 5.24, 5.30, 5.31). Trophy heads are also depicted in Wari Middle Horizon art (Cook 2001). On the north coast, trophy head iconography continues to appear through the Late Intermediate period in Lambayeque (Sicán) art and the Late Horizon in Chimú objects (Lapiner 1976) but is not seen elsewhere in these periods, at least in part because the emphasis shifts to geometric instead of realistic designs.

On the south coast, trophy head images begin to appear in the Late Paracas period as part of the spread of Chavín themes and ideology (Early Horizon, phases 9 and 10; see table 17.1). In the Late Paracas and Early Nasca phases (Early Intermediate period, phases 1–4; see table 17.1), trophy heads are often associated with mythical beings such as the "Killer Whale" and the "Oculate Being" (Menzel et al. 1964). Peters (1991:311) states that trophy head images in Late Paracas and Early Nasca iconography occur in three main contexts: "with hunter/warriors, with beans and feline/monkey figures, and with condors and images of human sacrifice." Townsend (1985) notes that Nasca iconographic depictions of death, rejuvenation, and human sacrifice reflect an association with agricultural fertility. Trophy head depictions are most prevalent in the Early Nasca epochs and begin to decline in frequency in the Nazca valley toward the end of Epoch 4 (Proulx 1968:89). A strong association between war images and trophy heads emerges in Middle Nasca (Epoch 5) and continues throughout the later phases and into the Middle Horizon (Roark 1965; Silverman 1993). Militaristic themes dominate these later phases, and trophy heads are depicted in or near battle scenes. The heads are also shown being held by individuals instead of mythical beings (Silverman and Proulx 2002:149). Many new ritual practices appear in the Wari culture of the subsequent Middle Horizon, such as the breaking of beautifully painted urns and jars for burial offerings, but the theme of sacrificers holding trophy heads remains an important image. Interestingly, Cook (2001) notes the presence of two different sacrificer images in Wari iconography: the front-facing staff deity also found on earlier Nasca textiles, and the profile staff figure found in altiplano Pucará and Tiwanaku iconography. She suggests that the presence of both images represents an integration of coastal and highland themes during this period.

Clearly, Nasca trophy head imagery changes over time, from earlier depictions that are associated with mythical and/or naturalistic themes to the militaristic themes that dominate the later periods. Silverman (1993) and Browne and colleagues (1993), noting this trend, have posited that the taking of trophy heads became "secularized" through time.

Physical Evidence

Most of the physical evidence for head taking comes from the south coast. Although some decapitated heads have been found in other parts of the Andes, most of the heads from other regions show no evidence of modification (Verano 2001a). Rare examples of modified crania have been recovered from several sites outside the Nazca region. For example, Verano et al. (1999) found two crania modified into bowls in the urban sector of the Moche pyramids. An Initial period bowl made from a fire-hardened human calva was found at Shillacoto (Izumi et al. 1972). Decapitated heads with perforations similar to those found in Nasca trophy heads were found at Aspero, a preceramic coastal site (Engel 1967). Wari trophy heads found at Conchapata have perforations at Bregma on the cranial vault instead of the forehead perforation typical of the Nasca type (Tung 2003).

Unlike the famous Jívaro shrunken heads of Amazonia, Nasca trophy heads retain the skull as well as the surrounding soft tissues. The frontal bone of the skull was perforated to allow a suspensory cord to be attached, and some portion of the base of the skull was removed, possibly to facilitate the removal of the brain and other soft tissues. Additional preparation of Nasca heads often included sealing the lips and/or eyelids of the individual with desert plant spines and inserting plain-weave cotton cloth into the eye sockets and beneath the skin of the cheeks and jaw.

Physical evidence of trophy head practices has been found in the Nazca valley, particularly at the important ceremonial site of Cahuachi (see figure 17.1), but also in other tributaries and adjacent valleys. These practices span a broader time

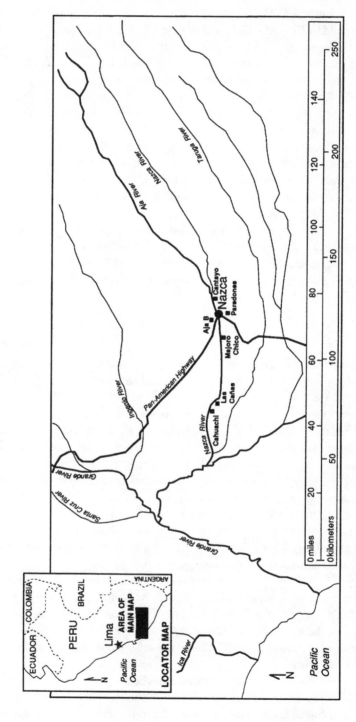

Figure 17.1. Map of the Nazca valley showing sites excavated by Kroeber where trophy heads were found (adapted from Silverman 1993).

Table 17.2. Summary of Trophy Head Information

Specimen number	Sex	Age	Deformation form
1	Male?	Young adult	Anteroposterior
2	Male	Young adult	Anteroposterior
3	Undetermined	Young adult	Anteroposterior vertical
4	Male	Young adult	Anteroposterior
5	Male	Young adult	Anteroposterior
6	Undetermined	Young adult	Anteroposterior
7	Undetermined	Young adult	Anteroposterior
8	Undetermined	Child, 4–6 years	Anteroposterior
9	Female	Young adult	Anteroposterior
10	Female	Young adult	Anteroposterior oblique
11	Undetermined	Subadult, 15–16 years	Anteroposterior oblique
12	Undetermined	Subadult, 14–18 years	Anteroposterior vertical
13	Undetermined	Child, 8–10 years	Anteroposterior oblique
14	Male	Young-middle adult	Anteroposterior oblique
15	Male	Young adult	Anteroposterior vertical
16	Male	Young adult	Anteroposterior vertical
17	Male	Young adult	Anteroposterior
18	Undetermined	Middle-older adult	Unknown

range than was previously believed. Several researchers recovered Nasca period trophy heads at Cahuachi (Doering 1958, 1966; Drusini and Baraybar 1991; Orefici 1993; Silverman 1993; Strong 1957:36, described more fully in Silverman 1993). A large cache of 48 trophy heads was found at Cerro Carapo in the valley of the Palpa River, a tributary of the Río Grande de Nazca drainage (Browne et al. 1993). Pezzia Assereto (1968) found two caches of trophy heads in the Ica valley. Frances Riddell (personal communication 2001) as well as Coelho and Neira Avedaño (Coelho 1972; Neira Avedaño and Coelho 1972) recovered trophy heads from excavations in the Acarí valley. Most of the heads date to the Early Intermediate period, but some come from the earlier Paracas period (Pezzia Assereto 1968; Verano 1995), and others date to the subsequent Middle Horizon and perhaps even the Late Intermediate period (this chapter).

The Kroeber Collection

During A. L. Kroeber's excavations in 1925 and 1926, 18 trophy heads were found (table 17.2). They were recovered from six sites: Aja (n=1), Cahuachi (n=10), Cantayo (n=2), Las Cañas (n=1), Majoro Chico (n=2), and Paredones (n=2) (see figure 17.1). Three of the 18 skulls Kroeber brought back to the United States (Specimens 1, 11, and 18) would not now be recognized as trophy heads because they are very incomplete, but we included them in our analysis because of his excellent descriptions. Kroeber's field notes (n.d.) demonstrate that he was well aware of the criteria necessary for a cranium to be labeled a trophy head.

Frontal perforation location and the extent of the posterior cranium removed were carefully recorded for each specimen collected during that trip. Specimen 18 is very fragmentary, however, so we deleted it from most of the summary statistics.

The Kroeber collection specimens described here are now primarily skeletalized, but the condition of most skulls is excellent. Shreds of soft tissues remain on the majority of the heads, but none is completely mummified. Verano (1995) has argued that these artifacts should be labeled trophy heads to indicate their original state as depicted in Paracas and Nasca iconography. The residual soft tissues that remain on these heads indicate that disintegration, not intentional removal, is responsible for their present condition. Therefore, the convention of referring to them as trophy heads will be followed here.

Methods

A series of standard observations was recorded following Buikstra and Ubelaker (1994). The absence of postcranial remains meant that age estimates were based primarily on dental eruption, with cranial suture closure and relative size used as corroborative evidence. Dental wear was observed but not weighted heavily because sample size was insufficient to permit an assessment of dental wear patterns in the population. Sex determination was based on cranial features, again because there were no postcranial remains. Buikstra and Ubelaker's guidelines were used to record demographic information. Anton's (1989) naming conventions for artificial cranial deformation patterns were followed. Cranial deformation was difficult to assess in many cases because the posterior half of the cranium had been removed as a part of the trophy-making process. We could usually assess the general category of deformation style, whether anteroposterior or circumferential, but subclassification as vertical or oblique was frequently impossible. Pathology assessment was based on visual inspection. Bone surfaces were easily observed in the majority of cases. No radiographs were taken of the specimens. Perimortem modification was described, and measurements were taken when possible. Descriptions of archaeological context were taken from Kroeber's unpublished field notes and Kroeber and Collier's then-unpublished manuscript (Kroeber and Collier 1998). Carmichael's analysis (1988) of the tomb contents from the Kroeber collection provided additional information about the cemeteries and several of the graves. Associated grave contents were studied and photographed when available. Detailed descriptions and photographs of each trophy head can be found in Williams and colleagues 2001.

Results

Demographic patterns, cranial deformation style, pathology and other features, perimortem modification practices, and archaeological context and associated

Table 17.3. Age and Sex Distribution of Trophy Heads

Site	Adult Male	Female	Unknown sex	Subadult	Child	Total
Aja	1	—	—	—	—	1
Cahuachi	3	2	3	1	1	10
Cantayo	—	—	—	1	1	2
Las Cañas	1	—	—	—	—	1
Majoro Chico	2	—	—	—	—	2
Paredones	1	—	1	—	—	2
Total	8	2	4	2	2	18

artifacts were surveyed in our osteological analyses. Each will be discussed in turn, with comparisons with findings from previous work.

Table 17.2 records age, sex, and cranial shape by individual. Table 17.3 summarizes the age and sex estimations for each of the trophy heads and presents them by site. The collection contained 14 adults, 2 subadults, and 2 children. Of the adults, 7 were male, 1 was probably male, and 2 were female; the sex of the remaining 4 adults could not be determined.

Trophy head sex and age distribution has been presented as evidence both for and against enemies as the source of the heads. Proulx (1989, 2001; Silverman and Proulx 2002) and others have argued that the predominance of young males indicates that warfare was the source of many trophy skulls. Verano (1995) presented the strongest case for this argument, reporting that 85 percent of the 84 trophy heads he studied were adult males. In contrast, Coelho (1972; Neira Avedaño and Coelho 1972), Tello (1918), and Drusini and Baraybar (1991) each described samples that included men, women, and children. Here, 6 (43 percent) of the 14 individuals whose age and sex could be determined were women and children. The presence of women and children in the sample does not necessarily mean that the heads were not obtained through warfare, however. Their presence instead may indicate that raiding was a common practice. For example, the Jívaro of Ecuador and the Iatmül of Papua New Guinea both considered taking heads of women and children during raids a legitimate practice, and in certain cases they were the preferred targets (Bateson 1932, 1958; Harner 1972; Trompf 1991).

Anteroposterior cranial deformation was recorded in the 17 individuals for which observation was possible (see table 17.2). Four specimens were assigned to the vertical subtype, and 4 were assigned to the oblique subtype. The remaining 9 specimens could not be specified to subtype.

Both Coelho (1972; Neira Avedaño and Coelho 1972) and Tello (1918) argued that the "Nasca" deformation style characteristic of the Nasca trophy heads demonstrates a shared ethnic identity, but in fact, this deformation style is ambiguously defined in the literature. Generally, researchers agree that Nasca

Table 17.4. Summary of Frontal Bone Perforation and Cranial Base Breakage Areas

Specimen number	Site	Relative size	Minimum diameter	Maximum diameter	Perforation to nasion	Nasion to bregma	Area removed
				Frontal bone perforation			Cranial base break
1	Aja	Small?	9.5	NP	NP	NP	Posterior cranium
2	Cahuachi	Small	7	8	33	124	Posterior cranium
3	Cahuachi	Large	21	24	9	104.5	Foramen magnum
4	Cahuachi	Small	5	9	44	109	Posterior cranium
5	Cahuachi	Small	7	8	31	100.5	Posterior cranium
6	Cahuachi	Small	8	9	19	107	Posterior cranium
7	Cahuachi	Small	9	9	39	102	Posterior cranium
8	Cahuachi	Small	7.5	9	21.5	91	Posterior cranium
9	Cahuachi	Small	8.5	10	34	112	Posterior cranium
10	Cahuachi	Large?	15.5	19?	NP	NP	Foramen magnum
11	Cahuachi	Large?	>10	NP	NP	NP	Inferior occipital b
12	Cantayo	Large	16	21.5	0	99.5	Foramen magnum
13	Cantayo	Small	8	12	23	100.5	Posterior cranium
14	Las Cañas	Small	6	8	63	113	Posterior cranium
15	Majoro Chico	Large	17.5	22	24	107.5	Inferior occipital b
16	Majoro Chico	Large	18	21	9	107	Foramen magnum
17	Paredones	Small	8	13	29.5	108.5	Posterior cranium
18	Paredones	Small?	NP	NP	NP	NP	Unknown

Note: NP = no posterior margin present. All measurements are in millimeters.

deformation is an anteroposterior form, but further classification differs according to the researcher (Allison et al. 1981; Drusini and Baraybar 1991; Orefici 1993; Pezzia Assereto 1968; Weiss 1961). Kroeber (n.d.:26) reported that Nasca frontal deformation reflected local and perhaps temporal variations of custom within the geographical and chronological limits of a larger culture. The trophy heads described here were uniformly anteroposterior but varied in subtype. Both subtypes were found at Cahuachi and Cantayo.

Nasca deformation encompasses too much variation for use as an ethnicity identifier without more careful study. Furthermore, even if a "Nasca" style can be identified, Verano (1995) rightly argues that warfare in this area could have been intraethnic in nature. Thus, groups could share the same cranial deformation style preferences and yet consider each other enemies.

Relatively little pathology or trauma was observed in this collection. The young age of many of the individuals in the sample contributed in part to the generally good levels of health. Healed porotic hyperostosis was observed on the posterior vault of one subadult, and no cases of cribra orbitalia were found. Inactive or healing lytic lesions were observed on the superior vault of one adult individual. Slight active periostitis was noted on an 8–10-year-old child's left mandibular notch, probably related to imminent dental eruption. Degenerative

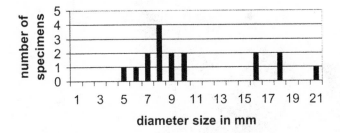

Figure 17.2. Chart showing distribution of frontal perforation diameter.

joint disease was observed in one adult individual, where slight porosity was present on both occipital condyles. Mild to pronounced periodontal disease and dental abscesses were observed in about 65 percent of the specimens. Fractures were identified on three crania: one antemortem, one postmortem, and one possibly perimortem.

Perimortem trauma often is cited as evidence of warfare, and high frequencies of perimortem cranial trauma in trophy head collections would be powerful evidence that the heads were taken in battle. However, few examples of perimortem trauma have been found in trophy heads. Only one of the 48 Cerro Carapo trophy heads exhibited a cranial fracture that occurred at or near the time of death (Silverman 1993:223). Likewise, only one of the three cranial fractures seen in the Kroeber collection exhibited the spiral fracture pattern typical of perimortem trauma. Its rarity in these collections is not strong evidence that warfare does not account for head-taking activities, though, because death can result from many violent acts that do not result in cranial trauma and classic compression fractures.

The size and placement of the frontal perforation and the amount of the posterior cranium that is removed varied in this sample (table 17.4). The perforations could be divided into two categories by perforation size. The small perforations averaged 7.6 millimeters in diameter, while the large perforations averaged 17.6 millimeters in diameter (figure 17.2). The small perforations were located in the center of the frontal bone, placed approximately on the midline of the bone. The large perforations were located roughly at glabella. The amount of bone removed from the base of each cranium ranged from a slight expansion of the foramen magnum to the complete removal of the posterior cranium. The foramen magnum was enlarged in 4 specimens by the removal of one or both of the occipital condyles and the posterior margin. The entire basioccipital and squamosal portions of the occipital bone were removed in 2 cases. The entire occipital bone and the posterior portions of the parietal and temporal bones (that is, the entire posterior portion) were removed in the remaining 11 crania.

The frontal bone and posterior cranium modifications observed in this sample were organized into three groups, based on the frontal perforation size and posi-

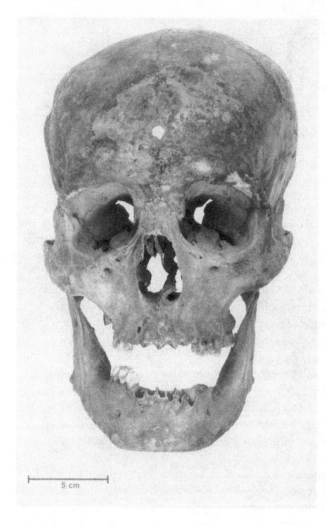

5 cm

Figure 17.3. Frontal perforation, preparation style 1. Specimen 2, FMNH 170222, neg. #A113611. Copyright by the Field Museum.

tion and the size of the posterior enlargement (see table 17.4). The first group was characterized by a very small frontal perforation about 10 millimeters in diameter in the middle of the forehead combined with the removal of most of the posterior cranium, including the posterior half of the parietal bones (figures 17.3 and 17.4). The second group was defined by a large hole about 20 millimeters in diameter at glabella combined with an enlargement of the foramen magnum and very little posterior region involvement (figures 17.5 and 17.6). The final group was characterized by a large hole similar to that found in group 2 but with the entire basioccipital portion of the occipital bone removed (figures 17.7 and 17.8). Eleven trophy heads were included in the first group, four heads were of the second type, and two heads were of the third style.

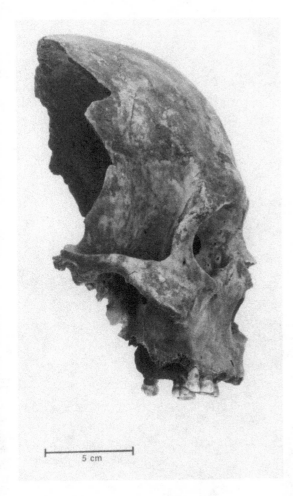

Figure 17.4. Lateral view of posterior enlargement, preparation style 1. Specimen 2, FMNH 170222, neg. #A113634. Copyright by the Field Museum.

5 cm

Most of Kroeber's trophy heads showed other evidence of processing, in addition to the frontal perforation and posterior enlargement, which is described in more detail elsewhere (Williams et al. 2001). Cut marks were present on the cranial vault and mandible surfaces of all but three of the trophy heads. Resin was applied to the cut bone margins of the posterior enlargement areas and the edges of the larger frontal perforations in six specimens. Application of resin to these margins would effectively seal them and prevent seepage of the spongy interior. Gauze pads were present in the orbits and/or nasal apertures of three specimens. During excavations, Kroeber and Collier (1998:50) noted the presence of gauze pads in the orbits of an additional specimen, but those pads are not present in the collection.

Evidence for prolonged use in some of these specimens suggests an ongoing ritual function. Wear on the frontal perforations where the cords rubbed against

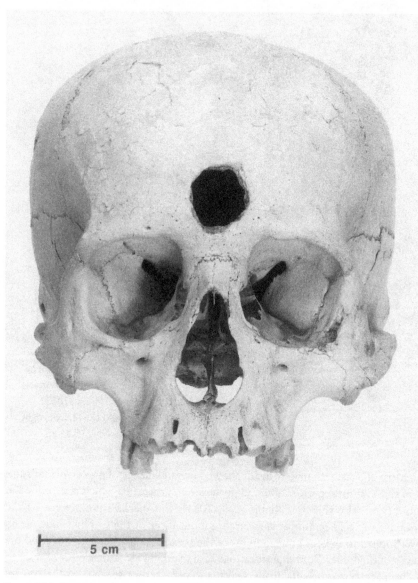

Figure 17.5. Frontal perforation, preparation style 2. Specimen 3, FMNH 170224, neg. #A113587. Copyright by the Field Museum.

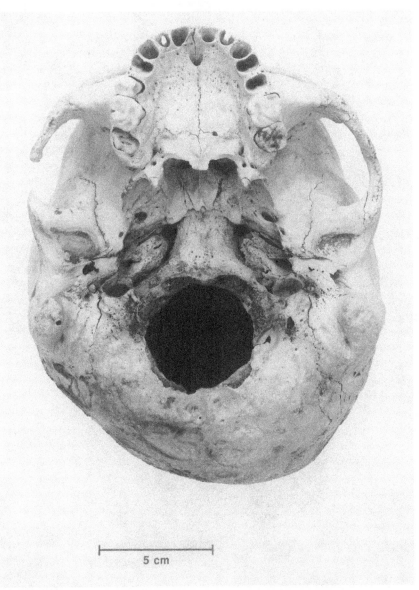

5 cm

Figure 17.6. Posterior enlargement, preparation style 2. Specimen 3, FMNH 170224, neg. #A11590. Copyright by the Field Museum.

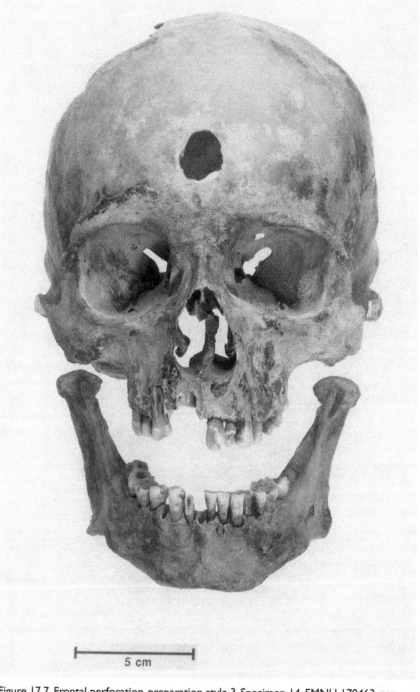

Figure 17.7. Frontal perforation, preparation style 3. Specimen 14, FMNH 170463, neg. #A11593. Copyright by the Field Museum.

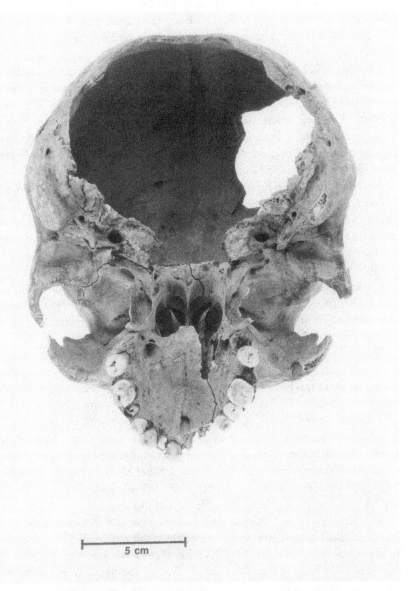

5 cm

Figure 17.8. Posterior enlargement, preparation style 3. Specimen 14, FMNH 170463, neg. #A11594. Copyright by the Field Museum.

the bone was observed in six cases and is most pronounced on the right edges. Wear polish was noted on the zygomatic arch of one specimen and the left gonial angle of another. The wig found attached to one of the trophy heads suggests prolonged use of that specimen. The discolored areas observed on two other specimens may be the remnants of the glues once used to attach similar items to those heads.

Guillén (1992) and Verano (1995) both emphasize the importance of the time and effort invested in the making of trophy heads. Guillén believes that this kind of attention would more likely be lavished on relatives than on enemies and suggests that these heads are better explained as evidence of an ancestor cult. Verano, by contrast, although agreeing that the heads hold ritual significance beyond that of a simple battle trophy, remains convinced that enemies are the most likely source of the heads.

Evidence for the careful preservation and display of remains taken from both ancestors and enemies is present in the ethnographic record (Bateson 1932, 1958; Haddon 1901; Harner 1972; Holmes 1924; Landtman 1927; Saville 1926; Seligmann 1910; Trompf 1991). The Jívaro made shrunken heads of warfare victims (Harner 1972). Melanesian groups, particularly those in Papua New Guinea and the Solomon Islands, made skulls with elaborate modeled faces made of clay, sap, and fiber from the heads of both ancestors and enemies (Bateson 1932, 1958; Forge 1973; Keesing 1982:#2215; Lewis 1951:201; Trompf 1991). In Mexico, ritual defleshing (Beck and Sievert, this volume) and the display of decapitated enemy skulls resulted in patterned modification (Miller 1999).

The elaborate preparation seen in the Nasca-area trophy heads is rare in the archaeological record of the Andes. For example, although the Nasca are often compared with the Early Intermediate period Moche of the north coast, where decapitated heads have been found as well, the Moche pattern is quite different. The Moche severed heads were found in association with cervical vertebrae, which often bore cut marks on their anterior and lateral surfaces. No evidence of further modification or preparation or of ongoing use in subsequent Moche ritual was present. Verano (2001a) comments that Moche imagery focuses more heavily on bloodletting and dismemberment and is seemingly less concerned with the taking of heads than with the collection of blood.

The Kroeber collection spans the periods from late Paracas to the Middle Horizon/Late Intermediate period, based on associated artifacts or those found in surrounding tombs (table 17.5). Neither the heads nor any of the other grave contents have been radiocarbon dated. Two of the heads were found on the surface, so little is known of their original context, but the remaining 16 heads are from undisturbed or minimally disturbed contexts. Roughly one-third of the sample (8 of the Kroeber trophy heads) can be placed in the Early Intermediate period, phases 1–4. The ceramics found in a Paredones tomb that contained 2 trophy heads date to the Late Nasca period (Kroeber and Collier 1998). The

Table 17.5. Archaeological Context of Trophy Heads

Specimen number	Site	Phase	Basis for date	Context	Disturbance
1	Aja	EIP 2–3	Sherd found in grave	Cache	Intact
2	Cahuachi	Unknown	N/A	Surface	Disturbed
3	Cahuachi	MH/LIP	Textile found in tomb	Tomb	Disturbed
4	Cahuachi	MH/LIP	Textile found in tomb	Tomb	Disturbed
5	Cahuachi	MH/LIP	Textile found in tomb	Tomb	Disturbed
6	Cahuachi	MH/LIP	Textile found in tomb	Tomb	Disturbed
7	Cahuachi	MH/LIP	Textile found in tomb	Tomb	Disturbed
8	Cahuachi	MH/LIP	Textile found in tomb	Tomb	Disturbed
9	Cahuachi	EIP 1–3?	Surrounding graves	Tomb	Disturbed
10	Cahuachi	EIP 1–3	Surrounding graves	Cache	Intact
11	Cahuachi	EIP 1–3	Surrounding graves	Cache	Intact
12	Cantayo	EIP 1–3	Sherds found in grave	Tomb?	Disturbed?
13	Cantayo	EIP 1–2	Grave contents	Structure?	Disturbed?
14	Las Cañas	Unknown	N/A	Surface	Disturbed
15	Majoro Chico	EIP 3	Sherds found in grave	Structure	Disturbed?
16	Majoro Chico	EIP	Surrounding graves	Structure	Intact
17	Paredones	LN	Tomb contents	Tomb	Disturbed
18	Paredones	LN	Tomb contents	Tomb	Disturbed

Note: EIP = Early Intermediate period; MH = Middle Horizon; LIP = Late Intermediate period; LN = Late Nasca.

remaining 6 heads were recovered from a large, rectangular Middle Horizon/ Late Intermediate period tomb like the ones described by Doering (1958, 1966).

The trophy heads were found in three main archaeological contexts (see table 17.5): (1) in architectural features; (2) included as grave goods in the burials of others; and (3) buried alone or in small caches in cemeteries. Three trophy heads were found in pits dug near walls like the ones that Coelho (1972) and Silverman (1993) described at Chaviña and Cahuachi, respectively. Ten of the trophy heads were found in tombs. Six of those were found in the Middle Horizon tomb described above. The last three trophy heads were recovered from two caches, unassociated with other grave goods. One head was buried in a pit beneath a large jar fragment in a cemetery at Aja. The second cache was located on the summit of Cahuachi Location A and contained three trophy heads (Kroeber and Collier 1998:78–79). One was left behind when it fragmented in the field.

Coelho (1972; Neira Avedaño and Coelho 1972) posited that burial context reveals aspects of the intentions of the makers of trophy heads. She believed that the Chaviña heads she studied were placed in a ceremonial structure, which she considered evidence of a ritual function not necessarily related to warfare. Coelho also noted that Nasca trophy heads often were accorded a burial treatment similar to Nasca individuals, which suggests a shared ethnic identity. Verano (1995) pointed out that many trophy heads were recovered from architectural features or caches. He argued that the fact that trophy heads were rarely buried in graves implies corporate ownership of the heads. This argument may prove true for some of the heads, but half of the heads in the Kroeber collection were found in graves.

Discussion

The patterns observed in our osteological analysis provide partial explanations for the great variability seen in trophy head iconography, physical attributes, and archaeological context. First, three lines of evidence (iconography, demographic composition, and disposal method) imply that the meaning and role that trophy heads held in Nasca society changed through time. Second, the patterned variation seen in trophy head preparation methods suggests that trophy heads were prepared by different means to serve different functions in different contexts.

Silverman (1993) and Browne and colleagues (1993) correlated changes in iconography through time with increasing trophy head prevalence. Trophy head images were associated with mythical beings in early periods but appeared with warriors and warfare in later periods. Trophy head image frequency is highest in the earlier periods and is inversely proportional to the number of actual trophy head finds, which increase through time. Silverman (1993:223) and Browne and colleagues (1993) suggested that headhunting became more "secularized" through time. They emphasized the association of trophy heads with "big men" or "chiefs" in Late Nasca iconography (for example, Silverman and Proulx 2002: Figure 9.1) and speculated that head taking was used to enhance the status and consolidate the power of these important persons.

Variation in other trophy head attributes also suggests that practices changed through time. For example, the demographic composition shows temporal differences. The earlier trophy heads described by Tello (1918), Coelho (1972), Drusini and Baraybar (1991), and this study contain men, women, and children. Later trophy head finds described by Strong (1957), Silverman (1993), and Browne and colleagues (1993; see also Verano 1995) are predominantly young males. These temporal differences in sample composition could be caused by changing warfare patterns but may indicate more significant shifts in the role and meaning of trophy heads in Nasca ideology. Brown (1995a) saw a logical connection between conserving the heads of valued ancestors and the act of taking a head from one's enemy, suggesting that the latter practice could have easily developed from the former.

In the Kroeber collection and elsewhere, trophy head disposal methods vary. Trophy heads have been found in caches, graves, and structures. Unfortunately, a number of factors combine to make the identification of temporal trends difficult. First, many trophy heads were recovered from looted contexts or were found many years ago, when field methods were different and documentation less detailed. Second, many trophy heads were buried in simple pits with no other grave goods, so diagnostic artifacts are rare. Finally, important cemeteries such as those at Cahuachi were used and reused through time, so accurate temporal assignments are even more difficult when diagnostic artifacts are absent.

Some temporal changes in disposal practices are suggested in the evidence published to date despite the previously mentioned problems. Head caches appear throughout the period, but the average number of heads found in them may increase through time, as DeLeonardis (2000) suggests. Placing trophy heads in structures seems to be more common in the earlier Nasca phases. The practice of including trophy heads in tombs may be more typical of the later phases, especially the Middle Horizon. If this trend continues as more heads are found, Verano's (1995) suggestion that burial in caches and structures implies corporate ownership of the trophy heads may be an appropriate model in the early phases. The burial of trophy heads as grave goods in later elite tombs may indicate that trophy heads were viewed as personal property by Late Nasca and Middle Horizon times, as Silverman's model of increasing secularism would suggest (Silverman 1993; Browne et al. 1993).

The three trophy head types observed in the Kroeber collection from the Nazca valley show no obvious geographic, contextual, or temporal trends, although intervalley differences in preparation style in an expanded sample have been observed. The common first type, with a small perforation and a large posterior enlargement, was found in all archaeological contexts and at every site except Majoro Chico. The less common second and third types were found at Cahuachi, Cantayo, and Majoro Chico. All three types were found in pits and caches. Types 1 and 2 were found in graves as well. Type 1 and 2 heads were found together in the Middle Horizon tomb. One head each of types 2 and 3 were found in the same cache on the summit of Cahuachi Mound A.

If trophy heads were preserved for long-term ritual use, any temporal trends could be obscured. However, the observed variation in preparation is also consistent with the use of trophy heads for more than one purpose (that is, serving multiple functions). Trophy heads may have been prepared differently for use or display in specific ceremonies or situations. Unfortunately, Nasca iconographic images provide little evidence for display method. People are most often depicted holding trophy heads by a cord or by the hair (for example, Lapiner 1976). Less commonly, trophy heads are shown attached to clothing, suspended from belts, or in one case suspended from a pole (Blasco Bosqued and Ramos Gomez 1985:24–25). Wear polish was most commonly observed on the small perforations where carrying cords had once been attached, as predicted by the iconography. No wear polish or damage was observed on any interior cranial surfaces that would suggest display on poles.

Researchers often cite ethnographic descriptions of human trophy making in other cultures, particularly the Jívaro of Ecuador and the numerous groups in Melanesia, especially those in Papua New Guinea. The Jívaro and many of the

Melanesian groups prepared elaborate artifacts from human heads. The Jívaro made shrunken heads from human skin (Harner 1972), while the Melanesian groups in the Solomon Islands and New Guinea constructed modeled clay heads over human skulls (Lewis 1951). Although the Jívaro and the Nasca are both South American groups, the Jívaro shrunken heads appear to have functioned quite differently in Jívaro society than the Nasca and Melanesian heads. The Jívaro shrunken heads played an important part of the feasts that followed a successful head-taking raid but were often discarded after the feasts ended (Harner 1972). Up de Graff (1923:283) found it surprising that the heads were often treated with complete indifference when the feasts were done and might be given to the children as playthings or lost in a nearby swamp or river. Furthermore, although headhunting was an important way to accrue personal power among Jívaro, the heads did not hold the fertility and regenerative symbolic value that is prevalent in Nasca iconography and Melanesian ethnographic accounts.

Melanesian modeled skulls were used in numerous ceremonies to promote prosperity and fertility, to perform sorcery, or to foretell the future (Bateson 1958; Beaver 1920; Lewis 1951). A skull's specific purpose could be based on the personal attributes that an individual held in life. For example, the skull of a woman who had been considered very beautiful in life was used in fertility ceremonies long after her death (Bateson 1958:Plate XXV). The skull of a young male who had a reputation as a lover and seducer of wives in life became an important relic of his clan after his death, believed to hold great love magic and increase sexual attraction (Bateson 1932:406). The heads of brave or outstanding leaders continued to exude the power those men had held in life (Bateson 1958:chapter 11; Trompf 1991:45). Some groups considered modeled skulls to be particularly powerful tools in sorcery (Seligman 1910). Heads were often used for divination and were consulted on a wide variety of topics, much like the mummified Inca rulers described in ethnohistoric documents (Guáman Poma de Ayala 1980; see Salomon 1995).

The Melanesian cultures are extraordinarily diverse, but one of the common features is the sense of community that includes both the living and the dead (Trompf 1991). Religion in places like the Solomon Islands revolved around relatives and the skulls of ancestors (Rivers 1914:258). The skulls were the subjects of numerous rites and mourning rituals that were entwined with fertility ceremonies (Deacon 1934:543–544; Rivers 1914:258). The heads of dead relatives might be taken initially as part of the process of remembering the recent dead, and many were buried or otherwise disposed of after a generation or two when those who remembered the individual no longer remained (Haddon 1901:91; Trompf 1991). Most dead relatives began their career with relatively minor status, remembered only by immediate family, and then passed into the "rank and file" membership of ancestors of an area after a few generations (Keesing 1982). A few went on to achieve great prominence and a permanent place in religious life. Keesing (1982:110) noted that the most powerful ancestors, quite apart from their powers in life, were distinguished by the success and proliferation of their descendants.

The Melanesians believed that the dead passed through stages, which they marked with special ceremonies, just as they did for the living (Haddon 1901:91; Keesing 1982). On Murray Island, the dead began their journey through the process of mummification. The skull was removed when the mummy crumbled and given to a specialist for clay modeling. The closest male relative then kept the modeled skull, both for sentimental reasons and to use for divination. In other societies, the modeled skulls were presented to the widows, who carried them in baskets either for a few weeks or until remarriage (Landtman 1927:160). Among the Iatmül, modeled skulls were kept, either in houses of relatives or in the men's house. This process of passing through stages in death (that is, of transformation) is also seen in Early Horizon Paracas textiles on the south coast, where images representing the recent dead transform into images of older ancestors and ultimately into magical creatures (Frame 2001).

Iatmül heads were used in a variety of ways, and the preparation they were given differed accordingly. Heads of both dead relatives and enemies were kept for use in ceremonies. The treatment the skulls received varied from minimal to elaborate. Enemy heads could be buried under the Mbwan, the ancestor stones in front of the men's house, or lined up on skull racks inside the men's house. Others were modeled with clay like those of dead relatives. The skulls used in special ceremonies received very elaborate treatment. They were modeled with clay, covered with all kinds of ornamentation, and placed on poles or life-sized wooden figures (Bateson 1932, 1958). Rivers (1914) noted that heads of enemies were just as important as those of ancestors but were used for different purposes, for example, as dedicatory offerings. Iatmül beliefs about the spirits of ancestors and slain enemies sometimes became intermingled by some vague sense that the victims also contributed to the village's prosperity through their participation in the act of headhunting.

In a final example of head taking in other cultures, ethnohistoric accounts from the Late Postclassic period in Mexico (A.D. 1200–1519), combined with archaeological evidence from late Classic (ca. A.D. 600) through Late Postclassic periods, provide insight into the function of ritualized display of trophy heads there (Miller 1999). The *tzompantli*, or skull rack, was used to display skulls throughout central Mexico and the Maya highlands (Miller 1999). Skulls, perforated through the coronal plane to be strung horizontally on wooden poles, were found associated with a collapsed wooden skull rack at the site of La Coyotera (Spencer 1982). At Alta Vista, Zacatecas, a number of skulls perforated in the sagittal plane, to be suspended vertically by ropes from a beam or rack, were found near the beam from which they had fallen (Kelley 1978; Pickering 1985). Skulls placed on these racks included men, women, and children (Spencer 1982). Some were warfare victims; others were defeated ballplayers. Still others may have been members of the community who were convicted of participating in local uprisings (Miller, personal communication 2003). Miller (1999) believes that the public display of decapitated heads provided a means to intimidate both enemies and the local population.

The Nasca heads show evidence of continued use and of a complex role similar to those described in these ethnographic and ethnohistoric examples. The variety of contexts in which the Nasca trophy heads are shown, at least in the earlier iconography, is similar to the fertility symbolism attributed to heads and head taking in Melanesia. Alternatively, ancestor veneration has not been proposed to explain the evidence of skull modification among the Maya, even though the Maya skull racks contained the skulls of men, women, and children and preparation methods varied, as they do with Nasca trophy heads. The Maya skull racks were used to intimidate both outsiders and their own populace. Similar intimidation practices may have been used in later Nasca phases or more likely by the Moche on the north coast.

Conclusion

Nasca trophy heads should not be envisioned as a homogeneous category of artifacts, all made from the same pattern, with only a small amount of variation introduced by individual choice during the trophy-making process. Substantial evidence of patterned variation exists, which we need to acknowledge if we are to understand their function and meaning. The variation in preparation method indicates specific ideas about trophy head construction determined by a number of variables.

Our analysis identifies some of the reasons for the great variability observed in trophy head preparation and explains why discrepancies were observed by previous researchers. It also demonstrates that standard osteological analyses cannot resolve adequately the question of whether Nasca trophy heads were made from heads taken from enemies or ancestors. Previous researchers attempted to use indirect information to infer trophy head origins, basing their arguments on demography, cause of death, burial context, shared cultural traits, and preparation methods. Unfortunately, none of these arguments can answer the fundamental questions about the source of the heads. A predominance of males is a good argument for war deaths, but the presence of women and children cannot be used to argue against warfare as the source. Evidence of violent death does suggest warfare, but the converse is not true. Warfare-related injuries and deaths frequently leave no trace in the osteological record. Context and the investment costs of trophy making both suggest a larger role for the heads than that of simple war trophy. Guillén (cited in Browne et al. 1993) believes that the elaborate preparation involved in trophy making indicates the importance of the trophy heads' role in ceremonial practices, specifically in ancestor cults, but many groups were known to lavish similar attention on the heads of their victims.

Nasca trophy heads are relatively rare and their archaeological context is often poor, so it has been difficult to determine their ethnic affiliation. Traditional biodistance studies based on metric and nonmetric traits are not possible because the remains are often very incomplete. The traits cannot be observed, either because they were removed during the trophy-making process or because they are covered by soft tissues. Theoretically, cranial deformation studies might be used to identify ethnic affiliation, but many of the crania are very incomplete, and current methods are not sufficiently standardized to permit the confident assessment of differences among groups.

Ancient DNA studies (see Kaestle and Horsburgh 2002 and Stone 2000 for recent reviews) would be an appropriate choice in this case because these methods are unaffected by missing or incomplete elements and DNA is likely to be well preserved in bone and teeth from this desert area. More important, such studies allow the direct measurement of genetic relationships among individuals and groups without complicating environmental and developmental factors. Stable isotope ratios of elements such as strontium or oxygen (which measure geological variation in chemical composition) could lend additional support to such a study if sufficient variation is present in this region (see review in Katzenberg 2000). However, expensive and labor-intensive technical studies such as these must be undertaken in conjunction with careful osteological analysis and archaeological documentation. The temporal and spatial variation identified by these latter means must be considered when choosing samples for genetic or isotopic analysis in order to minimize the variation attributable to change through time and across space. In fact, we undertook the current osteological study to assess the importance of these variables before beginning a DNA study of ancient material (now in progress).

Archaeological settlement patterns indicate that the Early Intermediate period was a time of dynamic change on the south coast. The iconographic record reflects a similar trend. This study provides new physical evidence for the characterization of the Early Intermediate period as a time of flux. Patterned variation in trophy head preparation indicates that temporal and possibly other factors governed the process of trophy making, suggesting that the role of trophy heads in Nasca society changed as well.

Our analysis of the Kroeber collection shows that past assumptions do not adequately explain the variability observed in this collection. The original source of the heads will be solved only by the application of methods uniquely suited to the study of biological identity. Ultimately, the combination of archaeological, osteological, and genetic methods will provide the most complete portrait of the complex function of trophy heads in Nasca society.

Acknowledgments

This research was supported through a cooperative agreement between the Departments of Anthropology at the University of Illinois at Chicago and the Field

Museum of Natural History. We wish to thank the following individuals for their contributions: Jonathan Haas, who gave us permission to study the collection; Will Grewe-Mullins and Janice Klein, who were helpful in providing us with access to the osteological and ethnographic material; and John Weinstein, Field Museum photographer.

Notes

1. The term "Nasca" will be used to designate the archaeological culture, and "Nazca" will be used to designate the geographic location and town.

2. Primary author's translation from Portuguese.

18

Human Sacrifice and Postmortem Modification at the Pyramid of the Moon, Moche Valley, Peru

John W. Verano

Recent advances in iconographic analysis and archaeological excavation have demonstrated that the Moche of ancient Peru (figure 18.1) sacrificed war prisoners at their major ceremonial centers in rituals directed by priests who impersonated Moche deities. Until 1995 the evidence was indirect—derived from new interpretations of Moche art based on grave goods found in elite tombs at the Moche sites of Sipán and San José de Moro (Alva and Donnan 1993; Donnan and Castillo 1992, 1994). In 1995, the first osteological evidence of prisoner sacrifice was found at the Pyramid of the Moon (figure 18.2) in the Moche River valley by Canadian archaeologist Steve Bourget, who discovered a sacrificial site (Plaza 3A) that would eventually produce the skeletal remains of more than 70 victims (Bourget 1997a, 1997b, 1998).

During the summers of 1995 and 1996, I conducted an osteological study of these remains to determine the age at death, sex, and physical characteristics of the victims, as well as to identify injuries and possible cause of death. The results of this analysis were consistent with Bourget's hypothesis that the victims were war captives, given their demographic profile (age and sex) and the presence of numerous healed fractures indicating prior experience with interpersonal violence (table 18.1). Moreover, the manner in which the victims were killed (slitting of the throat) was consistent with depictions of prisoner sacrifice in Moche art (Alva and Donnan 1993; Verano 1998a).

Bourget's excavations in Plaza 3A were important in demonstrating that the Moche indeed sacrificed captives at the Pyramid of the Moon. Similar activities probably occurred at other Moche ceremonial centers, as can be inferred from depictions of prisoner sacrifice in monumental and portable art at sites such as El Brujo, San José de Moro, Sipán, and Pañamarca (Alva and Donnan 1993; Donnan and Castillo 1992, 1994; Franco et al. 1994). The specific motivation for these sacrificial rituals is a subject of some debate, however. Bourget hypothesizes that the Moche offered captives during periods of environmental crisis—specifi-

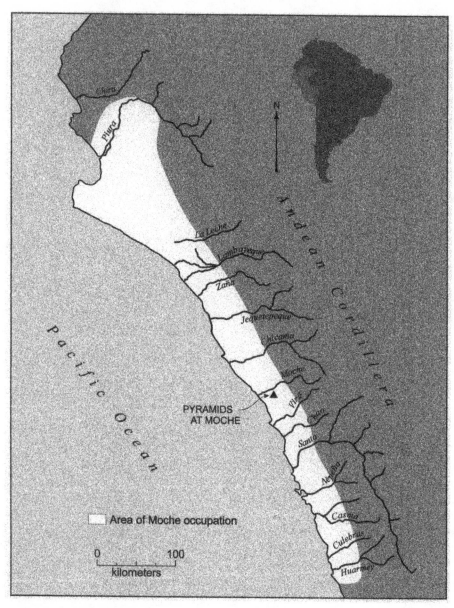

Figure 18.1. Map of the north coast of Peru showing the location of the pyramids at Moche. Illustration by Don McClelland.

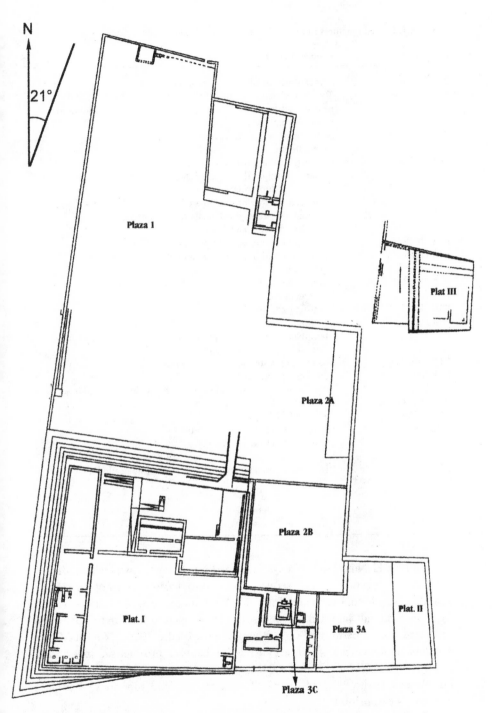

N

21°

Plaza 1

Plat III

Plaza 2A

Plaza 2B

Plat. I

Plat. II

Plaza 3A

Plaza 3C

Figure 18.2. Map of the Pyramid of the Moon. Plazas 3A and 3C are at lower right. Courtesy of the Proyecto Arqueológico Huaca de la Luna.

Table 18.1. Healed Fractures in the Plaza 3A (P3A) and Plaza 3C (P3C) Samples

Field number	Element/location
P3A Skeleton I	Left second rib; left radius and ulna midshaft
P3A Skeleton VI	Two healed depressed fractures: left frontal and left parietal; healed fracture, distal third of shaft of right radius and styloid process of right ulna
P3A Cranium VII	Four healed depressed fractures: two on left frontal, two on right parietal
P3A Skeleton XX	Left distal radius, articular surface; proximal and distal phalanges of right thumb fused in flexed position; depressed fracture, left superciliary arch
P3A Cranium XXVI	Depressed fracture on left superciliary arch, lateral third
P3A Skeleton XXX	Left humerus, distal third of shaft; anterior wedge fracture of bodies of vertebrae L1 and L2
P3A HG96-49	Depressed fracture on right parietal
P3A HG96-69	Three depressed fractures: one on right parietal, two on right frontal
P3A HG96-100	Anterior wedge fracture of seventh thoracic vertebra
P3A HG96-101	Left zygomatic
P3A HG96-104	Right first and second ribs
P3A HG96-178	Left fibula, distal third of shaft
P3A H96-211	Mandible, fractured through chin with chipping and fracture of left canine and three incisors
P3A H96-218	Nasal bones, with displacement to right side
P3A DS2 08 EN	Both ischiopubic rami
P3A DS2 08 EM-EN	Anterior wedge fracture of third and fourth lumbar vertebrae
P3A DS2 11 EM	Proximal phalanx of thumb
P3C HG99-3	Depressed fracture, left frontal
P3C H99-8	Depressed fracture, right frontal
P3C E2	Depressed fracture, left parietal
P3C E4	Depressed fracture, sagittal suture at Lambda
P3C E6	Right second metatarsal, shaft; right distal tibia, fibula, and talus
P3C E12	Possible fracture, midshaft of left fibula
P3C H6	Distal shaft of left radius
P3C H11	Left rib (3-10)

cally during El Niño Southern Oscillation (ENSO) events, which periodically bring devastating rains and subsequent droughts to the north coast of Peru (Nials et al. 1979a, 1979b; Uceda and Canziani 1993). Indeed, Bourget found evidence of intense rainfall in Plaza 3a, and some of the victims appear to have been sacrificed during periods of rain (Bourget and Millaire 2000). Not all Moche scholars are convinced of a direct correlation between prisoner sacrifice and El Niño events, however (Verano 2001b), and the stratigraphy of a second sacrificial deposit at the Pyramid of the Moon does not lend support to Bourget's hypothesis (see below).

The identity of Moche sacrificial captives and the way in which they were acquired is also a subject of debate at the present time. Some researchers argue that Moche combat was a ritual activity limited to the elite males of Moche society (Donnan 1997). Others suggest that Moche combat may have been analogous to the largely nonlethal ritual battles (*tinku*) still fought between some neighboring Andean highland communities today (Topic and Topic 1997). Still others have suggested that Moche art may depict secular warfare between different coastal valleys or between the coastal Moche and their highland neighbors (Shimada 1994). I agree with Shimada that this may well be the case, and in a recent study of the iconography of Moche combat (Verano 2001b), I caution against an overly literal interpretation of Moche iconography.

A Second Sacrificial Site at the Pyramid of the Moon

In 1996, a small test pit was excavated in nearby Plaza 3C, a courtyard located to the west of Bourget's excavations, in an attempt to locate a presumed access corridor between the sacrificial area and the principal platform of the Pyramid of the Moon (Orbegoso 1998). While a corridor was not found, more human remains appeared. I examined these remains in 1997 and found evidence of not only violent death, but also defleshing and partial dismemberment of the victims, suggesting a more complex sacrificial ritual than was seen in Bourget's sample (Verano 1998a). Further excavation was needed, however, to better define the relationship between the two plazas and to recover additional remains. In 1999, field-workers from the Proyecto Arqueológico Huaca de la Luna (National University of Trujillo) removed the overburden of windblown sand that had sealed Plaza 3C for some 1,500 years; they eventually reached the level where skeletal remains had been found in 1996. In doing so, they discovered a well-preserved temple decorated on its external surface with polychrome friezes and reliefs (Tufinio 2001). After exposure of the temple and removal of nine skeletons from the center of the plaza, the area was covered until sufficient funding could be obtained to allow the complete excavation of the sacrificial area. Such funding was obtained the following year, and excavation began in June of 2000 (Verano 2000).

Objectives and Methods

The objective of the 2000 field season was to fully excavate Plaza 3C down to its prepared clay floor and to remove and analyze all skeletal remains and associated cultural materials. Our primary goal was the reconstruction of activities that occurred within its walls, in particular those associated with the sacrifice and postmortem treatment of victims. Owing to the fragile nature of the human skeletal remains, excavation was conducted with wood and bamboo digging tools and paintbrushes. Excavators worked on boards raised above the sand to avoid damage to buried bone and artifacts. Excavation was done in arbitrary 20-centimeter levels, although sediment changes reflecting episodes of rainfall and any

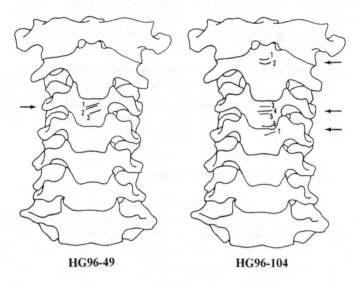

HG96-49   HG96-104

Figure 18.3. Examples of cut marks on cervical vertebrae from Plaza 3A.

shifts in color or composition of the plaza fill were noted and mapped in profiles. Skeletal material was analyzed in the project's osteology laboratory; ceramics were drawn and described by archaeologist José Armas of the Pyramid of the Moon Project.

Results

A detailed report on the 2000 season excavation is provided elsewhere (Verano and Tufinio 2005); here I provide a general overview of our results. The 2000 season excavations uncovered the remains of 15 complete or largely complete human skeletons, 16 sets of articulated elements including associated crania and mandibles, hands, feet, and limb segments, and hundreds of isolated bones. Most of the articulated remains show cut marks on the bodies of cervical vertebrae (figure 18.3) indicating cause of death (exsanguination following slitting of the throat), as well as complex postmortem treatment that included defleshing and dismemberment (see below). Some of the victims were found fully articulated, while others were missing the skull or one or more limbs. Others were represented only by articulated trunks or limbs. Some articulated skeletons, as well as isolated limbs and one foot, had the remains of rope associated with them. Preserved rope fragments, which were found encircling the wrists, ankles, or neck, were collected for radiocarbon dating by the accelerator mass spectrometry method.

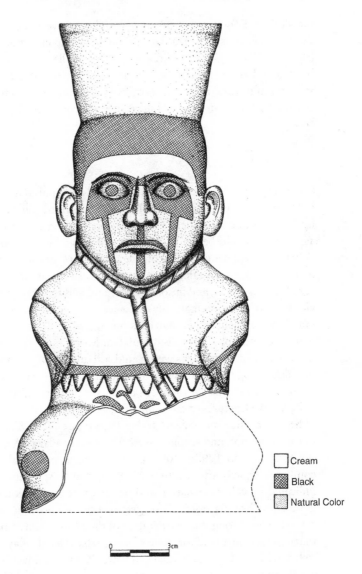

Figure 18.4. Prisoner figure from Plaza 3C, reconstructed from fragments. Illustration by José Armas.

Cream
Black
Natural Color

Also recovered in Plaza 3C were more than 650 fragments of ceramics, representing vessels of various forms. Some are fragments of undecorated utilitarian vessels that may represent occupational refuse or construction fill that accumulated in and around Plaza 3C. However, one complete example and numerous fragments were found of ceramic vessels in the form of seated prisoners (figure 18.4). These prisoner vessels presumably were used in the sacrificial rituals conducted in Plaza 3C and were then intentionally broken and deposited along with the victims. Fragments of prisoner vessels also were found associated with the sacrificial victims in Plaza 3A, although in this case the vessels were unfired (Bourget 1997a, 1998). Additional finds in Plaza 3C included fragments of burned and unburned textiles, a number of small gilded copper plates of a type sewn on tunics and other elite textiles as adornments, and food refuse consisting of camelid bones, marine and terrestrial gastropod shells, and carbonized corn-cobs.

Laboratory Findings

Skeletal remains were cleaned, inventoried, and analyzed in our field laboratory in Huanchaco. Age and sex determination was done following criteria published by Buikstra and Ubelaker (1994). All skeletal material for which sex and age assessments could be made are male and range in age from late adolescents to young adults (a demographic profile similar to that found in Plaza 3A). Labora-tory examination revealed a consistent pattern of cut marks on long bones, ribs, vertebrae, os coxae, and in some cases hand and foot bones, indicating that most victims had been systematically defleshed. Cut marks are concentrated in areas of muscle attachment rather than at joints (figure 18.5), indicating that bodies were defleshed and not simply disarticulated. More important, many skeletons with extensive defleshing marks were found still fully or largely articulated, suggesting that defleshing rather than disarticulation of bodies was the objective.

In addition to perimortem cut marks on the cervical vertebrae, several indi-viduals have fractures of the hand, arm, and shoulder that were in the early stages of healing at the time of death (table 18.2; figure 18.6). Similar healing fractures of forearms, ribs, and scapulae were found in the Plaza 3A material excavated by Bourget (Verano 1998a, 2001a). The fractures presumably were sustained in combat or shortly after capture. Most show at least several weeks of healing, as indicated by callus formation and periosteal reaction around the fracture mar-gins. These healing fractures suggest one of two possible scenarios: either that captives were brought to the Pyramid of the Moon from some distant location or that captives were held for some weeks, perhaps for display or other rituals prior to being killed. Eight individuals in Plaza 3C also had well-healed fractures sug-gestive of prior experience with combat, similar to what was found in the Plaza 3A victims (see table 18.1).

The specific motive for defleshing the Plaza 3C sacrificial victims is unknown. While ritual cannibalism could be proposed, the way in which the bodies were treated seems to suggest body processing for some purpose other than consump-tion, based on the following observations. Most skeletons, even those with cut marks on nearly all elements, were found fully or largely articulated and not systematically dismembered as would be expected in large-animal butchery. Moreover, no evidence was found of burning, cooking, or breaking open bones to extract marrow, as is the case in deposits of presumably cannibalized remains

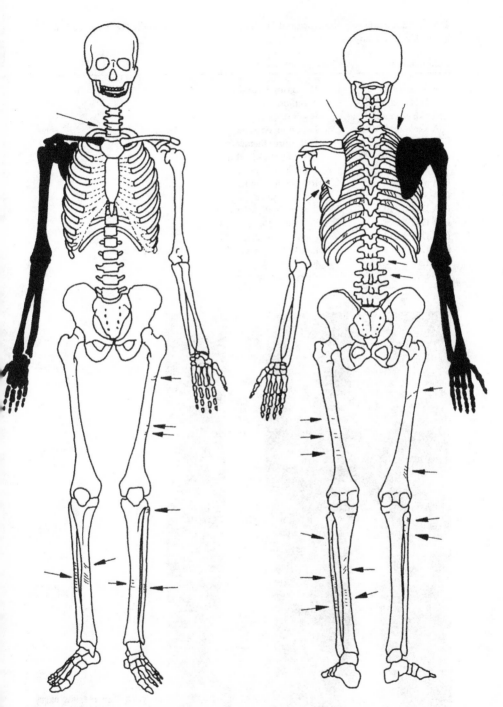

Figure 18.5. Locations of defleshing cut marks, skeleton E4. Dark shading indicates missing bone. Illustration by Carlos Ayesta.

Table 18.2. Fractures in the Process of Healing at Time of Death in the Plaza 3A (P3A) and Plaza 3C (P3C) Samples

Field number	Element/location
P3A Skeleton I	Right ribs 10 and 11, shafts
P3A Skeleton XVII	Nasal bones
P3A Skeleton XIX	Right scapula
P3A Skeleton XVIII	Lesion on occipital (triangular, 16 mm long)
P3A Skeleton "3"	Left fourth metacarpal shaft
P3A HG96-102	Parry fracture, left ulna
P3A H96-213	Rib (shaft fragment)
P3A SS2 08 EL	Rib (shaft fragment)
P3A SS2 09 EL	Left second rib
P3A DS2 08 EL	Left rib 3-10, sternal end
P3A DS2 08 EN	Left rib 3-10, vertebral end
P3A DS2 11 EL	Right rib 3-20, midshaft
P3C E5	Left fifth metacarpal, impacted fracture of head
P3C E5	Right scapula
P3C E6	Parry fracture, left ulna

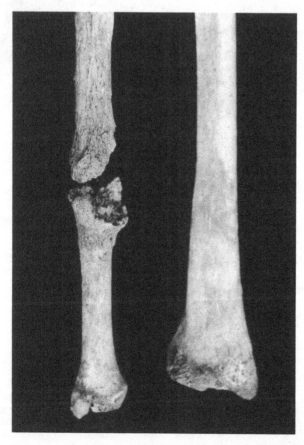

Figure 18.6. Healing parry fracture, left, distal ulna and radius, skeleton E6.

found at archaeological sites in the American Southwest (Turner and Turner 1999; White 1992) and central Mexico (Pijoan Aguadé and Mansilla Lory 1997). Our current working hypothesis is that the Moche may have been interested specifically in the defleshed skeletons of their victims, for display or other purposes. This is supported by the discovery of several isolated arms, a foot, and an articulated axial skeleton with ropes still tied around them, suggesting that they were originally suspended from some object—perhaps from the roof of the small temple in Plaza 3C or in some other location at the Pyramid of the Moon. Depictions of detached arms, legs, and feet with ropes encircling them are known from Moche art, appearing in scenes depicting the presentation and sacrifice of prisoners (Donnan 1978; Hocquenghem 1987). Our discoveries in Plaza 3C suggest that such images are not merely metaphorical but depict actual behavior. At some point the defleshed remains appear to have served their purpose, at which time they were deposited in a small walled patio adjacent to the Plaza 3C temple, where they were gradually buried in windblown sand and silt that was allowed to accumulate there. Two modified skulls found in the urban sector near the Pyramid of the Moon in 1996 provide additional osteological evidence of the intentional manipulation of human remains at the site (Verano et al. 1999).

Moche Warfare and Human Sacrifice

The ultimate reasons for sacrificing captives at the Pyramid of the Moon are not known. One of the objectives of our excavation of Plaza 3C was to test Bourget's hypothesis that sacrifices were performed in times of crisis associated with torrential El Niño rains. Some of the sacrificial victims in Plaza 3A appear to have been killed during episodes of heavy rainfall, as their bones were embedded in a stratum of hardened mud, but similar evidence was not found in Plaza 3C. We found indications of several episodes of rain that had deposited layers of silt over the plaza, but none of the skeletons was directly associated with these events. Although the sacrifice of captives in Plaza 3A may mark a period of environmental crisis and social strife associated with a major El Niño event, one must be cautious in assuming a direct correlation between sacrifice and rainfall, since multiple deposits of sacrificed victims are present in both Plaza 3A and Plaza 3C, whereas in only two strata of Plaza 3A are skeletons directly associated with rainfall (Bourget and Millaire 2000).

Major El Niño events could be expected to lead to destruction of agricultural fields and to be followed by drought years, as well as to result in short-term disruption of the marine food chain normally supported by coastal upwelling (Nials et al. 1979a, 1979b). Food shortages and epidemics could well have led to social disruption, warfare, and both intra- and intervalley competition for limited resources.

However, a direct linkage between prisoner sacrifices and El Niño events is less than convincing, given the lack of a consistent correlation between episodes of rainfall and prisoner sacrifices in Plaza 3C. While climatological phenomena may have played an occasional role in stimulating warfare and the taking of prisoners for sacrifice, perhaps these activities are better viewed within the larger context of Moche religion and political organization. The iconography of warfare, prisoner capture, and sacrifice were pervasive themes in Moche art for centuries, and this iconography is found at mortuary and monumental sites throughout their geographic range, from Piura in the north to the Nepeña River valley in the south (Alva and Donnan 1993; Verano 2001b). Given the widespread geographic and temporal distribution of this iconography, prisoner capture and sacrifice perhaps can be hypothesized to have been an important ritual that served to establish and reaffirm the religious and political power of major centers like the pyramids at Moche. While there continues to be debate over whether the Moche were a unified state-level society or a loosely affiliated group of rival polities, and over the nature of Moche warfare (whether ritual, secular, or both), conflicts between north coast polities did occur, apparently with increasing frequency in late Moche times (post A.D. 500). Evidence for this rise in conflict includes an increase in fortified sites in some valleys (Dillehay 2001), as well as the collapse and abandonment of major centers such as Galindo and Pampa Grande (Bawden 1982; Shimada 1994).

Sacrifice and Mortuary Behavior

The deposits of human remains excavated from Plazas 3A and 3C show no similarity to normal Moche burial practices. Moche funeral behavior is well documented (Donnan 1995; Donnan and Mackey 1978) and does not include defleshing and secondary burial. Primary burial in the extended dorsal position with the head oriented to the south is the rule. Cases of delayed interment have been identified at two Moche sites, indicated in one case by partially disarticulated remains in burial shrouds or cane coffins (Verano 1997), and in the other inferred from bone position in graves (Nelson 1998). No evidence of defleshing or other intentional modification of the body was observed in these cases, however, and their archaeological context (tombs with funerary offerings) conforms to the canons of Moche funerary practice. The archaeological context of Plazas 3A and 3C also is quite distinct from normal Moche mortuary sites, which range from simple communal cemeteries to elite tombs and burial platforms (Donnan 1995). As I have argued in the case of a mass grave of sacrificed individuals at the site of Pacatnamu (Verano 1986, 1995), the denial of proper burial of victims in Plazas 3A and 3C was no doubt a significant and intentional statement about the social status of the victims and the nature of their deaths. Donnan has noted that an important aspect of prisoner capture and presentation in Moche art was the humiliation of captives, who were stripped of their weapons and elaborate clothing, including all markers of rank such as ear and nose ornaments and headdresses, and were then publicly displayed by their captors as nude prisoners bound with ropes (Alva and Donnan 1993; Donnan 1997).

The subsequent execution of captives and the denial of proper burial as defined by the norms of Moche society are consistent with our hypothesis that the capture, display, and sacrifice of captives served to reaffirm the power and status of their captors and of the ceremonial center where the sacrifices occurred (in this case, the Pyramid of the Moon). The subsequent modification of victims' remains by defleshing, decapitation, and dismemberment constitutes additional osteological evidence of activities that previously were known only from Moche iconography.

Further research is needed to better understand Moche warfare, the taking of prisoners, and rituals associated with their sacrifice and postmortem treatment. We anticipate that further excavation and analysis of sacrificial contexts at the Pyramid of the Moon will contribute new data and lead to refinement of our current working hypotheses.

Acknowledgments

Financial support for aspects of research reported in this article came from a Summer Fellowship from the Tulane University Committee on Research (1995), a Fulbright Lectureship (1996) from the Council for the International Exchange of Scholars, and Summer Faculty Research Fellowships (1997, 1998) from the Roger Thayer Stone Center for Latin American Studies at Tulane University. The 2000 season excavations were made possible by a grant from the National Geographic Society (Grant Number 7024-01). The Proyecto Arqueológico Huaca de la Luna is grateful for financial support from the Unión de Cervecerías Peruanas Backus y Johnston, the Municipalidad Provincial de Trujillo, Gobierno Regional de La Libertad, and the Universidad Nacional de Trujillo. I am especially grateful for the collaboration and support of Santiago Uceda, co-director of the Proyecto Arqueológico Huaca de la Luna; for the collaboration of my co–field director, Moisés Tufinio, of the Huaca de la Luna Project; and for the assistance of graduate and undergraduate students from Tulane University, the University of Pennsylvania, the University of San Marcos, and the University of Trujillo, who assisted in excavation and laboratory analysis of the remains.

19

Mortuary Pathways Leading to the Cenote at Chichén Itzá

Lane A. Beck and April K. Sievert

Archaeological mythology is often more pervasive within the realm of archaeological science than we are aware. The names given to features of the archaeological landscape at times create or reinforce such myths. One such feature is the "Sacred Cenote" at Chichén Itzá. From earliest contact to the present day, this "Cenote of Sacrifice" has been described as a location where rituals of human sacrifice took place. In this chapter we first trace the history of archaeological recovery and analysis of human remains from the Cenote. We then use newly collected evidence derived from skeletons and from chipped stone artifacts recovered from the Cenote to explore the sacrifice "model" and also to consider alternative explanations. We therefore depart from previous studies in our broad definition of cenote-centered rituals and in our explicit concern for alternative routes by which the remains from the Cenote may have reached this disposal context.

History of Archaeological Recovery and Bioarchaeological Study at the Cenote

Stimulated in part by accounts of sacrifice in original Spanish *relaciónes* for Yucatán, Edward H. Thompson (U.S. consul and owner of a portion of the site) was the first to engage in systematic exploration of the Cenote (Coggins 1992:12–24; Thompson 1992:4–7; Tozzer 1957). He conducted dredging operations during the first decade of the twentieth century, beginning on March 5, 1904. The fifth dredge load on March 10 brought up the first human remains (Tozzer 1957:195). As a result of Thompson's efforts, objects of jade, copal, gold, stone, wood, and other materials were recovered along with human bones representing over 100 individuals. Public representations and scholarly reports, although varying in sensationalism, viewed his findings as confirmation that this Cenote was indeed a site where human sacrifice had occurred.

The Cenote as an open disposal environment could have been used at any time throughout occupation of the region. Although Tozzer (1957:200) reports that most artifactual materials recovered by Thompson date to the Postclassic period, Piña Chan (1970:54) and Coggins (1992) identify Late or Terminal Classic components as well, based on ceramics. It is also possible that the cenotes of Yucatán were used postcontact; Redfield and Villa Rojas (1934) state that people killed in the rebellion of 1920–1921 were reportedly thrown into cenotes. Even so, the bulk of the materials and individuals should derive from Terminal Classic or Early Postclassic events (Coggins 1984:27–28, Figure 21).

Although considerable speculation about dumping people into the Cenote had developed during the intervening years, scientific reporting of the human remains did not occur until Hooton's 1940 report. By that time, myths about virgin sacrifices (Arnold and Frost 1909) had gained currency. Edward Thompson had recounted his investigations to a writer, T. Willard, whose popularized volume (Willard 1926) spread such misinformation well beyond the scientific community. Hooton (1940) countered the "virgin sacrifice" myth by observing that age at death for the remains ranged from very young children to old adults. He also identified more male than female adults.

Reporting on crania recovered during excavations within the Cenote during the 1960s, Saul (1975) has identified 29 children, 19 adult males, and 10 adult females. The notion of "virgin sacrifices" was further weakened by Saul's observation that at least one of the adult females exhibited skeletal evidence of pregnancy, based upon the observation of "gestation pits" on the dorsal aspect of the pubic bone. While the proper interpretation of dorsal pitting remains controversial (Galloway 1985), Hooton's and Saul's studies have convincingly debunked the virgin sacrifice myth. No further skeletal biological investigations have been conducted on the Cenote remains.

As mentioned above, there are two collections of human remains from the Cenote at Chichén Itzá. The first set of remains, recovered by Edward Thompson, is at the Peabody Museum at Harvard University. Hooton's (1940) report on this series stated that it included the remains of at least 42 individuals. The second collection comes from excavations carried out in the 1960s and is located in the National Museum of Mexico (Piña Chan 1970). Although Saul's published analysis focuses on the more recently excavated series, he examined both collections and reports that the distribution of age, sex, and body parts is similar in the two series (Saul 1975). The current analysis includes only those remains from the early-twentieth-century project. All of the human remains from the Cenote in the collections of the Peabody Museum were examined and recorded by Beck in 1990. Her reanalysis of the Harvard Peabody materials anchors the following discussion.

At the time Hooton conducted his study of the Cenote materials, physical anthropology emphasized the analysis of skulls, especially those of adults. Hooton reported cranial remains from 13 adult males, 8 adult females, 7 children

Table 19.1. Skeletal Distribution by Age

Age	Number of cranial elements	Number of postcranial elements	Total number of elements
Infant	1	2	2
Child	3	6	6
2 to 4 years	1	5	5
4 to 8 years	12	6	12
8 to 12 years	15	4	15
Juvenile to subadult	5	11	11
Subadult total	37	34	51
Adult, male	33	5	33
Adult, female	10	1	10
Adult total[a]	50	14	50
Total	87	48	101

[a] Adult total includes individuals for whom sex could not be determined.

between the ages of 10 and 12, and 14 children around 6 years old. Although he referenced an assortment of long bones in passing, his report centers on cranial features and metric observations. Furthermore, his enumeration includes only postcranial remains from adults. Reanalysis of this collection included the total sample, thus increasing the minimum number of individuals (MNI) to 101, including 51 individuals under the age of 18. Owing to the depositional context of the Cenote and the manner of its excavation, reassociation of any of the cranial remains with any of the postcranial elements is impossible. The overall MNI was estimated by first establishing MNIs for each element, and then combining these, partitioned by age and sex (see table 19.1). It is probable that the actual number of individuals is greater than this MNI. Table 19.1 illustrates that the relative frequency of cranial and postcranial remains varies with age at death. To further examine this apparent age-related pattern, we consider subadult (<17.99 years) and adult (18+ years) separately.

Subadults

The subadults from the Cenote include a minimum of 51 individuals ranging from 2 infants under 2 years of age to 2 individuals in their midteens. The modal age is between the ages of 4 and 6 years old.

Thirty-seven juveniles are represented by cranial remains and 34 by postcranial elements. All portions of the postcranium are represented, distributed as might be expected given the manner of recovery. Larger skeletal elements are more frequently encountered than are smaller bones. For example, only 1 subadult clavicle was found, while 27 femora were present. The distribution by element is highly correlated with size, with the femur (n=27) being most commonly encountered, then the tibia (n=23), the humerus (n=20), the radius (n=16), the fibula (n=12), and the ulna (n=11) for the long bones. Only 5 bones were present from the hands and feet.

All bones were closely examined for any signs of perimortem modification. Marks from excavation were easily recognized as deep gouges or breaks that exposed bone of a lighter color than that of the exterior surfaces. Of the 37 individuals represented by cranial remains, 3 exhibited shallow cuts or scratches that may have been perimortem. All 3 displayed additional extensive postmortem damage. A child roughly 6 years old had dredge marks on the left parietal and both temporal bones. There were, in addition, two scratches near the right eye orbit that could have occurred near the time of death or at some other point after death but prior to excavation. A similar pattern was noted on the highly fragmentary skull of a child approximately 8 years of age who presented a series of shallow scratches on the frontal between the orbits. In both individuals the shallow cuts were vertically oriented. The third case involved a series of five or six short scratches, vertically oriented, on the left parietal of a child around age 10. It is possible that these scratches resulted from objects being dropped into the Cenote following initial decay and bone exposure, or they could have been produced by abrasion in the mud of the Cenote. The location of the scratches, however, is similar to that found on the crania of adult males. This would suggest that they occurred as part of the mortuary processing. The only cultural modifications noted among juvenile postcranial remains were small spots of red pigment located on two right humeri from young adolescents. Again, this could be either mortuary processing or depositional in origin.

In general, the skeletal elements from immature individuals appear to include body parts from throughout the skeleton, with the sample biased by the size of the individual bones. Skulls are common; the small bones of the hands and feet are rare. No cut marks that definitively demonstrate defleshing or other forms of perimortem processing were noted, although three sets of scratches are suggestive. Therefore, we conclude that these children—whether living or dead—entered the Cenote as complete bodies.

The ethnohistoric literature for Yucatán refers to the sacrifice of young children (Landa in Tozzer 1941:117; Tozzer 1941:fn. 946). Cenote usage, for example, is closely associated with rituals conducted at times of crop failure, famine, and drought, with the sacrifice being offered to gain favor from the rain gods or Chacs, who dwell in cenotes (see Tozzer 1941:180–181 for a discussion of various sources). McAnany (1995:122) points out that when sacrifices were needed, it made sense to offer a slave or orphaned child, a person who had some economic but marginal social value. Tozzer (1957:204), based on his reading of Landa and other relaciónes, relays that rain gods may have liked small things, including both children of 5 or 6 as well as miniature objects (this young age matches well with the modal age for the skeletal series from the Cenote).

At some towns the bodies of victims are said to have been thrown into cenotes for disposal following heart removal (see notes, Tozzer 1941:119). Robicsek and Hales (1984) list children among those customarily dispatched via heart excision, and Tozzer (1941:115 n. 531) reviews the ethnohistoric basis for this practice. Landa (Tozzer 1941:180) explicitly identifies the Cenote at Chichén Itzá as one in which victims were thrown in while alive (see also Tozzer 1957:199). As emphasized above, we have no definitive evidence for how the juveniles from Chichén Itzá's Cenote may have been killed; however, bone representation and the lack of cut marks would be consistent with death either through drowning or by some other means that leaves no visible skeletal record. Heart removal can be accomplished without compromising any bones (Robicsek and Hales 1984). Alternatively, cenotes could have simply been one of perhaps several disposal locations for dead juveniles.

Adults

Both Hooton (1940) and Saul (1975) reported a preponderance of male remains, a pattern reinforced by this study. Skeletal remains range in age from young adults in their late teens or early twenties to the elderly. They include 33 males, 10 females, and 7 individuals for whom sex could not be estimated. This determination is based upon cranial dimorphic features, although it is reinforced by pelvic observations, which identify 5 males and 1 female.

As illustrated in table 19.2, 50 different adult crania were observed, while a MNI of only 14 individuals could be identified postcranially. In contrast to the matter of immature remains, there was no apparent size-related bias in the recovery of adult postcranial elements. For example, a MNI of 8 is reached for elements of such different size as the femur, the cervical vertebrae, the radius, the humerus, and the tibia, while 9 individuals are represented by the fibula. The adult pattern of postcranial underrepresentation and lack of size bias in recovery contrasts with that for the juveniles and suggests that at least some of the adults entered the Cenote by a pathway that differs from that of the children.

Tozzer (1957:204) discusses a human sacrifice investigation conducted during the 1560s. The report from this inquiry states that of 168 human sacrifices, 80 percent of the victims were men or boys and only 20 percent were women or young girls. The demographic composition of the sexable Cenote series is roughly similar: 77 percent male and 23 percent female.

Patterns of body treatment appear to differ for males and females. Six women are represented by portions of the face and cranial vault, while an additional four female mandibles do not articulate with any of the skulls. Two of these mandibles exhibit cut marks on ascending rami, perhaps due to defleshing. Many of the long bones from the Cenote are rather gracile. None of the female postcranial remains exhibit any signs of perimortem modification. This suggests that most adult females entered the Cenote as complete bodies but that some experienced more extensive mortuary processing prior to their deposition.

Table 19.2. Cranial Representation of Adults

Age	Sex	Vault	Mandible	Total
Young adult	Unknown			
	Male	5	4	9
	Female		1	1
Young to mature adult	Unknown			
	Male	3	2	4
	Female	4		4
Mature adult	Unknown	2		2
	Male	4		4
	Female	1		1
Mature to older adult	Unknown	1		1
	Male	6		6
	Female	1		1
Older adult	Unknown			
	Male		1	1
	Female			
Adult of undetermined age	Unknown	4		4
	Male	3	6	9
	Female		3	3
Total		34	17	50

Tozzer (1941:180–182, 1957:193) reports that adult females were sometimes thrown into the Cenote as rain-related offerings, just as young children were. Although sacrifices of women are mentioned in ethnohistoric accounts, females are more commonly referred to as oracles or mediators between the living and the supernatural. Water is thus seen as an environment that unites the living with the gods (McGee 1990:64). According to Thompson (1970:180), "Adults and adolescents thrown in alive were expected to converse with the Chacs, the rain gods at the bottom of the pool." Both men and women were said to have entered cenotes alive for the purpose of bringing communications from the people to the gods and back from the gods to the people. The relación of Tomas Lopez (Tozzer 1941:fn. 948) tells of a young woman who escaped by telling the priests that if they threw her in she would refuse to speak to the gods on their behalf. (Another mediator was then chosen.) Being thrown into the Cenote was apparently not necessarily a death sentence, although many probably did not survive. The reports of time spent in the Cenote before a person could be brought back out ranges from a few hours to three days (Thompson 1970; Tozzer 1941). If they survived, after some interval they were rescued, brought back to the top of the Cenote, and asked to report on what the gods had told them. The most famous report involves Hunac Ceel, the ruler of Mayapan, who offered himself to be thrown into the Cenote at Chichén Itzá (Tozzer 1957). From surviving his time in the Cenote, he is reported to have returned with messages from the gods that supported his ascending to a leadership role. Death by drowning was considered to be desirable by the gods and to bring the person who drowns into their favor

(Sullivan 1974:91–92). Thus, even if the person did not survive to report back to the living, the death itself could be viewed as favorable. Perhaps for this reason, self-sacrifice in cenotes is reported for priests (Makemson 1951).

Suicide is another pathway that could take an individual into a cenote (Redfield 1941:119). An ethnography done at Chan Kom, located only 14 kilometers from Chichén Itzá, indicates that people who hurt tortoises (highly revered as inhabitants of cenotes) are at risk of becoming suicides and throwing themselves in. If people do fall in they meet an old couple who prepare them for the demons below (Redfield and Villa Rojas 1934:207). Belief in cenotes as places for suicides is still quite strong, as David Freidel found on a trip to Chichén Itzá, when his friend, a Maya elder, pointed into the Sacred Cenote and exclaimed that "young girls still kill themselves by jumping into cenotes" (Freidel et al. 1993:389). While it would be impossible to distinguish suicides from prognostication gone awry, the fact remains that some individuals undoubtedly died of drowning, and therefore we would expect no signs of trauma.

Adult males predominate in the Cenote collection. Twenty-one males are represented by portions of the face and cranial vault, while 12 are represented by isolated mandibles that do not articulate with these skulls and do not match maxillary occlusal planes. Of the 33 male crania, 16 exhibit cut marks, scratches, or chopping damage consistent with perimortem modifications. Ten of these modified male crania include portions of the face and/or vault, and 6 are isolated mandibles.

Modification of the mandibles includes destruction of the mandibular condyles, which were removed by chopping or breaking rather than by cutting. The bones often exhibit extensive cut marks on the posterior aspect of the ascending ramus with additional cuts or scratches on the anterior aspect of the ramus and on the dorsal aspect of the mentum. This pattern of modification could suggest removal of the jaw from a fleshed skull, followed by defleshing.

Many of the images of the gods symbolizing death include skeletal features. The death god images associated with sacrifice often show a hand in the position of the lower jaw. Additionally, "fleshless jawbones, symbols of death and, by extension, the underworld realm of the death god, replace normal jaws" (Thompson 1970:220). At other times, the jaw is simply depicted as missing (Thompson 1970:222). When the god Tlaloc is associated with representations of war, he is often pictured as being jawless (Schele and Mathews 1998:416). Landa (Tozzer 1941:123) explicitly refers to the use of mandibles removed by the victor from the vanquished in a conflict, defleshed and worn as trophies. Schele and Mathews (1998) describe Tlaloc in representations at ball courts, sites of ritual combat. They note that he is often depicted with his hand covering his lower jaw. Alternatively, it appears that perhaps the hand is not over the jaw but is hiding the absence of that element.

The 10 male crania with cut marks fall into two patterns. Six of the skulls have chopping or cutting damage to the temporals adjacent to the temporo-mandibular joint. This damage includes breakage of the zygomatic arch, cut marks around the auditory meatus, and slicing cuts on the mastoid process. Again, this type of modification could be associated with removal of the lower jaw from a fleshed body. The remaining four skulls and one of the skulls with this pattern have clusters of fine cut marks on the frontal with some cuts along the temporal line. The area exhibiting the greatest clustering of cut marks is the superior margin of the eye orbits. This pattern is consistent with sites of tissue attachment and could be explained as a result of defleshing. It is also consistent with cut marks recorded for cranial material from a Terminal Classic context at Colha, Belize (Massey and Steele 1997:72, Figures 9 and 10). In two cases, the base of the cranium shows damage near the foramen magnum. Although no cutting or chopping marks were observed, damage to this region of the skull would be consistent with decapitation.

Images identified as warriors are sometimes depicted wearing human heads or skulls (Schele and Miller 1986:250). Ball court symbolism also uses the disembodied head as a standard icon. In the largest Maya ball court at Chichén Itzá, a large relief panel at midfield clearly depicts an event culminating with a player being decapitated and his slayer holding his severed head in one hand and a large bipointed knife in the other (Schele and Miller 1986:Figure VI.3). This and the presence of a *tzompantli* (platform for displaying skulls) near the Great Ball Court gives credence to the idea that decapitation did occur at Chichén Itzá. The tzompantli at Chichén Itzá is embellished with rows of skulls carved in relief (Sievert 1992:Figure 5.2).

In addition, Roys, writing in 1943, reported that the colonial Itzas of Petén beheaded older men at about age 50 so they would not use their wisdom to become sorcerers (Roys 1962:27). Although this may be difficult to substantiate, special attitudes concerning powerful older men may be indicated by the following bone artifact.

The collection from the Cenote includes one very complete skull of a young to mature adult male with the mandible, cranial vault, and face present. This individual has a round hole measuring 80 millimeters in diameter cut in the crown of the skull. The interior of the skull is filled with resinous incense, and wooden plugs have been placed in the eye orbits (Moholy-Nagy and Ladd 1992:140). Examination of the endocranial vault confirms that the skull had been used as an incense burner or *incensario*.

The area from which the circular piece of bone was removed shows traces of perhaps false starts or slippage during the cutting process. The bone surrounding the perforation has been scraped and smoothed, and pores in the skull are filled with a claylike substance. Traces of orange or red pigment are visible on all aspects of the skull. In some areas of the face, the orange pigment appears to have been placed in stripes that alternate with a black or other dark-toned pigment. Although the mandibular condyles are intact, the posterior aspect of the ascending ramus is heavily scratched, as are the temporal bones in the region surrounding the external auditory meatus. The area with the greatest concentration of cut marks is the supraorbital aspect of the frontal bone. Clusters of scratches are also present along the temporal line, with more cut marks on the frontal portion of this line than on the parietal aspect. Few scratches or cut marks are present on the posterior portion of the skull, but both petrous temporals have been removed. Aspects of the cranial base are obscured by the resins that seal the foramen magnum and petrous region. There are also some striations that suggest that the cut section at the top of the skull may have been polished by a long strip of material passed in through the opening and out through the foramen magnum. Additional scattered scratches are visible on the zygomatic bones and maxillae.

This skull had clearly been used as an incense burner. "At the Spanish Conquest, the Maya of Yucatan had immense numbers of idols, most of them probably effigy incense burners which were both receptacles for burning copal and gods in their own right, as among the Lacandon of today" (Thompson 1970: 187). Incense burners are reported for this region from the Preclassic until modern times. Maya words that relate to effigy censers have been translated as "god pots," "lords of fire," and "lords of incense" (Rice 1999). Such terms clearly convey a high level of respect for the images used in effigy. McGee (1990:51), in his book on the ritual life of the Lacandon, discusses ceramic censers, or god pots, but points out that the pot, although presenting an image of a god, does not represent a god but rather a person through whom a god can be contacted. Perhaps this censer from the Cenote served a similar function. Among the Lacandon, bones located in shrines that contain both god pots and pre-Hispanic human remains are referred to as the actual remains of gods who once took human form (McGee 1990:57).

This individual could easily represent an ancestor and not in any way a victim (McAnany 1995:36). Landa reports as follows on the practice of modifying human crania for future use: "They used to cut off the heads of the old lords of Cocom, when they died, and after cooking them they cleaned off the flesh, and then sawed off half the crown on the back, leaving the front part with the jaws and teeth. Then they replaced the flesh which was gone from the half-skulls by a kind of bitumen, and gave them a perfect appearance characteristic of those whose skulls they were" (Landa in Tozzer 1941:131).

The clay and resins that cover portions of this incensario along with the applications of pigment appear similar to this description. Color choice likely reflects important Maya symbolic relationships. Red is often associated with the leaders of Maya communities, while black and blue are associated with sacrifice (Tozzer 1957). Red pigment also embodies ch'ulel, a sort of "soul force." Materials containing ch'ulel also comprise bone, jade, scepters, and bloodletters, among other items (Freidel et al. 1993:272). That the human skull remade into an incense burner might be imbued with ch'ulel would not be unexpected. Furthermore, such objects are potent, and when they cease to be used, their power needs to be either safely contained or released (Freidel et al. 1993:234) in a process that

Kunen and colleagues (2002) refer to as "kratophanous." This need to reduce potency might explain how such an artifact found its way into the Cenote in the first place. In most cases, however, such an object would be first destroyed; the censer shows no signs of having been ceremonially killed, although other artifacts from the Cenote, such as large bifaces, do appear to have been intentionally destroyed (Sievert 1992). Censers remain one of the most special types of ceremonial equipment (Vogt 1993), and censers falling into disuse become ceremonial trash that needs to be disposed of in a special place (Tozzer 1907:139–141).

The cut marks on this skull and on the skulls of other adult males in the collection cluster along the upper edge of the eye orbits and nasal region. Thompson (1970:180) reports, "There is a single reference to a form of sacrifice called in Yucatec *pech'ni*, 'squash the nose,' which is described as to bruise the nose and afterward slay the person." One of the passages from Chilam Balam is translated as "then was cut the membrane and the nose of the skeleton and then went the heart" (Edmonson 1982:47). Although attention to the supraorbital region is expected in any situation of cranial defleshing, an apparent special attention to the nasal region may more explicitly relate to rituals of sacrifice, flaying, and defleshing.

This pattern of cut marks, centered on the face, differs from that reported throughout North America in association with scalping. One possible interpretation would be that in the course of defleshing, perhaps following decapitation, the skin at the back of the head was sliced open and reflected forward, as is done in modern surgery. A major area of resistance to this peeling would occur at the anterior attachment of the temporals and around the ears and face, and this perhaps correlates with the cut marks observed in some of the male skulls. This could also be viewed as consistent with images that show somewhat distorted and limp severed heads being carried or worn. Flaying is reported in Mesoamerica (Tozzer 1957:29), and art does include images that could be interpreted as skins of the head. Elsewhere in Mesoamerica, flaying the head is linked with the killing of war captives; Tozzer (1941:fn. 568) cites the contact period accounts by Motolinia to this effect. Hassig (1988:121), in writing about Aztec postmortem processing, reports that heads destined for display on a skull rack (tzompantli) were first skinned. There is, of course, a tzompantli at Chichén Itzá, conveniently located near the Great Ball Court. The Temple of the Warriors at Chichén Itzá exhibits a fresco showing images of what appear to be death gods holding trophy heads by the hair (Morris et al. 1931:Plate 164; Tozzer 1957). These heads do appear somewhat limp (possibly a function of the painting style), as does that depicted on another frieze at Chichén Itzá (Proskouriakoff 1970:Figure 15). In this case the imagery reveals individuals in warrior dress, wielding a head along with hatchets and large bifaces.

Severed heads can also symbolize renewal and rebirth. Schele and Miller (1986:244) retell the *Popol Vuh* story of the desiccated head of 1 Hunapu impregnating the daughter of the Underworld from its position in a calabash tree.

Thompson (1970:181–182) notes that "the sun god . . . , having acquired skeletal characteristics during his journey each night through the underworld from west to east, needed to be reclothed with flesh when he emerged each dawn into the upper world." Clavigero (1826, cited in Tozzer 1941:123) reported that Mexicans retained the heads of some sacrificial victims captured as prisoners of war. To retain the head, some form of preservation might be required, especially considering the warm and humid climate of Yucatán. A protracted period of treatment whereby heads were retained for an interval after decapitation and later deposited in the Cenote could account for underrepresentation of postcranial remains in this collection.

Decapitation as a form of killing and dismemberment is commonly reported in association with the ball game. In the *Popol Vuh* origin myths, for example, the games were truly a matter of life and death, with decapitation figuring prominently in the story (Tozzer 1957; Schele and Freidel 1990:126). Many ball court images show the skull or bones inside the ball itself (Day 2001:Figure 74; Gillespie 1991:Figure 16.4; Morris et al. 1931; Tozzer 1957:Figure 474; Uriarte 2001:Figure 40; Wilkerson 1991; Wren 1991). Gillespie (1991:336) suggests that the ball court itself is metaphorically human, with the ball representing the head of the structure. Gillespie also makes the point that the separation of head and body may be more important symbolically than the actual killing of a man in a ball game ritual. Decapitation then becomes a mechanism for symbolic renewal of fundamental beliefs rather than just another method of dispatching a loser, captive, or victim. Regardless of whether or not decapitation and possibly flaying is related to the ball game or to warfare, the population of individuals so treated should be male, and this fits with the cut marks found on cranial bones from males recovered from the Cenote, as well as with the inequitable number of adult male crania compared to postcranial remains.

In addition to modified cranial remains, postcranial remains from adults include at least three tools made from human long bones. All appear to be made from rather robust femora. In each case, the articular ends of the bones have been removed so that only the diaphysis remains. Two are long tubes that have been cleared of internal trabeculae and polished on the outside. The other object is less finely worked. The proximal end of the bone is beveled and exhibits a polished surface on the tip, similar in appearance to a scraper.

This use of adult postcranial elements for creating artifacts may further explain the discrepancy in representation of different areas of the body for adults relative to children. That the manufacture of objects from human bone was not a rare occurrence is supported by remains recovered at Uaxactun (Kidder 1947:Figures 83 and 84). Several dozen fragments of human bone, representing the remains of at least eight individuals, were recovered from the plaza floor just outside of Structure A-V (Smith 1950:96). These are primarily the articular ends from adult long bones (table 19.3). Some diaphyseal fragments are also present. All show extensive cutting and incising, often with the removal of splinters of

Table 19.3. Distribution of Elements Recovered from Plaza Floor Outside Structure A-V, Uaxactun

Element	Side	Proximal	Diaphysis	Distal	Total	MNI
Humerus	Right	5	4	8	17	8
	Left	4	4	7	15	7
Radius	Right	0	1	2	3	3
	Left	2	0	0	2	2
Ulna	Right	6	0	0	6	6
	Left	4	1	1	6	6
Femur	Right	8	3	2	13	8
	Left	5	2	1	8	5
Tibia	Right	3	0	3	6	3
	Left	0	2	2	4	2
Fibula	Right	0	1	0	1	1
	Left	0	0	2	2	2

Notes: MNI = minimum number of individuals.

bone several inches in length. This cutting is deliberate and is consistent with patterns found as a product of the manufacture of bone tools (MacGregor 1985). One femur has had the proximal end removed, but the distal aspect is still attached. Linea aspera and other sites of muscle attachment have been smoothed, and the bone is partially polished. It appears to be a piece that was being made into a tube similar to those recovered from the Cenote at Chichén Itzá. The only cranial element included in this collection is a single mandibular condyle that has been broken or chopped in removal from the remainder of the bone.

Brasseur de Bourbourg's 1864 report of Quiche drama suggests that elements other than skulls and jaws were sometimes retained: "See then the bone of my arm; see then it is a rod mounted in silver, the noise of which will resound, as it excites the tumult within the walls of the great castle; see the bone of my leg, which will become the beater of the *teponovoz* (or *teponaztli,* the drum of hollow wood) and of the drum, and which will make the heaven and earth tremble" (Tozzer 1941:120 n. 548). Additionally, Landa (Tozzer 1941:120–121) reports, "If the victims were slaves captured in war, their master took their bones, to use them as a trophy in their dances as tokens of victory." In addition to the bone tubes from Chichén Itzá, carved human bones have been found in a variety of forms and places throughout Mesoamerica. They have been reported as hair ornaments (Schele and Miller 1986:186), musical rasps (Lumbholtz and Hrdlicka 1898), and handles (Moholy-Nagy and Ladd 1992:129; Schele and Miller 1986). Imagery at Chichén Itzá in the Temple of the Warriors includes depictions of an old man wearing a bone as a breast ornament. Morris and colleagues (1931) interpret this as a human femur. In one case the figure wears a similar bone in his headdress. One suspects that if the collections of bone tools from Maya sites were closely examined, a large number of additional items made from human bone might be identified.

A somewhat cryptic reference in Tozzer (1941:18 n. 97) says that "red cuzcas which is a kind of bone among them of great value" is likened to emeralds in its worth. Red is often referred to as a color associated with leaders or ancestors. In the well-known Burial 116 at Tikal, engravings in bones are filled with cinnabar, a red pigment that mimics blood (Coe 1967:33). Recent work at Copan has demonstrated some level of reentry of tombs, with red cinnabar being placed on the bones after the flesh had decayed. It is possible that red *cuzcas* were pieces of bone from ancestors that were retained among the living. Schele and Miller (1986:156) refer to stelae that record the cutting of bones and the use of ancestral bones as relics retained within the leading families. Crossed long bones, common in Maya art, may symbolize ancestors as well as the idea of death (McAnany 1995:46).

Heart sacrifice, another form of ritual death among the Maya, is also depicted in scenes from Chichén Itzá, in both architectural and artifactual contexts (see Tozzer 1957:Figures 292–295). Only one bone was recovered from the Cenote that might bear direct evidence of this practice (see Robicsek and Hales 1984 for a discussion of possible technique). A single rib from an adult of unknown age and sex had a slicing cut on its inferior surface. A cut of this type could have been made with a sharp and narrow tool. The appearance of the cut is consistent with perimortem sharp force trauma. Arrow sacrifice is also reported for Chichén Itzá (and this could also explain the cut rib from the Cenote). Relaciónes of Francisco Camal, Antonio Pech (cited in Tozzer 1941:116 n. 533), and Bartolomé Rojo (Tozzer 1941:119 n. 541) indicate that the bodies of individuals (in these cases probably subadults) were sometimes disposed of in cenotes after their hearts were removed (Makemson 1951). The skeletal elements that would be most likely to contain evidence of heart removal are among those that are seriously underrepresented in the Cenote collection. The fact that one rib (out of a sample of less than 50 ribs) shows a cut mark does hint that some victims of either heart excision or arrow wounding were placed in the Cenote after death.

Lithic Tools

If many of the human remains deposited in the Cenote resulted from forms of sacrificial offering, it follows that other materials, such as chipped stone tools, may support this interpretation. To assess tool function, Sievert (1992) analyzed over 160 chipped stone tools from the Peabody Museum collection for traces of use-related wear. The tools generally fall into three categories: projectile points, large bifaces, and high-precision craft-working tools for use on stone, wood, and bone. Actions most frequently represented are shooting and butchery, behaviors that would be expected if lithic tools were used for killing and perimortem modification of human remains.

Tozzer (1957:216–217) discusses arrow sacrifice based on Spanish relaciónes by Landa, Torquemada, and others. Arrow sacrifice is reported for both males and females. In the lithic assemblage are 25 very similar corner-notched points of high-quality white chalcedony (Sheets et al. 1992; Sievert 1992). The points still retain traces of a black hafting mastic at the base. Impressions left in the mastic of several points (C5932) match the tips of wooden atlatl dart foreshafts also recovered from the Cenote, suggesting that these points may have been used with atlatls (see Coggins and Ladd 1992:Figure 8.26). Considering that atlatls, atlatl darts, and dart points are pictured at Chichén Itzá (Coggins and Ladd 1992:Figure 8.3), there is no reason to think they could not have been used in killing people during rituals. These finely made points do bear traces of having been shot, as indicated by impact fractures and breaks, in addition to microscopic linear traces diagnostic of shooting (see Sievert 1992:Table 8.2 for a summary of wear traces associated with shooting). Although some points are broken and therefore exhausted, others are not, and overall, wear traces are light, as though the tools were used only a few times before being deposited in the Cenote. The fact that they are so similar in material and form leads us to assert that these were prepared in a single episode of tool manufacture for what may have been a single ceremonial event.

Butchery tools from the Cenote are of several types—some formal, others less so. There is one distinctive type, consisting of a probably bipointed chert blade over 25 centimeters long. Tools of this type exhibit conspicuous wear traces from extended contact with bone and flesh or meat. Of the eight tools of this type, seven are burned and broken, with smeared deposits of melted resin. These knives closely resemble a bipointed knife shown at Chichén Itzá in the frieze on the Great Ball Court (Schele and Miller 1986:Figure VI.3) and in relief sculpture on Structure 6E1 (Proskouriakoff 1970:Figure 15). The combination of wear patterns, morphology, and representation in a heart excision scene on one gold disk from the Cenote (Tozzer 1957:Figure 393) strongly supports designating these knives as a tool type used directly in ceremonial contexts involving dismemberment. They have also been destroyed—completely fractured—by fire, a characteristic that testifies to an episode of ceremonial killing for these artifacts.

Summary

The straight-walled "Sacred" Cenote at Chichén Itzá presents a complicated mortuary context. The various pathways leading to the Cenote allow for remains entering the context as living people, as dead individuals, or as dismembered portions. In general, it appears that the Cenote, while not always a venue for sacrifice, was often a place for ritual deposition of human remains. From comparison of the patterns of age, sex, skeletal recovery, and perimortem processing to the rich artistic and ethnohistoric records, at least four distinct ritual-related pathways have been tentatively identified. Children, living or dead, were offered into the Cenote as gifts to the rain gods. Men and women entered the Cenote alive, carrying messages from the living to the gods and hoping to return with replies for the community. War trophies or the killing of war captives add another component. Decapitations, perhaps related to ball game activity, represent an additional alternative. The incensario may represent the transformation of a man from a leader into a god, or it may represent a powerful ancestor. In addition, several pathways may be unrelated to ritual at all; these include suicide, body disposal in times of postcontact interpersonal strife, and simple accident. Given these multiple pathways, human sacrifice should be viewed as only one of many alternatives that must be considered in the evaluation of Maya mortuary contexts. The Cenote at Chichén Itzá, while clearly presenting a ritual context, presents much more—an archaeological microcosm of Maya social and cosmological attitudes about death and rebirth.

20

Putting the Dead to Work

An Examination of the Use of Human Bone in Prehistoric Guam

Judith R. McNeill

The Chamorro people, the indigenous inhabitants of the Mariana Islands in Micronesia, held their deceased ancestors in high regard, and these ancestors continued to play an important role in the life of their descendants. As documented in several early Spanish accounts written after Magellan's landing in the Marianas in 1521 and the arrival of the first permanent group of missionaries and settlers in 1668, this regard found expression in the continuing physical contact of the living with the remains of the deceased. The Chamorro especially revered the skulls of ancestors (parents and grandparents), which were kept in the house and honored. Possessing power, these relics could bring both good fortune and bad to the living (Driver 1983:214). Sanvitores, the leader of the first group of Spanish missionaries, says that the ancestors were sacred and powerful spirits—invisible guardians to their descendants, who venerated and feared them. Professional "sorcerers" (that is, shamans) also maintained skulls of the dead and invoked their spirits for aid in warfare, subsistence, illness, and so forth (Thompson 1945:20). This reverence for the ancestors is, of course, to be expected in a society that, at the time of contact, appears to have been a kin-based, village-centric society, lacking any evidence of political centralization and stratified strictly on the basis of kinship (Russell 1998:139–143).

The bodies of the dead were interred within the house compound of their lineage group, most commonly beneath or next to the most impressive of the compound's buildings: the *latte* structure (Driver 1983:215–216). Each latte structure was constructed of a set of latte stones, large stone pillars ranging from 60 centimeters to over 3 meters in height topped with semispherical capstones and arranged in two parallel rows of three to seven pairs. These served as the foundation for raised pole-and-thatch dwellings (Graves 1986; Morgan 1988). To be buried in front of the principal house was a mark of status, and it was in front of this house, on the beach side, that the lineage chiefs would be buried (Driver 1988:93). It can be inferred that burial within house compounds was intended to maintain a close connection between the living and the dead. The archaeological record generally supports the early Spanish documentation, with burials commonly found in association with a latte set, either beneath or in front of the structure (Graves 1986, 1991; Kurashina et al. 1989; Spoehr 1957; Thompson 1932).

One other type of interaction with the dead, the secondary processing of human bone remains into spear points, is alluded to in a few early Spanish accounts but is amply illustrated in an excavated burial area on the island of Guam, the largest of the Mariana Islands. It illustrates an unusual type of interaction that, while having its roots in ritual and the Chamorro belief in the power of the bones of the dead, found expression in the manufacture of functional tools.

Previous Documentation of Bone Spear Points

Early Spanish accounts report spears and sling stones as the primary weapons used by the Chamorro people. Although some spears had fire-hardened wooden tips or fishbone points, others used sharpened and barbed human bone at the tip. As described in 1904 by the German District Officer Fritz (1989:5), an avid student of Chamorro history, the Chamorro used the arm and leg bones from their own dead, as well as from the Spaniards that they killed, for making spear points. Thompson (1945:19) quotes Cowley's 1685 voyaging report that "the sharp ends of their launces [sic] are made of dead men's bones; for upon the decease of a person, his bones make eight launces, of his leg-bones two, of his thighs as many, and his arms afford four, which being cut like a scoop and jagged like the teeth of a saw or eel spear, if a man happens to be wounded with one of those launces, if he be not cured in seven days, he is a dead man."

Mammal bone projectile points, awls, and knives have been recovered from numerous prehistoric and early historic period sites in the Mariana Islands, including sites on Saipan (Jones and Tomonari-Tuggle 1994; Thompson 1932) and Rota (Butler 1988, 1997). Excavations on Guam by Hornbostel (Thompson 1932), Spoehr (1957), Reinman (1977), and more recently Graves (personal communication), Micronesian Archaeological Research Services (Amesbury et al. 1991), and Paul H. Rosendahl, Inc. (personal communication) have all recovered plain or barbed spear points. Although many of these points have been positively identified as having been made of human bone, the lack of other large mammals as potential source material has contributed to the assumption that all of the points are made of human bone. The systematically recovered spear points have generally been found in association with inhumation burials, for example, at Oleai, Saipan (Graves, personal communication) and San Antonio, Guam (Amesbury et al. 1991). Some of the excavators and later researchers have interpreted these as grave goods—offerings deliberately placed in the grave with the deceased. They are unusual, because grave goods are seldom found associated with Chamorro burials. In contrast, other researchers have suggested that the presence of the points is an indication that some individuals died a violent death.

Complementing the historic and archaeological record for the use of human bone spear points is an observed pattern of bone collection from Chamorro burials. Supporting early Spanish accounts that the Chamorro used the long bones of their dead for weapons manufacture, modern archaeological burial excavations frequently encounter interments with missing arm or leg bones and sometimes crania (Hanson 1988; Hornbostel 1921–1923; Thompson 1932; Tayles and Roy 1989). Referring back to the Spanish accounts, researchers interpret the missing long bones as having been used for weapons manufacture, while the missing crania are presumed to have been used for worship or sorcery (Hunter-Anderson and Butler 1995).

East Hagåtña Bay Excavations

In 1990 International Archaeological Research Institute, Inc. (IARII) conducted a multiphase program of testing and data recovery at a site on east Hagåtña[1] Bay on the island of Guam. The site lies in sand deposits along a coastal strip between the shoreline and steep limestone cliffs that rise abruptly a few hundred meters inland. Habitation and cemetery areas identified at the site appear to correspond with the late prehistoric Latte period Chamorro village of Apotguan[2] identified on early Spanish maps of the island. In the 1920s Hornbostel (1921–1923) recorded two latte sets at this site and excavated several inhumation burials associated with the sets. On the basis of the IARII findings, it seems probable that the cemetery identified in 1990 was associated with at least one other no-longer-extant latte set.

The primary burial area at the Apotguan site is situated approximately 125 meters from the shore and inland of village habitation remains. Covering approximately 500 square meters, the cemetery contains over 175 individuals in three distinct groups of inhumation burials. Group A, the largest of these, has 88 burial features and over 125 individuals in an area measuring 106 square meters. Group B, with 7 burial pits and at least an equal number of individuals, is located just west of Group A. To the north of Group A, 34 burial features containing the remains of at least 37 individuals are identified as Group C. Groups A (possibly together with Group B) and C probably represent separate population samples. Rib fragments from 6 individuals were submitted for radiocarbon dating. Five of these samples, from Group A, yield calibrated dates in the range cal A.D. 1300 to 1700. The sixth sample, from Group C, dates to cal A.D. 1030 to 1270. The dates are consistent with 13 other dates obtained from the habitation deposits and with the Latte period ceramic materials recovered in the burial area.

Because of the size and composition of the cemetery sample, the excavations by IARII provide an excellent opportunity to examine and clarify the patterns of prehistoric bone removal and the nature of the association between barbed bone points and the individuals from whose interments these points were recovered. In fact, at Apotguan the findings document the complete use history of human bone projectile points in prehistoric Guam: from procurement of the raw material to manufacture, use, and disposal of the resulting artifacts.

Procurement

The skeletons of 20 individuals at Apotguan are identified as possibly or definitely the objects of bone acquisition activities. Five adults (4 female and 1 male) are represented only by isolated crania, 3 of which were recovered together in a tight cluster in Burial Group A. Because of postdepositional disturbances, it is not possible to be certain if the missing long bones of 2 other individuals were deliberately removed, but this explanation seems likely. The missing arm and leg bones of the remaining 13 individuals appear to have been deliberately removed. This interpretation is based on the observation of individuals with the bones of the hands, feet, knees, and pelvis all in correct anatomical position but no femora, tibiae, humeri, or other long bones (figure 20.1).

At Apotguan, several bones had been removed: the femur, tibia, fibula, humerus, ulna, and radius. No individual was identified as having had his skull removed, although, as previously noted, 5 individuals are represented only by crania. Long bones of the leg were removed from 14 individuals, 6 of whom also had missing arm elements. The remaining individual was missing only the left humerus.

Hanson (1988) examined the remains of 25 individuals recovered from seven excavation areas on the north coast of Rota and reported a pattern of sex-based distinctions for bone removal among 7 disarticulated individuals, characterized by males with missing crania and females with missing long bones. In his analysis of the 18 burials from the San Antonio site on Guam (Hanson 1991), he found a similar pattern. However, the pattern of sex-based distinctions in the Apotguan population is not the same.

Of the 5 isolated crania, 4 are female. Further, these 4 females are all mature (one aged 35 to 40, one "middle-aged," and two older than 50 years). This pattern may reflect the high status of females, especially older ones, in traditional Chamorro society (Russell 1998:150–151). The male, in contrast, is aged only 20 to 25 years and is perhaps a fallen warrior.

The distribution of removed long bones at Apotguan also contrasts with Hanson's observations. Of the individuals with missing long bones, 4 are female, 1 is an adolescent of undetermined sex, and the remaining 10 are males. Obviously the reports of early Europeans that Chamorro warriors used the leg bones of men killed in battle for their spear points (Russell 1998:209) may indicate either a European bias or simply insufficient knowledge of the procurement system and tool use. As with the isolated crania, 60 percent of those with missing

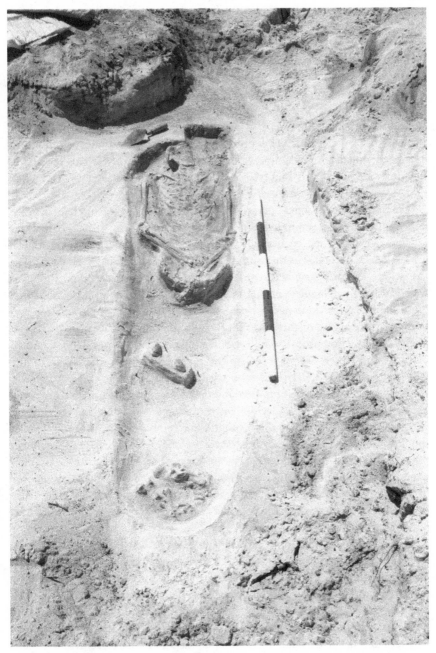

Figure 20.1. Burial 25 at Apotguan. Note the presence of both patella and feet but the absence of any of the long bones of the legs.

long bones are at least 35 years of age. The youngest individuals are adolescents in the 15–20-year-old age range (one female and the other of undetermined sex).

Although at Apotguan 89 different bones were removed from the burial sample, all (that is, less than 10 percent of the total cemetery population) came from only 15 individuals. As would be expected from historical accounts, there is a bias toward older individuals, particularly males (over 50 percent of males and approximately 30 percent of combined males and females over age 35 were selected). Additionally, there is a four-to-one (71:18) ratio of missing leg bone elements to arm elements. This ratio, however, like the spatial distribution of donor individuals, presents no readily interpretable pattern. Perhaps the preference for the lower limbs simply reflects an assessment that they provide more suitable raw material.

The findings at Apotguan permit speculation on the timing and nature of the bone removal. For seven individuals, the bones that directly articulate with the missing elements were left in place with only minor disturbance (for example, hips, knees, and feet just as they should be but no long bones between them). The ease with which the bone was removed would indicate that decomposition was well advanced or complete at the time of removal. Also, it would suggest that those removing the bone had a clear knowledge of the grave pit location and outline—there are no disturbances that would indicate random probing or digging. Cowley (Thompson 1945:27, from a 1685 account) states that Chamorro corpses were merely left exposed on the surface until they decomposed, and Hanson (Butler 1988:401–402) reports skeletal remains that were in variable states of decomposition prior to final interment. However, at least one historical account (Coomans 2000:25, written in 1673) suggests how bodies were buried, with the bone still made readily available for removal: "To make the former [human bone spear points], they despoil corpses of their leg bones, and the longer ones are the most desirable ones. For instance, should they want to get their hands on longer leg bones, they bury the corpses of the dead at a site, so that the earth would hardly cover the legs from the hips down to the heels, to which they tie small cords, so that, when the ligaments have already putrefied, they pull them out intact from the rest of the body."

The Apotguan burial groups represent at least two distinct cemetery samples. On the basis of a pattern of alignment of the burial pits of 10 individuals and a corresponding alignment of probable shaft support stones, Burial Group A is interpreted as having been directly associated with a former latte set. While no comparable patterns of association were observed in Burial Group C, it is quite possible that it too was associated with a no-longer-extant latte set. In addition, a pattern of post molds indicative of several pole-and-thatch structures was identified just seaward of the burial groups. In both instances, it seems likely that the kin group associated with each burial area would have been living in very close proximity. Thus the opportunity for bone removal belonged with the cemeteries' kin-based "owners." The postmortem timing of bone removal and the lack of

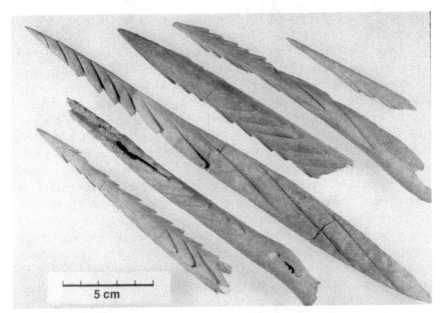

Figure 20.2. A selection of the human bone points recovered with Burial 57 at Apotguan.

evidence that graves were disrespectfully robbed supports the supposition that the bones were removed and used by the decedents' kin. This is further supported by the early Spanish accounts of Chamorros using the bones of *their own* dead (Ledesma 1975:23, written in 1669–1670; Fritz 1989:5).

Manufacture

Most of the reported bone projectile points recovered from archaeological contexts in the Marianas have been fragmentary. They range in length from 3 or 4 centimeters up to 40 centimeters. Typically, the points have two or three rows of finely formed barbs cut and polished along the length of the projectile, with each barb and the tip ending in a sharp point. According to historical sources (for example, Coomans 2000:25), the points were barbed so that they would break off inside the victim and be difficult to remove. The tibia is the most common source bone cited in the archaeological literature.

Eleven bone points were recovered from the Apotguan excavations (figure 20.2). Five of the points were fashioned from human tibia. Four of these utilized portions of the anterior crest, and the fifth used the medial side. Two of the points were formed of human fibula and one each of human humerus and radius. The remaining two points could not be securely attributed to particular elements or species. The ratio of leg to arm elements represented in the points is consistent with the ratio of leg to arm elements removed from the interments; however, it is interesting to note that none of the artifacts appears to have been formed from the femur.

An incomplete artifact from Rota formed from an adult femur provides evidence of the early stages of tool manufacture (Hanson 1997). Preliminary shaping was done, probably with a shell or chert tool, while the bone remained substantially intact, thus affording the tool-maker a gripping handle. A tip and rows of barbs were then cut, incising added, and the edges and remainder of the point well smoothed, usually on both the exterior and the intracortical surfaces. In cross-section the Apotguan implements vary considerably, primarily as a function of the raw material; for example, points formed from the anterior crest of the tibia are V-shaped in cross-section. All of the implements are finely barbed, exhibiting several different tri- , bi- or unilateral patterns. The longest point, measuring approximately 25 centimeters, is from the medial side of the tibia and is flat to slightly oval in cross-section. It is barbed and incised along its entire length. However from the midshaft onward the point is unmodified on the intracortical surface; its form suggests that it may have been used unhafted, as a dagger. Another of the points, although well barbed, is an almost complete human radius—still round and hollow in cross-section with the point at the distal end. On virtually all of the points, the fine tips of the barbs have been broken off, presumably as a result of use. None of the points shows evidence of having been modified or retouched, which might indicate previous use. The points therefore appear to have been manufactured as single-use implements.

Use

The contexts of previous finds of bone projectile points did not clearly indicate the nature of the association between the points and the individuals with whom they were found—whether these were grave offerings or the cause of injury or death. At Apotguan, the 11 recovered points came from two burial features. Burial 1 was identified during backhoe trenching at the site and produced a single, fragmentary point. As at other Mariana sites, no clear association between the point and the individual interred, a young adult male, could be made. However, since grave goods are uncommon at the site, the point cannot be assumed to represent an intentional offering.

All of the remaining 10 bone points were recovered from Burial 57, a male, aged 25 to 30 years. This is the first, and I believe only, case archaeologically documenting the use of human bone implements as weapons in prehistoric Micronesia. All of the points were found in situ within the body of this individual (figure 20.3). The positions of the points indicate that this individual received five wounds in the back, one in each side, one in the groin and two, most likely lethal, wounds in the head. After examining the skeletal remains, the osteologists concluded that "the lack of bone reaction suggests that this individual died within 12 days of injury, if not at the time of the injuries" (Pietrusewsky et al. 2003:36).

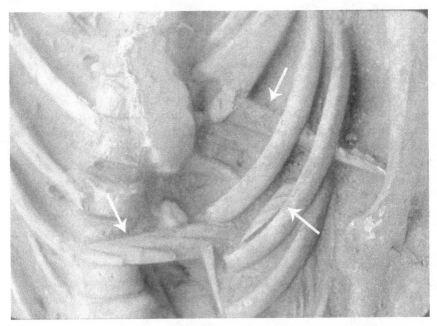

Figure 20.3. A close-up view of Burial 57 showing points in situ within the chest cavity.

Knowing the cause of death in this instance still leaves us with questions regarding how to explain this death. Other than the presence of the 10 points, nothing distinguishes this individual from those around him. His interment is one of an alignment of 10 supine, extended burials that I have interpreted as having been interred directly under a now-missing latte structure. This location is generally associated with individuals of higher, rather than diminished, status (Driver 1983:215, 1988:93). The most ready supposition is that this individual was a warrior killed in battle. However, traditional Chamorro warfare involved little bloodshed; typically, once two or three warriors were killed or wounded, the fighting ended (Russell 1998:211–213). Under these circumstances inflicting so many wounds on a single individual in battle would be highly unusual. There are also no reports of executions, even of murderers, who typically were able to escape punishment by paying restitution to the family of the dead (Driver 1983:214; Russell 1998:211). Further, the number of points and the location of the wounds suggest to the modern Western observer an emotional, vengeful act rather than a restrained, judicial one. The rarity of the points and their high production costs would suggest a special significance for this death.

Conclusion

Several of the Apotguan burials, and especially Burial 57, document stages in the entire cycle from raw material procurement to disposal of a particular artifact.

This cycle involves an unusual set of interactions between the members of the living society and their ancestral dead. Interpreting and explaining the evidence raises questions about how these interactions between the living and the dead complement the Chamorro belief system and how we explain the events that are represented in the archaeological record.

In the selection of human bone for the manufacture of spear points, we see at work a mixture of pragmatic concerns and spiritual beliefs. On the one hand, the choice of human bone seems to reflect the scarcity of other appropriate raw materials within an isolated island archipelago with no other large land mammals, no metal, and limited quantities of good quality stone. On the other hand, the belief that spiritual power resided in human skeletal remains probably influenced both their selection as a raw material for tools and the ways in which these tools were used. The most reliable of the early Spanish accounts indicate that displays of reverence for and propitiation of one's direct and immediate ancestors were the most obvious expressions of Chamorro spiritual belief. This manifested itself in the retention of the skulls of ancestors in the upper story of the houses that rested on the latte stones. Religious specialists, essentially shamans, were those who were believed to be most adept at utilizing the power of the ancestors; they kept a large number of skulls in their houses. They used this power to make rain, cure illness, and foresee the future, but we don't know the extent to which it may have been used for purposes of sorcery.

While the skulls were the focus of ancestral respect and ritual, power also resided in the limb bones, which were selected from one's own group's dead, not from the enemy or some other group. In addition, the bias toward the use of older individuals suggests a concern with using the bones of those with the greatest spiritual power. Thus, spiritual as well as pragmatic concerns factored in the selection of human bone for the making of these artifacts.

Belief in the power inherent in the bones may have influenced the purposes for which the spears tipped with these points were used. There is no evidence, archaeologically or ethnohistorically, that these weapons were used in hunting. All of the securely documented points have been recovered from burial contexts. Although the points have been interpreted both as grave goods and as weapons, the unambiguous nature of the Burial 57 association suggests that previous finds may best be similarly explained (that is, as having been embedded at the time of burial in the body of the deceased). Generally, ethnographic references connect these weapons with killing or wounding humans. The presence of human bone points in burial contexts is thus the archaeological evidence of this practice.

Using the available evidence, how do we explain the death of the individual with 10 spear points and his burial in a place of honor? Although the spears were used in warfare between villages, death in battle seems unlikely, given that a single wound or death was usually enough to end a battle. While the delivery of so many wounds could suggest a ritual aspect to his death, there is nothing else in the archaeological record or the ethnohistoric accounts to suggest that ritual killing was a part of Chamorro culture. Killing in response to an insult, however, seems to have been common. For example, the Spanish sailor Sancho, marooned on Rota in 1601, died as a result of a bone spear point wound delivered by a neighbor, who felt that Sancho had insulted him (Driver 1988). Adultery was punished by death, with the offended husband justified in killing the lover (but not the wife); according to the first Spanish missionaries, such punishments were a frequent occurrence (Lévesque 1995:472). The missionaries also mention that groups of women were known to have used spears tipped with bone points to threaten men who engaged in adulterous behavior (Russell 1998:150; Ledesma 1975:23). Perhaps in this instance they did more than threaten. Certainly the number of wounds suggests that if this man's killing was a response to an insult or adultery, the act offended more than a single individual and offended those people in a serious way. For now the best we can do is to conclude that the death was likely the result of an act that reflected a typical pattern of dispute settlement in such kin- and village-based societies. Whoever killed him, in the end he was returned to his own family, where he could be buried in the place accorded to him by his position within his kin group and receive the reverence due to an ancestor of that family.

Chamorro interactions with the dead reflect a family/kin-centered relationship in which the spiritual was intimately associated with the practical. Their use of the ancestral skulls, which Spanish observers attributed to spiritual life, seems also to reflect very practical concerns: harnessing the power of the ancestors to cure illness, bring rain to the rice fields, and protect fishermen while improving their catch. The use of the limb bones in the making of spears went one step further, investing the power of the ancestors in a tool that could be used as a weapon in war, in revenge, and in the escalation or resolution of disputes.

Acknowledgments

The International Archaeological Research Institute investigations upon which this chapter is based were carried out by a number of individuals. Bertell Davis directed the testing and data recovery excavations (Beardsley 2003); the author directed the burial recovery excavations (McNeill, in preparation), and Michael Pietrusewsky, Michele Toomay Douglas, and Rona Ikehara-Quebral (Pietrusewsky et al. 1997, 2003; Douglas et al. 1997) conducted the osteological analysis of the recovered human remains.

Notes

1. Hagåtña is the official spelling of the locality previously identified on maps as Agana or Agaña.

2. Apotguan is the official spelling of the locality previously identified on maps as Apurguan or Apotgun.

References Cited

Acosta, J. D.
1954 [1590] *Historia Natural y Moral de las Indias*. Biblioteca de Autores Espanoles, Madrid.

Adams, E. C.
1994 The Katsina Cult: A Western Pueblo Perspective. In *Kachinas in the Pueblo World*, edited by P. Schaafsma, pp. 35–46. University of New Mexico Press, Albuquerque.

Ahearn, L. M.
2001 Language and Agency. *Annual Review of Anthropology* 30:109–137.

Ahern, E.
1973 *The Cult of the Dead in a Chinese Village*. Stanford University Press, Stanford, Calif.

Allison, M. J.
1983 The Chinchorro Mummies. *National Geographic Reports* 21:1–3.
1984 Paleopathology in Peruvian and Chilean Populations. In *Paleopathology at the Origins of Agriculture*, edited by M. N. Cohen and G. J. Armelagos, pp. 515–529. Academic Press, Orlando, Fla.

Allison, M. J., G. Facacci, B. Arriaza, V. Standen, M. Rivera, and J. Lowenstein
1984 Chinchorro Momias de Preparacion Complicada: Methodos de Momificacion. *Chungará* 13:155–174.

Allison, M. J., E. Gerszten, A. J. Martinez, and D. M. Klurfeld
1977 Generalized Connective Tissue Disease in a Mummy of the Huari Culture. *Bulletin of the New York Academy of Medicine* 53:292–301.

Allison, M. J., E. Gerszten, J. Munizaga, C. Santoro, and G. Focacci
1981 La Práctica de la Deformación Craneana entre los Pueblos Andinos Precolombinos. *Chungará* 7:238–260.

Allison, M. J., A. Hossaini, J. Munizaga, and R. Fung
1978 ABO Blood Groups in Chilean and Peruvian Mummies. Part II: Results of Agglutination Inhibition Technique. *American Journal of Physical Anthropology* 49:139–142.

Allison, M. J., and A. Pezzia
1973 Preparation of the Dead in Precolumbian Coastal Peru. Part I. *Paleopathology Newsletter* 4(December):10–12.

Allison, M. J., A. Pezzia, E. Gerszten, and D. Mendoza
1974 A Case of Carrion's Disease Associated with Human Sacrifice from the Huari Culture of Southern Peru. *American Journal of Physical Anthropology* 41(2):295–300.

Alva, W., and C. B. Donnan
1993   *Royal Tombs of Sipan.* Fowler Museum of Cultural History, Los Angeles.

Ambrose, S. H.
1993   Isotopic Analysis of Paleodiets: Methodological and Inerpretive Considerations. In *Investigations of Ancient Human Tissue: Chemical Analyses in Anthropology,* edited by M. K. Sandford, pp. 59–130. Gordon and Breach, Langhorne, Penn.

Ambrose, S. H., B. M. Butler, D. B. Hanson, R. L. Hunter-Anderson, and H. W. Krueger
1997   Stable Isotopic Analysis of Human Diet in the Marianas Archipelago, Western Pacific. *American Journal of Physical Anthropology* 104(3):343–361.

Ambrose, S. H., and L. Norr
1993   Experimental Evidence for the Relationsip of the Carbon Isotope Ratios of Whole Diet and Dietary Protein to Those of Bone Collagen and Carbonate. In *Prehistoric Human Bone: Archaeology at the Molecular Level,* edited by J. B. Lambert and G. Grupe, pp. 1–38. Springer-Verlag, Berlin.

Amesbury, J. R., R. L. Hunter-Anderson, and D. R. Moore
1991   *An Archaeological Study of the San Antonio Burial Trench and a Report on the Archaeological Monitoring of Road Construction along Marine Drive between Rts. 8 and 4, Agana, Guam.* Report prepared for Government of Guam Public Works, Division of Highway Engineering, Agana, Guam and Black Construction Corporation, Guam. Micronesian Archaeological Research Services, Mangilao, Guam.

Anton, S. C.
1989   Intentional Cranial Vault Deformation and Induced Changes of the Cranial Base and Face. *American Journal of Physical Anthropology* 79:253–267.

Ariès, P.
1974   *Western Attitudes towards Death.* Johns Hopkins University Press, Baltimore, Md.
1977   *L'homme devant la mort.* L'Univers Historique, Paris.
1981   *The Hour of Our Death.* Alfred A. Knopf, New York.

Arnold, B.
2001   The Limits of Agency in the Analysis of Elite Iron Age Celtic Burials. *Journal of Social Archaeology* 1:210–224.

Arnold, B., and N. L. Wicker
2001   Introduction. In *Gender and the Archeology of Death,* edited by B. Arnold and N. L. Wicker, pp. vii–xxi. Altamira Press, Walnut Creek, Calif.

Arnold, C.
1980   Wealth and Social Structure: A Matter of Life and Death. In *Anglo-Saxon Cemeteries,* edited by Philip Rahtz, T. Dickinson, and L. Watts, pp. 81–142. BAR British Series 82. British Archaeological Reports, Oxford.

Arnold, C., and F. J. T. Frost
1909   *The American Egypt, a Record of Travel in Yucatan.* Hutchinson, London.

Arriaza, B. T.
1995   *Beyond Death: The Chinchorro Mummies of Ancient Chile.* Smithsonian Institution Press, Washington, D.C.

Arriaza, B. T., F. Cardenas-Arroyo, E. Kleiss, and J. W. Verano
1998   South American Mummies: Culture and Disease. In *Mummies, Disease, and Ancient Cultures,* edited by A. Cockburn, E. Cockburn, and T. A. Reyman, pp. 190–234. Cambridge University Press, Cambridge.

Ashmore, W.
1989   Construction and Cosmology: Politics and Ideology in Lowland Maya Settlement Patterns. In *Word and Image in Maya Culture: Explorations in Language, Writing, and Representation*, edited by W. F. Hanks and D. S. Rice, pp. 272–286. University of Utah Press, Salt Lake City.
1991   Site-Planning Principles and Concepts of Directionality among the Ancient Maya. *Latin American Antiquity* 2:199–226.
2002   Encountering Maya Women. In *Ancient Maya Women*, edited by T. Ardren, pp. 229–245. Altamira Press, Walnut Creek, Calif.
2005   The Idea of a Maya Town. In *Structure and Meaning in Human Settlement*, edited by T. Atkin and J. Rykwert. University of Pennsylvania Museum Press, Philadelphia.

Ashmore, W., and A. Knapp (editors)
1999   *Archaeologies of Landscape: Contemporary Perspectives*. Blackwell, Oxford.

Aufderheide, A. C., and M. L. Aufderheide
1991   Taphonomy of Spontaneous ("Natural") Mummification with Applications to the Mummies of Venzone, Italy. In *Human Paleopathology: Current Syntheses and Future Options*, edited by D. Ortner and A. C. Aufderheide, pp. 79–86. Smithsonian Institution Press, Washington, D.C.

Aufderheide, A. C., I. Muñoz, and B. Arriaza
1993   Seven Chinchorro Mummies and the Prehistory of Northern Chile. *American Journal of Physical Anthropology* 91(2):189–202.

Augustin [Saint]
1869   Enchiridion. In *Oeuvres Complètes de Saint Augustin*, edited by X. Raul, vol. 12, pp. 1–43. Bar-le Duc.
1948   De Cura Gerenda pro Mortuis. In *Oeuvres de Saint Augustin*, translated by G. Combes, vol. 2, pp. 457–523. Bibliothèque Augustinienne. Desclée de Brouwer, Paris.
1949   De Civitate Dei. In *Oeuvres de Saint Augustin*, translated by G. Combes, vol. 37, pp. 521–719. Bibliothèque Augustinienne. Desclée de Brouwer, Paris.
1984   *Selected Writings of Augustine of Hippo*, translated by M. T. Clark. Paulist Press, New York.

Austen, L.
1939   Megalithic Structures in the Trobriand Islands. *Oceania* 10:30–53.

Baby, R. S.
1954   *Hopewell Cremation Practices*. Papers in Archaeology No. 1. Ohio Historical Society, Columbus.

Bada, J., B. Herrmann, I. L. Payan, and E. H. Man
1989   Amino Acid Racemization in Bone and the Boiling of the German Emperor Lothar I. *Applied Geochemistry* 4:325–327.

Bartel, B.
1982   A Historical Review of Ethnological and Archaeological Analyses of Mortuary Practices. *Journal of Anthropological Archaeology* 1:32–58.
1989   Comment on "The Historical Dimension in Mortuary Expressions of Status and Sentiment," by Aubrey Cannon. *Current Anthropology* 30:447–448.

Bartlett, M. L., and P. A. McAnany
2000   "Crafting" Communities: The Materialization of Formative Maya Identities. In

The Archaeology of Communities: A New World Perspective, edited by M. A.
Canuto and J. Yaeger, pp. 102–122. Routledge, London.

Bass, W. M.
1971   *Human Osteology: A Laboratory and Field Manual of the Human Skeleton.* 2nd
ed. Missouri Archaeological Society, Columbia.

Batchelor, S.
1998   *The Tibet Guide: Central and Western Tibet.* Wisdom Publications, Somerville,
Mass.

Bateson, G.
1932   Social Structure of the Iatmül People of the Sepik River. *Oceania* 2(3):245–291,
401–453.
1958   *Naven: A Survey of the Problems Suggested by a Composite Picture of the Culture
of a New Guinea Tribe Drawn from Three Points of View.* 2nd ed. Stanford University Press, Stanford, Calif.

Bawden, G. L.
1982   Galindo: A Study in Cultural Transition during the Middle Horizon. In *Chan
Chan: Andean Desert City,* edited by M. E. Moseley and K. C. Day, pp. 285–320.
University of New Mexico Press, Albuquerque.
1989   Settlement Survey and Ecological Dynamics on the Peruvian South Coast. *Andean
Past* 2:39–67.
2000   Burial: The Deus Ex Machina of Social Transformation? *Current Anthropology*
41(1):145–147.

Beardsley, F. R.
2003   *Archaeological Investigations in Apotguan, Guam: Agana Beach Condominium
Site.* Volume 1: *Testing, Data Recovery, and Monitoring.* Draft report prepared for
Hanil Development Co., Hagåtña, Guam. International Archaeological Research
Institute, Honolulu, Hawaii.

Beauchamp, W. M.
1900   Iroquois Women. *Journal of American Folklore* 13:81–91.

Beaver, W. N.
1920   *Unexplored New Guinea: A Record of the Travels, Adventures, and Experiences of
a Resident Magistrate amongst the Head-hunting Savages and Cannibals of the
Unexplored Interior of New Guinea.* Seeley, Service and Co., London.

Beck, L. A.
1995   (editor) *Regional Approaches to Mortuary Analysis.* Plenum Press, New York.
2000   Cremation Deposits from Sunset Mesa. In *Excavation at Sunset Mesa Ruin,* edited
by M. W. Lindeman, pp. 215–228. Desert Archaeology Research Series, Technical
Report 2000–02. Desert Archaeology, Tucson, Ariz.

Becker, M. J.
1988   Burials as Caches; Caches as Burials: The Meaning of Ritual Deposits among the
Classic Period Lowland Maya. In *Recent Studies in Pre-Columbian Archaeology,*
edited by N. J. Saunders and O. de Montmollin, pp. 117–142. BAR International
Series 421. British Archaeological Reports, Oxford.
1992   Caches as Burials; Burials as Caches: A New Interpretation of the Meaning of
Ritual Deposits among the Classic Period Lowland Maya. In *New Theories on the
Ancient Maya,* edited by E. C. Danien and R. J. Sharer, pp. 185–196. University
Museum Monographs 77. University of Pennsylvania, Philadelphia.

1993   Earth Offering among the Classic Period Lowland Maya: Burials and Caches as Ritual Deposits. In *Perspectivas Antropologicas en el Mundo Maya*, edited by M. Josefa, I. Ponce de Leon, and F. L. Perramon, pp. 45–74. Publicaciones de la SEEM No. 2. Sociedad Española de Estudios, Barcelona.

Beer, R.
1999   *The Encyclopedia of Tibetan Symbols and Motifs.* Shambala Publications, Boston.

Behrensmeyer, A. K.
1978   Taphonomic and Ecologic Information from Bone Weathering. *Paleobiology* 4:150–162.

Belan Franco, L. A.
1981a   *Chiribaya: Apuntes para el Conocimiento de la Arqueología Surperuana.* Editorial "Arqueos," Arequipa, Peru.
1981b   Estudio Sobre Chiribaya. *Arqueos Peru* 2(2–3):23–30.

Bell, C.
1992   *Ritual Theory, Ritual Practice.* Oxford University Press, Oxford.
1997   *Ritual: Perspectives and Dimensions.* Oxford University Press, New York.

Bell, E. E., R. J. Sharer, L. P. Traxler, D. W. Sedat, C. W. Carrelli, and L. A. Grant
2004   Tombs and Burials in the Early Classic Acropolis at Copan. In *Understanding Early Classic Copan*, edited by E. E. Bell, M. A. Canuto, and R. J. Sharer, pp. 131–157. University of Pennsylvania Museum of Anthropology and Archaeology, Philadelphia.

Bell, E. E., L. P. Traxler, D. W. Sedat, and R. J. Sharer
1999   Uncovering Copán's Earliest Royal Tombs. *Expedition* 41:29–35.

Bendann, E.
1930   *Death Customs: An Analytical Study of Burial Rites.* Alfred A. Knopf, New York.

Benson, E. P.
2001   Why Sacrifice? In *Ritual Sacrifice in Ancient Peru*, edited by E. P. Benson and A. G. Cook, pp. 1–20. University of Texas Press, Austin.

Berryman, H. E.
2002   Disarticulation Pattern and Tooth Mark Artifacts Associated with Pig Scavenging of Human Remains: A Case Study. In *Advances in Forensic Taphonomy: Method, Theory, and Archaeological Perspectives*, edited by W. D. Haglund and M. H. Sorg, pp. 490–495. CRC Press, Boca Raton, Fla.

Besom, T.
1991   Another Mummy. *Natural History* 4(April):66–68.

Bill, C. R., C. L. Hernandez, and V. R. Bricker
2000   The Relationship between Early Colonial Maya New Year's Ceremonies and Some Almanacs in the Madrid Codex. *Ancient Mesoamerica* 11(1):149–168.

Billman, B. R., and G. M. Feinman (editors)
1999   *Settlement Pattern Studies in the Americas: Fifty Years since Virú.* Smithsonian Institution Press, Washington, D.C.

Billman, B. R., P. M. Lambert, and L. Banks
2000   Cannibalism, Warfare, and Drought in the Mesa Verde Region in the Twelfth Century A.D. *American Antiquity* 65(1):145–178.

Billoin, D., and A. Gape
1997   Sépulture Médiévales de l'Église Saint-Symphorien de Thibie (Marne) et Étude des

Carreaux Vernissés (fin XIIe–debut XIVe siècle). *Bulletin de la Société Archéologique Champenoise* 90(2): 83–96.

Binford, L. R.
1962   Archaeology as Anthropology. *American Antiquity* 28:217–225.
1963   An Analysis of Cremations from Three Michigan Sites. *Wisconsin Archaeologist* 44:98–110.
1971   Mortuary Practices: Their Study and Their Potential. In *Approaches to the Social Dimensions of Mortuary Practices*, edited by J. A. Brown, pp. 6–29. Society for American Archaeology, Washington, D.C.

Birkby, W. H.
1976   Cremated Human Remains. In *The Hohokam: Desert Farmers and Craftsmen*, edited by E. W. Haury, pp. 380–384. University of Arizona Press, Tucson.

Bláhová, M.
1997   Die königlichen Begräbniszeremonien im spätmittelalterlichen Böhmen. In *Der Tod des Mächtigen*, edited by L. Kolmer, pp. 89–111. Schöningh, Paderborn, Germany.

Blance, B. M.
1964   The Argaric Bronze Age in Iberia. *Revista de Guimarães* 74:129–142.
1971   *Die Anfänge der Metallurgie auf der Iberischen Halbinsel.* Studien zu den Anfängen der Metallurgie 4. Römisch-Germanisches Zentralmuseum, Berlin.

Blasco Bosqued, M. C., and L. J. Ramos Gomez
1974   Cabezas Cortadas en la Cerámica Nazca Según la Collección del Museo de América de Madrid. In *Cuadernos Prehispanicos*, vol. 2, pp. 29–79. Seminario Americanista de la Universidad, Valladolid, Spain.
1985   *Catalogo de la Ceramica Nazca del Museo de America*, vol. 1. 1st ed. Ministerio de Cultura, Madrid.

Bloch, M.
1971   *Placing the Dead: Tombs, Ancestral Villages, and Kinship Organization in Madagascar.* Seminar Press, New York.
1982   Death, Women, and Power. In *Death and the Regeneration of Life*, edited by M. Bloch and J. Parry, pp. 211–230. Cambridge University Press, New York.
1992   *Prey into Hunter: The Politics of Religious Experience.* Lewis Henry Morgan Lectures. Cambridge University Press, New York.

Bloch, M., and J. Parry
1982   Introduction: Death and the Regeneration of Life. In *Death and the Regeneration of Life*, edited by M. Bloch and J. Parry, pp. 1–44. Cambridge University Press, Cambridge.

Bloch, M., and J. Parry (editors)
1982   *Death and the Regeneration of Life.* Cambridge University Press, Cambridge.

Blofeld, J.
1970   *The Tantric Mysticism of Tibet.* Dutton, New York.

Boase, T. S. R.
1972   *Death in the Middle Ages.* McGraw-Hill, New York.

Bodde, D.
1967 [1950]   *Peking Diary.* Fawcett, New York.

Bonde, S., E. Boyden, and C. Maines
1990   Centrality and Community: Liturgy and Gothic Chapter Room Design at the Augustinian Abbey of Saint-Jean-des-Vignes, Soissons. *Gesta* 29(2):189–213.

Bonde, S., and C. Maines
1994   L'Abbaye Augustinienne de Saint-Jean-des-Vignes à Soissons. In *Congrès de l'Aisne Méridionale*, pp. 589–632. Société Française d'Archéologie, Paris.
1999   Saint-Jean-des-Vignes à Soissons, Fouilles Programmées du Grand Cloître de l'Abbaye. *Rapport Préliminaire des Fouilles de 1999*. www.wesleyan.edu/MonArch.
2000   *Rapport Annuel des Fouilles de 2000*. www.wesleyan.edu/MonArch.
2001   Saint-Jean-des-Vignes à Soissons, Fouilles Programmées du Grand Cloître de l'Abbaye. *Rapport Annuel des Fouilles de 2001*. www.wesleyan.edu/MonArch.

Boot, E.
1995   Kan Ek' at Chich'en Itsa: A Quest into Possible Itsa Heartland in the Central Peten, Guatemala. *Yumtzilob* 7(4):333–339.

Bordua, L.
1997   Mendicants. In *Atlas of Medieval Europe*, edited by A. MacKay and D. Ditchburn, pp. 116–117. Routledge, London.

Boremanse, D.
1998   *Hach Winik: The Lacandon Maya of Chiapas, Southern Mexico*. Institute for Mesoamerican Studies 11. University of Texas Press, Austin.

Bourget, S.
1997a   Las Excavaciones en la Plaza 3a. In *Investigaciones en la Huaca de la Luna 1995*, edited by S. Uceda, E. Mujica, and R. Morales, pp. 51–59. Universidad Nacional de Trujillo, Trujillo, Peru.
1997b   La Colère des Ancêtres: Découverte d'un Site Sacrificiel à la Huaca de la Luna, Vallé de Moche. In *À l'Ombre du Cerro Blanco, Nouvelles Découvertes sur la Culture Moche, Côte Nord du Pérou*, edited by C. Chapdelaine. Les Cahiers d'Anthropologie No 1. Université de Montréal, Montréal.
1998   Excavaciones en la Plaza 3a y en la Plataforma II de la Huaca de la Luna durante 1996. In *Investigaciones en la Huaca de la Luna 1996*, edited by S. Uceda, E. Mujica, and R. Morales, pp. 43–64. Universidad Nacional de Trujillo, Trujillo, Peru.

Bourget, S., and J. F. Millaire
2000   Excavaciones en la Plaza 3A y Plataforma II de la Huaca de la Luna. In *Investigaciones en la Huaca de la Luna 1997*, edited by S. Uceda, E. Mujica, and R. Morales, pp. 47–60. Universidad Nacional de Trujillo, Trujillo, Peru.

Bradley, R.
1995   Foreword. Trial and Error in the Study of Mortuary Practices—Exploring the Regional Dimension. In *Regional Approaches to Mortuary Analysis*, edited by L. A. Beck, pp. v–ix. Plenum Press, New York.

Brady, J. E.
1988   The Sexual Connotation of Caves in Mesoamerican Ideology. *Mexicon* 10:51–55.

Brady, J. E., and W. Ashmore
1999   Caves, Mountains, Water: Ancient Maya Ideational Landscapes. In *Archaeologies of Landscape: Contemporary Perspectives*, edited by W. Ashmore and A. B. Knapp, pp. 124–145. Blackwell, Oxford.

Brandherm, D.

2000   El Poblamiento Argárico de las Herrerías (Cuevas de Almanzora, Almería), según la Documentación Indédita de L. Siret. *Trabajos de Prehistoria* 57(1):157–172.

Braudel, F.

1972   *The Mediterranean and the Mediterranean World in the Age of Phillip II.* Translated by S. Reynolds. Harper and Row, New York.

Braun, D. P.

1977   *Middle Woodland–Early Late Woodland Social Change in the Prehistoric Central Midwestern U.S.* Ph.D. dissertation, University of Michigan, Ann Arbor.

1979   Illinois Hopewell Burial Practices and Social Organization: A Reexamination of the Klunk-Gibson Mound Group. In *Hopewell Archaeology: The Chillicothe Conference*, edited by D. S. Brose and N. Greber, pp. 66–79. Kent State University Press, Kent, Ohio.

1981   A Critique of Some Recent North American Mortuary Studies. *American Antiquity* 46:398–416.

1987   Coevolution of Sedentism, Pottery Technology, and Horticulture in the Central Midwest, 200 B.C.–A.D. 600. In *Emergent Horticultural Economies of the Eastern Woodlands*, edited by W. F. Keegan, pp. 153–181. Center for Archaeological Investigations Occasional Paper No. 7. Southern Illinois University at Carbondale, Carbondale.

Breton, G. le

1867   *Description de Paris sous Charles VI.* Histoire Générale de Paris. Leroux de Liney, L. Tisserand, Paris.

Briggs, C.

1992   "Since I Am a Woman, I Will Chastise My Relatives": Gender, Reported Speech, and the (Re) Production of Social Relations in Warao Ritual Wailing. *American Ethnologist* 19:337–361.

1993   Personal Sentiments and Polyphonic Voices in Warao Women's Ritual Wailing: Music and Poetics in a Critical and Collective Discourse. *American Anthropologist* 95:929–957.

Brown, E. A. R.

1978   The Ceremonial of Royal Succession in Capetian France: The Double Funeral of Louis X. *Traditio* 34:227–271.

1980   Philippe le Bel and the Remains of Saint Louis. *Gazette de Beaux-Arts* 115(May–June):175–182.

1981   Death and the Human Body in the Later Middle Ages: The Legislation of Boniface VIII on the Division of the Corpse. *Viator* 12:221–270.

1985   Burying and Unburying the Kings of France. In *Persons in Groups*, edited by R. C. Trexler, pp. 241–266. Medieval and Renaissance Texts and Studies 36. Binghamton, N.Y.

1991   *The Monarchy of Capetian France and Royal Ceremonial.* Variorum, Hampshire.

Brown, J. A.

1971a   (editor)*Approaches to the Social Dimensions of Mortuary Practices.* Memoirs of the Society for American Archaeology 25. Washington, D.C.

1971b   The Dimension of Status in the Burials at Spiro. In *Approaches to the Social Dimensions of Mortuary Practices*, edited by J. A. Brown, pp. 92–111. Memoirs of the Society for American Archaeology, Washington, D.C.

1979   Charnel House and Mortuary Crypts: Disposal of the Dead in the Middle Wood-
         land Period. In *Hopewell Archaeology: The Chillicothe Conference*, edited by D. S.
         Brose and N. Greber, pp. 211–219. Kent State University Press, Kent, Ohio.
1981   The Search for Rank in Prehistoric Burials. In *The Archaeology of Death*, edited by
         R. Chapman, I. Kinnes, and K. Randsborg, pp. 25–37. Cambridge University Press,
         Cambridge.
1985   Long-Term Trends to Sedentism and the Emergence of Complexity in the American
         Midwest. In *Prehistoric Hunter-Gatherers: The Emergence of Complexity*, edited
         by T. D. Price and J. A. Brown, pp. 201–231. Academic Press, Orlando, Fla.
1995a   Andean Mortuary Practices in Perspective. In *Tombs for the Living: Andean Mor-
         tuary Practices*, edited by T. D. Dillehay, pp. 391–405. Dumbarton Oaks, Washing-
         ton, D.C.
1995b   On Mortuary Analysis—with Special Reference to the Saxe-Binford Research Pro-
         gram. In *Regional Approaches to Mortuary Analysis*, edited by L. A. Beck, pp. 3–
         26. Plenum Press, New York.
Brown, P., and D. Tuzin (editors)
1983   *The Ethnography of Cannibalism*. Society for Psychological Anthropology, Wash-
         ington, D.C.
Browne, D. M., H. Silverman, and R. García
1993   A Cache of 48 Nasca Trophy Heads from Cerro Carapo, Peru. *Latin American
         Antiquity* 4(3):274–294.
Brunson, J.
1989   *The Social Organization of the Los Muertos Hohokam: A Reanalysis of Cushing's
         Hemenway Expedition Data*. Ph.D. dissertation, Arizona State University, Tempe.
Buikstra, J. E.
1976   *Hopewell in the Lower Illinois Valley: A Regional Approach to the Study of Hu-
         man Biological Variability and Prehistoric Behavior*. Scientific Papers No. 2.
         Northwestern University Archaeological Program, Evanston, Ill.
1981   Mortuary Practices, Palaeodemography, and Palaeopathology: A Case Study from
         the Koster Site (Illinois). In *The Archaeology of Death*, edited by R. Chapman, I.
         Kinnes, and K. Randsborg, pp. 123–132. Cambridge University Press, Cambridge.
1988   *Chiribaya: An Integrated Approach to the Biological and Cultural Development of
         an Andean Society*. Proposal for research support to the Archaeology Program,
         National Science Foundation, Washington, D.C.
1995   Tombs for the Living . . . or . . . for the Dead: The Osmore Ancestors. In *Tombs for
         the Living: Andean Mortuary Practices*, edited by T. D. Dillehay, pp. 229–280.
         Dumbarton Oaks, Washington, D.C.
2000   *Never Anything so Solemn: An Archaeological, Biological, and Historical Investi-
         gation of the 19th Century Grafton Cemetery*. Center for American Archeology,
         Kampsville, Ill.
2001   Discussion for the Symposium "New Directions in Bioarchaeology: Case Studies in
         Meaning and Interpretation." Paper presented at the Society for American Archae-
         ology, New Orleans, La.
Buikstra, J. E., P. Castro, R. Chapman, P. G. Marcen, L. Hoshower, V. Lull, R. Mico, M.
         Picazo, R. Risch, M. Ruiz, and M. E. S. Yll
1995   Approaches to Class Inequalities in the Later Prehistory of South-East Iberia: The
         Gatas Project. In *The Origins of Complex Societies in Late Prehistoric Iberia*,

edited by K. T. Lillios, pp. 153–168. Archaeological Series 8. International Monographs in Prehistory, Ann Arbor, Mich.

Buikstra, J. E., and D. K. Charles

1999   Centering the Ancestors: Cemeteries, Mounds, and Sacred Landscapes of the Ancient North American Midcontinent. In *Archaeologies of Landscape: Contemporary Perspectives,* edited by W. Ashmore and A. B. Knapp, pp. 201–228. Blackwell, Oxford.

Buikstra, J. E., D. K. Charles, and G. F. M. Rakita

1998   *Staging Ritual: Hopewell Ceremonialism at the Mound House Site, Greene County, Illinois.* Kampsville Studies in Archaeology and History 1. Center for American Archeology, Kampsville, Ill.

Buikstra, J. E., and L. Hoshower

1994   Análisis de los Restos Humanos de la Necrópolis de Gatas. In *Proyecto Gatas: Sociedad y Economía en el Sudeste de España c.2500–90 cal ANE,* edited by P. Castro, R. Chapman, E. Colomer, S. Gili, P. G. Marcén, V. Lull, R. Micó, S. Montón, C. Rihuete, R. Risch, M. R. Parra, M. E. Sanahuja, and M. Tenas, pp. 339–361. Memoria de la Junta de Andalucía. Presentada a la Consejería de Cultura de la Junta de Andalucía, Seville.

Buikstra, J. E., M. C. Lozada Cerna, G. F. M. Rakita, and P. D. Tomczak

2001   Fechados Radiocarbónicos de Sitios Chiribaya en la Cuenca del Río Osmore. Manuscript, University of New Mexico, Albuquerque.

Buikstra, J. E., and K. Nystrom

2003   Mummies, Bones, and Liminality: Hertz Revisited. In *Papers in Honor of James A. Brown,* edited by R. Jeske and D. K. Charles, pp. 29–48. Greenwood Press, Westport, Conn.

Buikstra, J. E., and D. H. Ubelaker (editors)

1994   *Standards for Data Collection from Human Skeletal Remains: Proceedings of a Seminar at the Field Museum of Natural History, organized by Jonathan Haas.* Arkansas Archeological Survey No. 44. Fayetteville.

Bullard, W.

1970   *Topoxte: A Postclassic Maya Site in Petén, Guatemala.* Papers of the Peabody Museum of Archaeology and Ethnology, Harvard University, Cambridge, Mass. Copies available from Vol. 61.

Bulmer, R.

1976   Selectivity in Hunting and Disposal of Animals by the Kalam of the New Guinea Highlands. In *Problems in Economic and Social Archaeology,* edited by G. Sieveking, I. Longworth, and K. Wilson, pp. 169–186. Duckworth, London.

Bulmer, S.

1975   Settlement and Economy in Prehistoric Papua New Guinea: A Review of the Archaeological Evidence. *Journal de la Societe des Oceanistes* 31(46):7–75.

Bunzel, R.

1930   Introduction to Zuni Ceremonialism, Zuni Origin Myths, Zuni Ritual Poetry, Zuni Katcinas. In *Forty-seventh Annual Report of the Bureau of American Ethnology, 1929–1930,* pp. 467–1086. Government Printing Office, Washington, D.C.

Burger, R.

1992   *Chavín and the Origins of Andean Civilization.* Thames and Hudson, New York.

Burgess, F.
1963   *English Churchyard Memorials*. Lutterworth Press, London.
Butler, B. M. (editor)
1988   *Archaeological Investigations on the North Coast of Rota, Mariana Islands*. No. 23. Center for Archaeological Investigations Occasional Paper No. 8. Southern Illinois University, Carbondale.
1997   *An Archaeological Survey of the East and Southeast Coast of Rota, Mariana Islands*. Prepared for the Division of Historic Preservation, Department of Community and Cultural Affairs, Saipan, Marianas Protectorate.
Byers, A. M.
1987   *The Earthwork Enclosures of the Central Ohio Valley: A Temporal and Structural Analysis of Woodland Society and Culture*. Ph.D. dissertation, State University of New York at Albany. University Microfilms, Ann Arbor, Mich.
1998   Is the Newark Circle-Octagon the Ohio Hopewell "Rosetta Stone"? In *Ancient Earthen Enclosures of the Eastern Woodlands*, edited by R. C. Mainfort Jr. and L. P. Sullivan, pp. 135–153. University Press of Florida, Gainesville.
1999   Intentionality, Symbolic Pragmatics, and Material Culture: Revisiting Binford's View of the Old Copper Complex. *American Antiquity* 64(2):265–287.
2004   *The Ohio Hopewell Episode: Paradigm Lost and Paradigm Gained*. University of Akron Press, Akron, Ohio.
Cabrol, F., and H. Leclercq
1924–1953   *Dictionnaire d'Archéologie Chrétienne et de Liturgie*. 15 vols. Letouzey, Paris.
Cannon, A.
1989   The Historical Dimension in Mortuary Expressions of Status and Sentiment. *Current Anthropology* 30(4):437–458.
1991   Gender, Status, and the Focus of Material Display. In *The Archaeology of Gender: Proceedings of the Twenty-second Annual Conference of the Archaeological Association of the University of Calgary*, edited by D. Walde and N. D. Willows, pp. 144–149. University of Calgary, Archaeological Association, Calgary.
1995   Two Faces of Power: Communal and Individual Modes of Mortuary Expression. *ARX World Journal of Prehistoric and Ancient Studies* 1(1):3–8.
1996   Trends and Motivations: Scaling the Dimensions of Material Complexity. In *Debating Complexity: Proceedings of the Twenty-sixth Annual Chacmool Conference*, edited by D. A. Meyer, P. C. Dawson, and D. T. Hanna. University of Calgary Archaeological Association, Calgary.
1998   The Cultural and Historical Contexts of Fashion. In *Consuming Fashion: Adorning the Transnational Body*, edited by A. Brydon and S. Niessen, pp. 23–38. Berg, Oxford.
2002   Spatial Narratives of Death, Memory, and Transcendence. In *The Space and Place of Death*, edited by H. Silverman and D. Small, pp. 191–199. Archaeological Publications of the American Anthropological Association No. 11. Arlington, Va.
Carlsen, R., and M. Prechtel
1991   The Flowering of the Dead: An Interpretation of Highland Maya Culture. *Man* 26:23–42.
Carmichael, P. H.
1988   *Nasca Mortuary Customs: Death and Ancient Society on the South Coast of Peru*. Ph.D. dissertation, University of Calgary, Calgary.

1995   Nasca Burial Patterns: Social Structure and Mortuary Ideology. In *Tombs for the Living: Andean Mortuary Practices,* edited by T. D. Dillehay, pp. 161–187. Dumbarton Oaks, Washington, D.C.

Carneiro da Cunha, M.

1978   *Os Mortos e os Otros.* Hucitec, São Paulo.

Carneiro da Cunha, M., and E. Viveiros de Castro

1985   Vingança e Temporalidade: Os Tupinambá. *Journal de la Société des Américanistes* 71:191–208.

Carr, C.

1995   Mortuary Practices: Their Social, Philosophical-Religious, Circumstantial, and Physical Determinants. *Journal of Archaeological Method and Theory* 2(2):105–200.

Carrelli, C. W.

1990   *Mortuary Practices in Groups 8L-10 and 8L-12, Copán, Honduras.* Unpublished B.A. honors thesis, Rutgers University, New Brunswick, N.J.

Castro, P., R. Chapman, S. Gili, V. Lull, R. Micó, C. Rihuete, R. Risch, and M. E. Sanahuja

1993–1994   Tiempos Sociales de los Contextos Funerarios Argáricos. *Anales de Prehistoria de la Universidad de Murcia* 9–10:77–107.

1999a   *Proyecto Gatas.* Vol. 2: *La Dinámica Arqueoecológica de la Ocupación Prehistórica.* Junta de Andalucía, Consejería de Cultura, Seville.

1999b   Agricultural Production and Social Change in the Bronze Age of Southeast Spain: The Gatas Project. *Antiquity* 73:846–856.

2000   Archaeology and Desertification in the Vera Basin (Almería, South-East Spain). *European Journal of Archaeology* 3(2):147–166.

Catholic University of America

1967   *New Catholic Encyclopaedia.* McGraw-Hill, New York.

Cecil, L.

2001   *The Technological Styles of Late Postclassic Slipped Pottery Groups in the Petén Lakes Region, El Petén, Guatemala.* Ph.D. dissertation, Southern Illinois University at Carbondale.

Chan, V.

1994   *Tibet Handbook.* Moon Publications, Chico, Calif.

Chapdelaine, C.

1998   Excavaciones en la Zona Urbana de Moche durante 1996. In *Investigaciones en la Huaca de la Luna 1996,* edited by S. Uceda, E. Mujica, and R. Morales, pp. 85–115. Universidad Nacional de Trujillo, Trujillo, Peru.

Chapman, J.

2000   Tension at Funerals: Social Practices and the Subversion of Community Structure in Later Hungarian Prehistory. In *Agency in Archaeology,* edited by M.-A. Dobres and J. E. Robb, pp. 169–195. Routledge, London.

Chapman, R.

1977   Burial Practice: An Area of Mutual Interests. In *Archaeology and Anthropology: Areas of Mutual Interest,* edited by M. Spriggs, pp. 19–33. Supplement 19. British Archaeological Reports, Oxford.

1981   Archaeological Theory and Communal Burial in Prehistoric Europe. In *Patterns of the Past: Studies in Honor of David Clarke,* edited by I. Hodder, G. Isaac, and N. Hammond, pp. 387–411. Cambridge University Press, Cambridge.

1990   *Emerging Complexity: The Later Prehistory of South-East Spain, Iberia, and the West Mediterranean.* Cambridge University Press, Cambridge.

2003   *Archaeologies of Complexity.* Routledge, London.

Chapman, R., I. Kinnes, and K. Randsborg (editors)

1981   *The Archaeology of Death.* Cambridge University Press, Cambridge.

Chapman, R., V. Lull, M. Picazo, and M. Encarna Sanahuja (editors)

1987   *Proyecto Gatas: Sociedad y Economía en el Sudeste de España c. 2500–800 a.n.e.* BAR International Series 348. British Archaeological Reports, Oxford.

Charles, D. K.

1992   Woodland Demographic and Social Dynamics in the American Midwest: Analysis of a Burial Mound Survey. *World Archaeology* 24(2):175–197.

1995   Diachronic Regional Social Dynamics: Mortuary Sites in the Illinois Valley/American Bottom Region. In *Regional Approaches to Mortuary Analysis,* edited by L. A. Beck, pp. 77–99. Plenum Press, New York.

1998a   *Sex and Gender at the End of Hopewell.* Paper presented at the 14th International Congress of Anthropological and Ethnological Sciences, Williamsburg, Va.

1998b   *Women, Men, and the Hopewell Climax.* Paper presented at the 63rd Annual Meeting of the Society for American Archaeology, Seattle, Wash.

2000   *Reconstructing Hopewell: Gender, Economics, and Politics.* Paper presented at the Perspectives on Middle Woodland at the Millennium Conference, Pere Marquette State Park, Ill.

Charles, D. K., and J. E. Buikstra

1983   Archaic Mortuary Sites in the Central Mississippi Drainage: Distribution, Structure, and Behavioral Implications. In *Archaic Hunters and Gatherers in the American Midwest,* edited by J. L. Phillips and J. A. Brown, pp. 117–145. Academic Press, New York.

2002   Siting, Sighting, and Citing the Dead. In *The Space and Place of Death,* edited by H. Silverman and D. Small, pp. 13–25. Archeological Papers of the American Anthropological Association No. 11. Arlington, Va.

Charles, D. K., J. E. Buikstra, and L. W. Konigsberg

1986   Behavioral Implications of Terminal Archaic and Early Woodland Mortuary Practices in the Lower Illinois Valley. In *Early Woodland Archaeology,* edited by K. B. Farnsworth and T. E. Emerson, pp. 458–474. Center for American Archeology, Kampsville, Ill.

Charles, D. K., S. R. Leigh, and J. E. Buikstra

1988   *The Archaic and Woodland Cemeteries at the Elizabeth Site in the Lower Illinois River Valley.* Center for American Archeology, Kampsville, Ill.

Chase, D. Z., and A. F. Chase

1996   Maya Multiples: Individuals, Entries, and Tombs in Structure A34 of Caracol, Belize. *Latin American Antiquity* 7:61–79.

1998   The Architectural Context of Caches, Burials, and Other Ritual Activities for the Classic Period Maya (as Reflected at Caracol, Belize). In *Function and Meaning in Classic Maya Architecture,* edited by S. D. Houston, pp. 299–332. Dumbarton Oaks, Washington, D.C.

Chavez, S.

1992   *The Conventionalized Rules in Pucara Pottery Technology and Iconography: Im-*

plications for Socio-political Development in the Northern Lake Titicaca Basin. Ph.D. dissertation, Michigan State University, East Lansing.

Checura, J.

1977   Funebria Incaica en el Cerro Esmeralda (Iquique, I Region). *Estudios Atacamenos* 5:125–141.

Chesson, M. S. (editor)

2001   *Social Memory, Identity, and Death: Anthropological Perspectives on Mortuary Rituals.* American Anthropological Association, Washington, D.C.

Chiles, L.

1997   *Aitape in Context: A Reanalysis of the Evidence and a Discussion of Its Place in Pacific Prehistory.* B.A. honors thesis, University of Otago, New Zealand.

Chisholm, B. S., D. E. Nelson, and H. P. Schwarcz

1982   Stable-Carbon Isotope Ratios as a Measure of Marine Versus Terrestrial Protein in Ancient Diets. *Science* 216:1131–1132.

Chowning, A.

1986   Melanesian Religions: An Overview. In *Encyclopedia of Religion,* edited by M. Eliade, vol. 9, pp. 349–359. 17 vols. Macmillan, New York.

1991   Pigs, Dogs, and Children in Molima. In *Man and a Half: Essays in Pacific Anthropology and Ethnobiology in Honour of Ralph Bulmer,* edited by A. Pawley, pp. 182–187. Polynesian Society Memoirs 48. Polynesian Society, Auckland.

Clark, J. E., and M. Blake

1994   The Power of Prestige: Competitive Generosity and the Emergence of Rank Societies in Lowland Mesoamerica. In *Factional Competition and Political Development in the New World,* edited by E. M. Brumfiel and J. W. Fox, pp. 17–30. Cambridge University Press, Cambridge.

Clark, K.

1962   *The Gothic Revival: An Essay in the History of Taste.* Harper and Row, New York.

Clay, R. B.

1991   Adena Ritual Development: An Organizational Type in Temporal Perspective. In *The Human Landscape in Kentucky's Past: Site Structure and Settlement Patterns,* edited by C. Stout and C. K. Hensley, pp. 30–39. Kentucky Heritage Council, Lexington.

1992   Chiefs, Big Men or What? Economy, Settlement Patterns, and Their Bearing on Adena Political Models. In *Cultural Variability in Context: Woodland Settlements in the Mid-Ohio Valley,* edited by M. F. Seeman, pp. 77–80. Midcontinental Journal of Archaeology Special Paper No. 7. Kent State University Press, Kent, Ohio.

1998   The Essential Features of Adena Ritual and Their Implications. *Southeastern Archaeology* 17(1):1–21.

Cobb, C. R.

1991   Social Reproduction and the Longue Durée in the Prehistory of the Midcontinental United States. In *Processual and Postprocessual Archaeologies: Multiple Ways of Knowing the Past,* edited by R. W. Pruecel, pp. 168–182. Center for Archaeological Investigations Occasional Paper No. 10. Southern Illinois University at Carbondale, Carbondale.

Cobo, B.

1964 [1653]   *Historia del Nuevo Mundo.* Biblioteca de Autores Espanoles, Madrid.

1990   *Inca Religion and Customs.* Translated by R. Hamilton. University of Texas Press, Austin.

Cockburn, A., and E. Cockburn (editors)
1980   *Mummies, Disease, and Ancient Cultures.* Abridged ed. Cambridge University Press, Cambridge.

Coe, M. D.
1956   The Funerary Temple among the Ancient Maya. *Southwestern Journal of Anthropology* 12:387–394.
1975   Death and the Ancient Maya. In *Death and the Afterlife in Pre-Columbian America,* edited by E. P. Benson, pp. 87–104. Dumbarton Oaks, Washington, D.C.
1988   Ideology of the Maya Tomb. In *Maya Iconography,* edited by E. P. Benson and G. G. Griffin, pp. 222–235. Princeton University Press, Princeton, N.J.

Coe, W. R.
1967   *Tikal: A Handbook of the Ancient Maya Ruins.* University Museum, Philadelphia, Penn.

Coelho, V.
1972   *Enterramentos de Cabeças da Cultura Nasca.* Ph.D. dissertation, Universidad de São Paulo.

Coffin, M. M.
1976   *Death in Early America: The History and Folklore of Customs and Superstitions of Early Medicine, Funerals, Burials, and Mourning.* Elsevier/Nelson Books, New York.

Coggins, C. C.
1980   The Shape of Time: Some Political Implications of a Four-Part Figure. *American Antiquity* 45:727–739.
1984   The Cenote of Sacrifice: Catalogue. In *Cenote of Sacrifice: Maya Treasures from the Sacred Well at Chichén Itzá,* edited by C. C. Coggins and O. Shane III, pp. 23–165. University of Texas, Austin.
1992   Dredging the Cenote. In *Artifacts from the Cenote of Sacrifice, Chichen Itza, Yucatan: Textiles, Basketry, Stone, Bone, Shell, Ceramics, Wood, Copal, Rubber, Other Organic Materials, and Mammalian Remains,* edited by C. C. Coggins, pp. 9–32. Memoirs of the Peabody Museum of Archaeology and Ethnology, Vol. 3, No. 10. Harvard University, Cambridge, Mass.

Coggins, C. C., and J. M. Ladd
1992   Wooden Artifacts. In *Artifacts from the Cenote of Sacrifice, Chichen Itza, Yucatan: Textiles, Basketry, Stone, Bone, Shell, Ceramics, Wood, Copal, Rubber, Other Organic Materials, and Mammalian Remains,* edited by C. C. Coggins, pp. 235–344. Memoirs of the Peabody Museum, Vol. 3, No. 10. Harvard University, Cambridge, Mass.

Colardelle, M.
1981   Archéologie Religieuse du Haut Moyen Age en Milieu Rural: Méthodes et Problèmes. *Bulletin de Liaison de l'Association Française d'Archéologie Mérovingienne* 4:29–33.
1989   Eglises et Sépultures dans les Alpes du Nord (Aoste, Genève, Grenoble, Lyon et Vienne). Paper presented at the Actes du 11 Congrée International d'Archéologie Chrétienne, Lyon, France.

Conkey, M. W., and J. D. Spector
1984   Archaeology and the Study of Gender. In *Advances in Archaeological Method and Theory*, vol. 7, edited by M. B. Schiffer, pp. 10–38. Academic Press, Orlando, Fla.

Conklin, B. A.
1995   "Thus Are Our Bodies, Thus Was Our Custom": Mortuary Cannibalism in an Amazonian Society. *American Ethnologist* 22(1):75–101.
2001   *Consuming Grief.* University of Texas Press, Austin.

Conrad, G. W., and A. A. Demarest
1984   *Religion and Empire: The Dynamics of Aztec and Inca Expansionism.* Cambridge University Press, New York.

Cook, A. G.
2001   Huari D-Shaped Structures, Sacrificial Offerings, and Divine Rulership. In *Ritual Sacrifice in Ancient Peru*, edited by E. P. Benson and A. G. Cook, pp. 137–164. University of Texas Press, Austin.

Coomans, P.
2000   *History of the Mission in the Mariana Islands: 1667–1673*, translated and edited by R. Lévesque. Occasional Historical Papers Series 4. Division of Historic Preservation, Saipan.

Cordy-Collins, A.
1992   Archaism or Tradition?: The Decapitation Theme in Cupisnique and Moche Iconography. *Latin American Antiquity* 3(3):206–220.

Cotton, G. E., A. C. Aufderheide, and V. G. Goldschmidt
1987   Preservation of Human Tissue Immersed for Five Years in Fresh Water of Known Temperature. *Journal of Forensic Sciences* 32(4):1125–1130.

Coudart, A.
1999   Is Post-Processualism Bound to Happen Everywhere? The French Case. *Antiquity* 73:161–167.

Cowell, A.
1974   *The Tribe that Hides from Man.* Stein and Day, New York.

Cowgill, G. L.
1963   *Postclassic Period Culture in the Vicinity of Flores, Petén, Guatemala.* Ph.D. dissertation, Harvard University, Cambridge, Mass.
2000   "Rationality" and Contexts in Agency Theory. In *Agency in Archaeology*, edited by M.-A. Dobres and J. E. Robb, pp. 51–60. Routledge, London.

Creel, D.
1989   A Primary Cremation at the NAN Ranch Ruin, with Comparative Data on Other Cremations in the Mimbres Area, New Mexico. *Journal of Field Archaeology* 16:309–329.

Crown, P. L.
1991   The Hohokam: Current Views of Prehistory and the Regional System. In *Chaco and Hohokam: Prehistoric Regional Systems in the American Southwest*, edited by P. L. Crown and W. J. Judge, pp. 135–157. School of American Research, Santa Fe, N.Mex.

Crown, P. L., and S. K. Fish
1996   Gender and Status in the Hohokam Pre-Classic to Classic Transition. *American Anthropologist* 98(4):803–817.

Cunningham, W. M.
1948   *A Study of the Glacial Kame Culture in Michigan, Ohio, and Indiana.* Occasional Contributions from the Museum of Anthropology of the University of Michigan No. 12. University of Michigan Press, Ann Arbor.

Curet, L. A., and J. R. Oliver
1998   Mortuary Practices, Social Development, and Ideology in Precolumbian Puerto Rico. *Latin American Antiquity* 9(3):217–239.

Dale, T. E. A.
2000   Stolen Property: St Mark's First Venetian Tomb and the Politics of Communal Memory. In *Memory and the Medieval Tomb,* edited by E. Valdez del Alamo and C. S. Pendergast, pp. 51–88. Ashgate, Brookfield, Vt.

Dancey, W. S., and P. J. Pacheco
1997   A Community Model of Ohio Hopewell Settlement. In *Ohio Hopewell Community Organization,* edited by W. S. Dancey and P. J. Pacheco, pp. 3–40. Kent State University Press, Kent, Ohio.

Daniell, C.
1997   *Death and Burial in Medieval England: 1066–1550.* Routledge, London.

Darling, A.
1998   Mass Inhumation and the Execution of Witches in the American Southwest. *American Anthropologist* 100:732–752.

Dauelsberg, P.
1972–1973a Carta Respuesta a Luis Guillermo Lumbreras, "Sobre la Problemática Arqueológica de Arica." *Chungará* 1–2:32–37.
1972–1973b La Cerámica de Arica y su Situación Cronológica. *Chungará* 1–2:17–24.

David-Neel, A.
1986 [1927] *My Journey to Lhasa.* (Originally published as *Voyage d'une Parisienne à Lhassa* by Harper and Brothers, New York.) Beacon Press, Boston.

Davis, E. H.
1921   *Early Cremation Ceremonies of the Luiseno and Diegueno Indians of Southern California.* Indian Notes and Monographs, Vol. 7, No. 3. Museum of the American Indian, Heye Foundation, New York.

Davis, S. H.
1977   *Victims of the Miracle.* Cambridge University Press, Cambridge.

Day, J. S.
2001   Performing on the Court. In *The Sport of Life and Death: The Mesoamerican Ballgame,* edited by E. M. Whittington, pp. 64–77. Mint Museum of Art, Charlotte, N.C.

Deacon, A. B.
1934   *Malekula, A Vanishing People in the New Hebrides.* George Routledge and Sons, London.

DeGusta, D.
1999   Fijian Cannibalism: Osteological Evidence from Navatu. *American Journal of Physical Anthropology* 110:215–241.
2000   Fijian Cannibalism and Mortuary Ritual: Bioarchaeological Evidence from Vunda. *International Journal of Osteoarchaeology* 10:76–92.

DeLeonardis, L.
2000   The Body Context: Interpreting Early Nasca Decapitated Burials. *Latin American Antiquity* 11(4):363–386.

Demarest, A.
1984   Overview: Mesoamerican Human Sacrifice in Evolutionary Perspective. In *Ritual Human Sacrifice in Mesoamerica: A Conference at Dumbarton Oaks*, edited by E. H. Boone, pp. 227–242. Dumbarton Oaks, Washington, D.C.

Denziger, H.
1963   *Enchiridion Symbolorum*. 32nd ed. Herder, Freiburg, Germany.

Descola, P.
1992   Societies of Nature and the Nature of Societies. In *Conceptualizing Society*, edited by A. Kuper, pp. 107–126. Routledge, London.
1996   Constructing Natures: Symbolic Ecology and Social Practice. In *Nature and Society*, edited by P. Descola and G. Pálsson, pp. 82–102. Routledge, New York.

Dillehay, T. D.
2001   Town and Country in Late Moche Times: A View from Two Northern Valleys. In *Moche Art and Archaeology in Ancient Peru*, edited by J. Pillsbury, pp. 259–284. National Gallery of Art, Washington, D.C.

Dobres, M.-A., and J. E. Robb
2000   Agency in Archaeology: Paradigm or Platitude? In *Agency in Archaeology*, edited by M.-A. Dobres and J. E. Robb, pp. 3–17. Routledge, London.

Dockall, H. D., J. F. Powell, and D. G. Steele
1996   *Home Hereafter: Archaeological and Bioarchaeological Investigations at an Historic African-American Cemetery (41GV125)*. Report of Investigations No. 5. Center for Environmental Archaeology, Texas A&M University, College Station.

Dodson, A.
1994   The King Is Dead. In *The Unbroken Reed*, edited by C. Eyre, A. Leahy, and L. M. Leahy, pp. 71–95. Egypt Exploration Society, London.

Doering, H. U.
1958   Bericht über Archaologische Feldarbeiten in Perú. *Ethnos* 23(2–4):67–99.
1966   *On the Royal Highways of the Inca*. Praeger, New York.

Dongoske, K. E., D. L. Martin, and T. J. Ferguson
2000   Critique of the Claim of Cannibalism at Cowboy Wash. *American Antiquity* 65(1):179–190.

Donnan, C. B.
1978   *Moche Art of Peru: Pre-Columbian Symbolic Communication*. Museum of Cultural History, University of California, Los Angeles.
1995   Moche Funerary Practice. In *Tombs for the Living: Andean Mortuary Practices*, edited by T. D. Dillehay, pp. 111–160. Dumbarton Oaks, Washington, D.C.
1997   Deer Hunting and Combat: Parallel Activities in the Moche World. In *The Spirit of Ancient Peru: Treasures from the Museo Arqueológico Rafael Larco Herrera*, edited by K. Berrin, pp. 51–59. Thames and Hudson, New York.

Donnan, C. B., and L. J. Castillo
1992   Finding the Tomb of a Moche Priestess. *Archaeology* 45(6):39–42.
1994   Excavaciones de Tumbas de Sacerdotisas Moche en San José de Moro, Jequetepeque. In *Moche, Propuestas y Perspectivas: Actas del Primer Coloquio sobre la*

Cultura Moche, edited by S. Uceda and E. Mujica, pp. 415–424. Universidad Nacional de Trujillo, Peru.

Donnan, C. B., and C. J. Mackey
1978   *Ancient Burial Patterns of the Moche Valley, Peru.* University of Texas Press, Austin.

Dorsey, G. A.
1897   Observations on a Collection of Papuan Crania. *Field Columbian Museum Publication 21.* Anthropological Series, Vol. 2, No. 1, pp. 1–39. Chicago.

Douglas, M.
1966   *Purity and Danger.* Praeger, New York.
1982   *In the Active Voice.* Routledge Kegan and Paul, London.

Douglas, M. T., M. Pietrusewsky, and R. M. Ikehara-Quebral
1997   Skeletal Biology of Apurguan: A Precontact Chamorro Site on Guam. *American Journal of Physical Anthropology* 104:291–313.

Douglass, W. A.
1969   *Death in Murelaga: Funerary Ritual in a Spanish Basque Village.* University of Washington Press, Seattle.

Downs, H. R.
1980   *Rhythms of a Himalayan Village.* Harper and Row, New York.

Dragoo, D. W.
1963   *Mounds for the Dead: An Analysis of the Adena Culture.* Annals of the Carnegie Museum 37. Pittsburgh, Penn.

Driver, M. G.
1983   Fray Juan Pobre de Zamora and His Account of the Mariana Islands. *Journal of Pacific History* 18(3):198–216.
1988   Fray Juan Pobre de Zamora. *Journal of Pacific History* 23:86–94.

Drusini, A. G., and J. P. Baraybar
1991   Anthropological Study of Nasca Trophy Heads. *Homo* 41(3):251–265.

Duby, G.
1967   *L'An Mil.* Collection Archives. Julliard, Paris.

Duday, H.
1985   Observation Ostéologique et Décomposition du Cadavre: Sépulture Colmatée ou en Espace Vide? Paper presented at the Comptes-rendu de la Table Ronde Tenue à Saint-Germain-en-Laye, Paris.

Duday, H., P. Courtaus, E. Crubezy, P. Sellier, and A. M. Tiller
1990   L'Anthropologie "de Terrain": Reconnaissance et Interprétation des Gestes Funéraires. *Bulletin et Mémoire de la Société d'Anthropologique de Paris* 2(3–4):29–50.

Duday, H., and P. Sellier
1990   L'Archéologie des Gestes Funéraires et la Taphonomie. *Les Nouvelles de l'Archéologie* 40:12–14.

Duke, P.
1991   *Points in Time: Structure and Event in a Late Northern Plains Hunting Society.* University Press of Colorado, Niwot.

Duncan, W. N.
1999   Postclassic Mortuary Practice in Civic/Ceremonial Contexts in Petén, Guatemala. Paper presented at the 64th Annual Meeting of the Society for American Archaeology, Chicago.

2000   Soul Termination and Regeneration among the Maya. Paper presented at the American Anthropological Association, San Francisco, Calif.

Dunn, M.

1997   Cistercians, Premonstratensians, and Others. In *Atlas of Medieval Europe*, edited by A. MacKay and D. Ditchburn, pp. 114–115. Routledge, London.

Durand, M.

1988   Archéologie du Cimetière Médiéval au Sud-Est de l'Oise. *Revue Archéologique de Picardie* (special issue):1–208.

1991   Un Prieuré Moyen de l'Ordre de Cluny dans l'Oise: Saint-Nicolas d'Acy (XIe–XVIIe Siecles). *Revue Archéologique de Picardie* 1–2:21–160.

Durand de Mende, G.

1854 [1284]   *Rational ou Manuel des Divins Offices.* Vol. 1. Translated by C. Barthelemy. 5 vols. Vives, Paris.

Edmonson, M.

1982   *The Ancient Future of the Itza: The Book of Chilam Balam of Tizimin.* University of Texas Press, Austin.

1984   Human Sacrifice in the Books of Chilam Balam of Tizimin and Chumayel. In *Ritual Human Sacrifice in Mesoamerica*, edited by E. P. Boone, pp. 91–100. Dumbarton Oaks, Washington, D.C.

Egloff, B.

1972   The Sepulchral Pottery of Nuamata Island, Papua. *Archaeology and Physical Anthropology in Oceania* 7(2):145–163.

1979   *Recent Prehistory in Southeast Papua.* Terra Australis 4. Department of Prehistory, Research School of Pacific Studies, Australian National University, Canberra.

Ehlers, J., H. Müller, and B. Schneidmüller (editors)

1996   *Die französischen Könige des Mittelalters: Von Odo bis Karl VIII, 888–1498.* C. H. Beck, Munich.

Eliade, M.

1959   *The Sacred and the Profane.* Harcourt, Brace, and World, New York.

1974 [1951]   *Shamanism: Archaic Techniques of Ecstasy.* Translated by W. R. Trask. Bollingen Series 76. (Originally published as *Le Chamanisme et les Techniques Archaïques de l'Extase* by Librairie Payot, Paris.) Princeton University Press, Princeton, N.J.

Engel, F.

1967   *A Preceramic Settlement on the Coast of Peru: Asia, Unit I.* Transactions of the American Philosophical Society Vol. 53, No. 3. Philadelphia, Penn.

Ernst, T. M.

1999   Onobasulu Cannibalism and the Moral Agents of Misfortune. In *The Anthropology of Cannibalism*, edited by L. Goldman, pp. 143–160. Bergin and Garvey, Westport, Conn.

Faison, S.

1999   Lirong Journal: Tibetans and Vultures Keep Ancient Burial Rite. *The New York Times*, July 3.

Farnsworth, K. B., and D. L. Asch

1986   Early Woodland Chronology, Artifact Styles, and Settlement Distribution in the Lower Illinois Valley Region. In *Early Woodland Archaeology*, edited by K. B.

Farnsworth and T. E. Emerson, pp. 326–457. Center for American Archaeology, Kampsville, Ill.

Farnsworth, K. B., and M. D. Wiant (editors)
2005   *Gregory Perino's Excavations at Certain Hopewell and Late Woodland Sites in West-Central Illinois, 1951–1974.* Illinois Transportation Archaeological Research Program, Studies in Archaeology 3. University of Illinois Press, Urbana.

Fausto, C.
1999   Of Enemies and Pets: Warfare and Shamanism in Amazonia. *American Ethnologist* 26:933–956.

2001   *Inimigos Fieis: Historia, Guerra, e Xamanismo na Amazônia.* Universidade de São Paulo, São Paulo.

Fenner, F. J.
1941   Fossil Human Skull Fragments of Probable Pleistocene Age, from Aitape, New Guinea. *Records of the South Australian Museum* 6:335–354.

Finucane, R. C.
1981   Sacred Corpse, Profane Carrion: Social Ideals and Death Rituals in the Later Middle Ages. In *Mirrors of Mortality,* edited by J. Whaley, pp. 40–60. Europa Publications, London.

Foccaci Aste, G.
1981   Nuevos Fechados para la Época del Tiahuanaco en la Arqueología de Norte de Chile. *Chungará* 8:63–77.

1983   El Tiwanaku Clásico en el Valle de Azapa. In *Asentamientos Aldeanos en los Valles Costeros de Arica: Documentos de Trabajo,* vol. 3, pp. 94–124. Instituto de Antropología y Arquelogia, Universidad de Tarapacá, Arica, Chile.

Forde, C. D.
1931   *Ethnography of the Yuma Indians.* University of California Publications in American Archaeology and Ethnology, Vol. 28, No. 4. University of California, Berkeley.

Forde, D.
1962   Death and Succession: An Analysis of Yako Mortuary Ritual. In *Essays on the Ritual of Social Relations,* edited by M. Gluckman, pp. 89–123. Manchester University Press, Manchester.

Forenbaher, S.
1993   Radiocarbon Dates and Absolute Chronology of the Central European Early Bronze Age. *Antiquity* 67:235–256.

Forge, A.
1973   Style and Meaning in Sepik Art. In *Primitive Art and Society,* edited by A. Forge, pp. 169–192. Oxford University Press, London.

Fortes, M.
1945   *The Dynamics of Clanship among the Tallensi.* Oxford University Press, London.

Foster, R. J.
1990   Nurture and Force Feeding: Mortuary Feasting and the Construction of Collective Individuals in a New Ireland Society. *American Ethnologist* 17:431–448.

Foucault, M.
1995 [1977]   *Discipline and Punish: The Birth of the Prison.* Vintage Books, New York.

Frame, M.
2001   Blood, Fertility, and Transformation: Interwoven Themes in the Paracas Necro-

polis Embroideries. In *Ritual Sacrifice in Ancient Peru*, edited by E. P. Benson and A. G. Cook, pp. 55–92. University of Texas Press, Austin.

Franco, R., C. Gálvez, and S. Vásquez

1994   Arquitectura y Decoración Mochica en La Huaca Cao Viejo, Complejo El Brujo: Resultados Preliminares. In *Moche, Propuestas y Perspectivas: Actas del Primer Coloquio sobre la Cultura Moche*, edited by S. Uceda and E. Mujica, pp. 147–180. Universidad Nacional de Trujillo, Trujillo, Peru.

Freedman, M.

1966   *Chinese Lineage and Society: Fukien and Kwangtung*. Athlone Press, New York.

Freemantle, F., and C. Trungpa (translators)

1975   *The Tibetan Book of the Dead: The Great Liberation through Hearing in the Bardo*. Shambala Publications, Boulder, Colo.

Freidel, D., L. Schele, and J. Parker

1993   *Maya Cosmos: Three Thousand Years on the Shaman's Path*. William Morrow, New York.

Fritz, G.

1989   *The Chamorro: A History and Ethnography of the Marianas*. 2nd ed. Edited by Scott Russell. Translated by Elfriede Craddock. Originally published in German in 1904. First English edition 1986. Division of Historic Preservation, Saipan, Commonwealth of the Northern Mariana Islands.

Fuland, L.

1989   *Morning Breeze: A True Story of China's Cultural Revolution*. China Books, San Francisco, Calif.

Furst, J. L.

1995   *The Natural History of the Soul in Ancient Mexico*. Yale University Press, New Haven, Conn.

Galloway, A.

1985   Determination of Parity from the Maternal Skeleton: An Appraisal. *Rivista di Anthropologia (Roma)* 73:83–98.

García Márquez, M.

1988   *Excavaciones de dos Viviendas Chiribaya en El Yaral, Valle de Moquegua*. Bachelor's thesis, Facultad de Ciencias Histórico Arqueológicas, Universidad Católica "Santa María."

Garcilaso de la Vega, E. I.

1987 [1609]   *Royal Commentaries of the Incas and General History of Peru*, Part 1. Translated by H. V. Livermore. University of Texas Press, Austin.

Gardner, D.

1999   Anthropophagy, Myth, and the Subtle Ways of Ethnocentrism. In *The Anthropology of Cannibalism*, edited by L. Goldman, pp. 26–50. Bergin and Garvey, Westport, Conn.

Geertz, C.

1983   *Local Knowledge*. Basic Books, New York.

Geller, P. L.

1998   *Analysis of Sex and Gender in a Maya Mortuary Context at Preclassic Cuello, Belize*. Unpublished Master's thesis, University of Chicago.

2000   Sex and Gender at Preclassic Cuello: A Mortuary Analysis. Paper presented at the 65th Annual Meeting of the Society for American Archaeology, Philadelphia, Penn.

2001   *Maya Mortuary Spaces as Cosmological Metaphors.* 2001 Chacmool Conference, An Odyssey of Space, University of Calgary, Calgary.

2004   *Transforming Bodies, Transforming Identities: A Consideration of Pre-Columbian Maya Corporal Beliefs and Practices.* Ph.D. dissertation, University of Pennsylvania, Philadelphia.

Gerber, J., and E. Schecter

2002   Mollusks from Archaeological Excavations in Northwestern Papua New Guinea. Paper presented at the 68th Annual Meeting of the American Malacological Society, Charleston, South Carolina.

Gerbert, M., M. Herrgott, and R. Heer

1772   *Taphographia Principium Austriae, Monumenta Augustae Domus Austriae,* vol. 2, part 2. St. Blasien, Germany.

Ghersi Barrera, H.

1956   Informe Sobre las Excavaciones en Chiribaya. *Revista del Museo Nacional* 25:89–119.

Gibbs, L.

1987   Identifying Gender Representation in the Archaeological Record: A Contextual Study. In *The Archaeology of Contextual Meanings,* edited by I. Hodder, pp. 79–89. Cambridge University Press, Cambridge.

Giesey, R. E.

1960   *The Royal Funeral Ceremony in Renaissance France.* Libraire E. Droz, Geneva.

Gillespie, S.

1991   Ballgames and Boundaries. In *The Mesoamerican Ballgame,* edited by V. L. Scarborough and D. R. Wilcox, pp. 317–345. University of Arizona Press, Tucson.

2000   Maya "Nested Houses": The Ritual Construction of Place. In *Beyond Kinship: Social and Material Reproduction in House Societies,* edited by R. A. Joyce and S. D. Gillespie, pp. 135–160. University of Pennsylvania Press, Philadelphia.

2001   Personhood, Agency, and Mortuary Ritual: A Case Study from the Ancient Maya. *Journal of Anthropological Archaeology* 20:73–112.

2002   Body and Soul among the Maya: Keeping the Spirits in Place. In *The Space and Place of Death,* edited by H. Silverman and D. Small, pp. 67–78. Archeological Papers of the American Anthropological Association No. 11. Arlington, Va.

Gilman, A.

1981   The Development of Social Stratification in Bronze Age Europe. *Current Anthropology* 22:1–23.

Gladikas, B.

1978   Orangutan Death and Scavenging by Pigs. *Science* 200:68–70.

Gluckman, M.

1937   Mortuary Customs and the Belief in Survival after Death among the South-Eastern Bantu. *Bantu* 11:117–136.

Golden, C.

1997   Social Position, Burial Position: The Ideological Implications of Skeletal Position in the Maya Lowlands. Paper presented at the 62nd Annual Meetings of the Society for American Archaeology, Nashville, Tenn.

Goldman, L.

1999   From Pot to Polemic: Uses and Abuses of Cannibalism. In *The Anthropology of*

Cannibalism, edited by L. Goldman, pp. 1–26. Bergin and Garvey, Westport, Conn.

Goldstein, L. G.

1976   *Spatial Structure and Social Organization: Regional Manifestations of Mississippian Society*. Ph.D. dissertation, Northwestern University, Evanston, Ill.

1980   *Mississippian Mortuary Practices: A Case Study of Two Cemeteries in the Lower Illinois Valley*. Northwestern University Archaeological Program, Evanston, Ill.

1981   One-Dimensional Archaeology and Multi-Dimensional People: Spatial Organization and Mortuary Analysis. In *The Archaeology of Death*, edited by R. Chapman, I. Kinnes, and K. Randsborg, pp. 53–69. Cambridge University Press, Cambridge.

1995   Landscapes and Mortuary Practices: A Case for Regional Perspectives. In *Regional Approaches to Mortuary Analysis*, edited by Lane A. Beck, pp. 101–121. Plenum Press, New York.

Goldstein, P. S.

1989a   *Omo, A Tiwanaku Provincial Center in Moquegua, Peru*. Ph.D. dissertation, Department of Anthropology, University of Chicago.

1989b   The Tiwanaku Occupation of Moquegua. In *Ecology, Settlement, and History in the Osmore Drainage, Peru*, edited by D. S. Rice, C. Stanish, and P. R. Scarr, pp. 219–255. International Series 545. British Archaeological Reports, Oxford.

1990a   La Cultura Tiwanaku y la Relación de Sus Fases Cerámicas en Moquegua. In *Trabajos Arqueológicos en Moquegua, Peru*, edited by L. K. Watanabe, M. E. Moseley, and F. Cabieses, vol. 2, pp. 31–58. 3 vols. Programa Contisuyo del Museo Peruano de Ciencias de la Salud Southern Peru Copper Corporation, Lima.

1990b   La Occupación Tiwanaku en Moquegua. *Gaceta Arqueológica Andina* 5(18–19):75–104.

1993   Tiwanaku Temples and State Expansion: A Tiwanaku Sunken-Court Temple in Moquegua, Peru. *Latin American Antiquity* 4(1):22–47.

2000   Exotic Goods and Everyday Chiefs: Long-Distance Exchange and Indigenous Sociopolitical Development in the South. *Latin American Antiquity* 11(4):335–361.

Goldstein, P. S., and B. D. Owen

2000   Tiwanaku en Moquegua: Las Colonias Altiplánicas. Paper presented at the III Simposio Internacional de Arqueología, Wary, i Tiwanaku: Modelos vs. Evidencias. Pontificia Universidad Católica del Perú, Lima.

Goodale, J. C.

1985   Pig's Teeth and Skull Cycles: Both Sides of the Face of Humanity. *American Ethnologist* 12:228–244.

1995   *To Sing with Pigs Is Human*. University of Washington Press, Seattle.

Goody, J.

1962   *Death Property and the Ancestors: A Study of the Mortuary Customs of the Lodagaa of West Africa*. Stanford University Press, Stanford, Calif.

Gordon, B., and P. Marshall

2000   Introduction: Placing the Dead in Late Medieval and Early Modern Europe. In *The Place of the Dead*, edited by B. Gordon and P. Marshall, pp. 1–17. Cambridge University Press, Cambridge.

Gorecki, P.

1979   Disposal of Human Remains in the New Guinea Highlands. *Archaeology and Physical Anthropology in Oceania* 14(2):107–117.

Gorecki, P., and D. S. Gillieson (editors)
1989   A Crack in the Spine: Prehistory and Ecology in the Jimi-Yuat Valley, Papua New Guinea. James Cook University of North Queensland, Townsville, Australia.

Gorecki, P., M. Mabin, and J. Campbell
1991   Archaeology and Geomorphology of the Vanimo Coast, Papua New Guinea: Preliminary Results. Archaeology in Oceania 26:119–122.

Gorecki, P., and J. Pernetta
1989   Hunting in the Lowland Rainforest of the Jimi. In A Crack in the Spine: Prehistory and Ecology in the Jimi-Yuat Valley, Papua New Guinea, edited by P. Gorecki and D. S. Gillieson, pp. 80–99. James Cook University of North Queensland, Townsville, Australia.

Gossen, G. H.
1986   Mesoamerican Ideas as a Foundation for Regional Synthesis. In Symbol and Meaning beyond the Closed Community: Essays in Mesoamerican Ideas, edited by G. H. Gossen, pp. 1–8. Institute for Mesoamerican Studies, State University of New York, Albany.

Gow, P.
2000   Helpless—The Affective Preconditions of Piro Social Life. In The Anthropology of Love and Anger, edited by J. Overing and A. Passes, pp. 46–63. Routledge, New York.

Graeber, D.
1995   Dancing with Corpses Reconsidered: an Interpretation of Famadihana (in Arivonimamo Madagascar). American Ethnologist 22(2):252–278.

Grauer, A. L. (editor)
1995   Bodies of Evidence: Reconstructing History through Skeletal Analysis. Wiley-Liss, New York.

Graves, M. W.
1986   Organization and Differentiation within Late Prehistoric Ranked Social Units, Mariana Islands, Western Pacific. Journal of Field Archaeology 13:139–154.
1991   Architectural and Mortuary Diversity in Late Prehistoric Settlements at Tumon Bay, Guam. Micronesica 24(2):169–194.

Greber, N.
1976   Within Ohio Hopewell: Analyses of Burial Patterns from Several Classic Sites. Ph.D. dissertation, Case Western Reserve University, Cleveland, Ohio. University Microfilms.
1979a   A Comparative Study of Site Morphology and Burial Patterns at Edwin Harness Mound and Seip Mounds 1 and 2. In Hopewell Archaeology: The Chillicothe Conference, edited by D. S. Brose and N. Greber, pp. 27–38. Kent State University Press, Kent, Ohio.
1979b   Variations in Social Structure of Ohio Hopewell Peoples. Mid-Continental Journal of Archaeology 4(1):35–57.
1983   Recent Excavations at the Edwin Harness Mound, Liberty Works, Ross County. Ohio Special Paper No. 5. Midcontinental Journal of Archaeology. Kent State University Press, Kent, Ohio.

Greber, N., and K. C. Ruhl
1989   The Hopewell Site: A Contemporary Analysis Based on the Work of Charles C.

Willoughby. Investigations in American Archaeology. Westview Press, Boulder, Colo.

Green, M. K.

1990   *Prehistoric Cranial Variation in Papua New Guinea.* Ph.D. dissertation, Australian National University.

Green, R. C., and D. Anson

2000   Excavations at Kainapirina (SAC), Watom Island, Papua New Guinea. *New Zealand Journal of Archaeology* 20(1998):29–94.

Greenfield, H.

1988   Bone Consumption by Pigs in a Contemporary Serbian Village: Implications for the Interpretation of Prehistoric Faunal Assemblages. *Journal of Field Archaeology* 15:473–479.

Griffin, P. B.

1998   An Ethnographic View of the Pig in Selected Traditional Southeast Asian Societies. In *Ancestors for the Pigs: Pigs in Prehistory,* edited by S. Nelson, pp. 27–37. Museum Applied Science Center for Archaeology Research Papers in Science and Archaeology 15. University of Pennsylvania Museum, Philadelphia.

Grünberg, G.

1970   Contribuições para a Etnologia dos Kayabi do Brasil Central, trans. E. Wenzel. Manuscript, Centro Ecumênico de Documentação e Informação, São Paulo. (Originally published as "Beiträge zur Ethnographie der Kayabí Zentralbrasiliens," *Archiv für Völkerkunde* 24:21–186.)

Guáman Poma de Ayala, F.

1956 [c.1613]   *La Nueva Coronica y Buen Gobierno.* Editorial Cultura, Dirreccion de Cultura, Arqueologia e Historia del Ministerio de Educacion Publica del Peru, Lima.

1980   *El Primer Nueva Corónica y Buen Gobierno por Felipe Guaman Poma de Ayala.* Siglo XXI Editores, Mexico City.

Guillén, S. E.

1992   *The Chinchorro Culture: Mummies and Crania in the Reconstruction of Prehistoric Coastal Adaptation in the South Central Andes.* Ph.D. dissertation, University of Michigan, Ann Arbor.

1998   Laguna de los Cóndores: Donde Viven los Muertos. *BienVenida* 6:43–48.

Gut, J.

1999   Memorialorte der Habsburger im Südwesten des Alten Reiches. Politische Hintergründe und Aspekte. In *Vorderösterreich,* edited by Württembergisches Landesmuseum Stuttgart, pp. 94–113. Süddeutsche Verlagsgesellschaft, Ulm, Germany.

Haddon, A. C.

1901   *Head-Hunters: Black, White, and Brown.* Methuen, London.

Hall, G. D.

1989   *Realm of Death: Royal Mortuary Customs and Polity Interaction in the Classic Maya Lowlands.* Ph.D. dissertation, Harvard University, Cambridge, Mass.

Hall, R. L.

1979   In Search of the Ideology of the Adena-Hopewell Climax. In *Hopewell Archaeology: The Chillicothe Conference,* edited by D. S. Brose and N. Greber, pp. 258–265. Kent State University Press, Kent, Ohio.

1984   The Cultural Background of Mississippian Symbolism. In *The Southwestern Cer-*

emonial Complex: Artifacts and Analysis—The Cottonlandia Conference, edited by P. Galloway, pp. 239–278. University of Nebraska Press, Lincoln.

1997　*An Archaeology of the Soul: North American Indian Belief and Ritual.* University of Illinois Press, Urbana.

2000　Sacrificed Foursomes and Green Corn Ceremonialism. In *Mounds, Modoc, and Mesoamerica: Papers in Honor of Melvin L. Fowler,* edited by S. R. Ahler, pp. 245–253. Illinois State Museum Scientific Papers Series 28. Springfield.

Halsall, G.

1996　Female Status and Power in Early Merovingian Central Austrasia: The Burial Evidence. *Early Medieval Europe* 5:1–24.

Hammond, N., K. Pretty, and F. P. Saul

1975　A Royal Maya Family Tomb. *World Archaeology* 7:57–78.

Hanson, D. B.

1988　Mortuary Practices and Human Biology. In *Archaeological Investigations on the North Coast of Rota, Mariana Islands,* edited by B. M. Butler, pp. 375–436. Micronesian Archaeological Survey Report No. 23. Center for Archaeological Investigations Occasional Paper No. 8. Southern Illinois University, Carbondale.

1991　Appendix B: Mortuary and Skeletal Analysis of Human Remains Recovered from the San Antonio Burial Trench, Agana, Guam. In *An Archaeological Study of the San Antonio Burial Trench and a Report on the Archaeological Monitoring of Road Construction along Marine Drive between Rts. 8 and 4, Agana, Guam,* edited by J. R. Amesbury, R. L. Hunter-Anderson, and D. R. Moore, pp. 160–200. Report prepared for Government of Guam Public Works, Division of Highway Engineering, Agana, Guam and Black Construction Corporation, Guam. Micronesian Archaeological Research Services, Mangilao, Guam.

1997　Human Bone Artifact. In *An Archaeological Survey of the East and Southeast Coast of Rota, Mariana Islands,* edited by B. M. Butler, pp. 306–314. Report prepared for Division of Historic Preservation, Commonwealth of the Northern Mariana Islands, Contract No. C50296. Center for Archaeological Investigations, Southern Illinois University, Carbondale.

Harding, V.

2000　Whose Body? A Study of Attitudes towards the Dead Body in Early Modern Paris. In *The Place of the Dead,* edited by B. Gordon and P. Marshall, pp. 170–187. Cambridge University Press, Cambridge.

Härke, H.

1990　"Warrior Graves"? The Background of the Anglo-Saxon Weapon Burial Rite. *Past and Present* 126:22–43.

1992　Changing Symbols in a Changing Society: The Anglo-Saxon Weapon Burial Rite in the Seventh Century. In *The Age of Sutton Hoo,* edited by M. O. H. Carver, pp. 149–165. Boydell Press, Woodbridge, U.K.

1994　Data Types in Burial Analysis. In *Prehistoric Graves as a Source of Information,* edited by B. Stjernquist, pp. 31–39. Konferenser 29, Kungl. Vitterhets Historie och Antikvitets Akademien, Stockholm.

1997　The Nature of Burial Data. In *Burial and Society: The Chronological and Social Analysis of Archaeological Burial Data,* edited by C. K. Jensen and K. H. Nielsen, pp. 19–27. Aarhus University Press, Aarhus, Denmark.

Harner, M. J.
1972   *The Jívaro, People of the Sacred Waterfalls.* Doubleday/Natural History Press, Garden City, New York

Hart Hansen, J. P., J. Meldgaard, and J. Nordqvist
1985   The Mummies of Qilakitsoq. *National Geographic* 167(2):190–207.

Hassig, R.
1988   *Aztec Warfare: Imperial Expansion and Political Control.* University of Oklahoma Press, Norman.

Haury, E. W.
1957   An Alluvial Site on the San Carlos Indian Reservation, Arizona. *American Antiquity* 23:2–27.
1976   *The Hohokam, Desert Farmers and Craftsmen: Excavations at Snaketown, 1964–1965.* University of Arizona Press, Tucson.

Häusler, A.
1968   Kritische Bemerkungen zum Versuch soziologischer Deutungen ur- und frühgeschichtlicher Gräberfelder—erläutert am Beispiel des Gräberfeldes von Hallstadt. *Ethnographisch-Archäologische Zeitschrift* 9:1–30.

Haviland, W. A.
1997   The Rise and Fall of Sexual Inequality: Death and Gender at Tikal, Guatemala. *Ancient Mesoamerica* 8:1–12.

Hawlik–van de Water, M.
1993   *Die Kapuzinergruft.* Herder, Vienna.

Hayes, A. C., J. N. Young, and A. H. Warren
1981   *Excavation of Mound 7, Gran Quivira National Monument, New Mexico.* Publications in Archeology 16. National Park Service, Washington, D.C.

Helms, M. W.
1998   *Access to Origins: Affines, Ancestors, and Aristocrats.* University of Texas Press, Austin.

Herring, S. W.
1976   The Dynamics of Mastication in Pigs. *Archives of Oral Biology* 21:473–480.

Hertlein, E.
1997   Das Grabmal Friedrich III im Lichte der Tradition. In *Der Tod des Mächtigen,* edited by L. Kolmer, pp. 137–163. Schöningh, Paderborn, Germany.

Hertz, R.
1907   Contribution à Une Étude sur la Représentation Collective de la Mort. *Année Sociologique* 10:48–137.
1960 [1907]   *Death and the Right Hand: A Contribution to the Study of the Collective Representation of Death.* Free Press, Glencoe, Ill.

Heyden, D.
1981   Caves, Gods, and Myths: World-View and Planning in Teotihuacan. In *Mesoamerican Sites and World-Views,* edited by E. P. Benson, pp. 1–39. Dumbarton Oaks, Washington, D.C.

Heyerdahl, T., D. Sandweiss, A. Narvaez, and L. Millones
1996   *Tucume.* Banco de Credito del Peru, Lima.

Hill, E.
1998   Death as a Rite of Passage: The Iconography of the Moche Burial Theme. *Antiquity* 72:528–538.

Hingley, R.

1996   Ancestors and Identity in the Later Prehistory of Atlantic Scotland: The Reuse and Reinterpretation of Neolithic Monuments and Material Culture. *World Archaeology* 28:231–243.

Hirst, S. M.

1985   *An Anglo-Saxon Inhumation Cemetery at Sewerby, East Yorkshire.* York University Archaeological Publications 4. York, U.K.

Hocquenghem, A. M.

1987   *Iconografía Mochica.* Universidad Católica del Perú, Lima.

Hodder, I.

1980   Social Structure and Cemeteries: A Critical Appraisal. In *Anglo-Saxon Cemeteries,* edited by P. Rahtz, T. Dickinson, and L. Watts, pp. 161–169. BAR British Series 82. British Archaeological Reports, Oxford.

1982a   *Symbolic and Structural Archaeology.* Cambridge University Press, Cambridge.

1982b   The Identification and Interpretation of Ranking in Prehistory: A Contextual Perspective. In *Ranking, Resource, and Exchange: Aspects of the Archaeology of Early European Society,* edited by C. Renfrew and S. J. Shennan, pp. 150–154. Cambridge University Press, Cambridge.

1982c   *Symbols in Action.* Cambridge University Press, Cambridge.

1983   *The Present Past: An Introduction to Anthropology for Archaeologists.* Pica Press, New York.

1984   Burials, Houses, Women, and Men in the European Neolithic. In *Ideology, Power, and Prehistory,* edited by D. Miller and C. Tilley, pp. 51–68. Cambridge University Press, Cambridge.

1987   The Contribution of the Long Term. In *Archaeology as Long Term History,* edited by I. Hodder, pp. 1–8. Cambridge University Press, Cambridge.

1990   *The Domestication of Europe: Structure and Contingency in Neolithic Societies.* Blackwell, Oxford.

1991   Interpretive Archaeology and Its Role. *American Antiquity* 56(1):7–18.

Hodge, F. W.

1920   The Age of the Zuni Pueblo of Kechipauan. *Indian Notes and Monographs* 3(2):45–60.

Hohmann, J. W.

1982   *Sinagua Social Differentiation: Inferences Based on Prehistoric Mortuary Practices.* Arizona Archaeological Society, Phoenix.

2001   A Study of Sinagua Mortuary Practices and Their Implications. In *Ancient Burial Practices in the American Southwest: Archaeology, Physical Anthropology, and Native American Perspectives,* edited by D. R. Mitchell and J. L. Brunson-Hadley, pp. 97–122. University of New Mexico Press, Albuquerque.

Holmes, J. H.

1924   *In Primitive New Guinea, An Account of a Quarter of a Century Spent amongst the Primitive Tribes of Ipi and Namau, Groups of Tribes of the Gulf of Papua, with an Interesting Description of their Manner of Living, their Customs and Habits, Feasts and Festivals, Totems and Cults.* G. P. Putnam's Sons, New York.

Holmes, W. H.

1897   Preservation and Decorative Features in Papuan Crania. *Field Columbian Museum Publication 21.* Anthropological Series Vol. 2, No. 1, pp. 41–49. Chicago.

Hooton, E. A.

1940   Skeletons from the Cenote of Sacrifice at Chichen Itza. In *The Maya and Their Neighbors: Essays on Middle American Anthropology and Archaeology*, edited by C. L. Hay, R. L. Linton, S. K. Lothrop, H. L. Shapiro, and G. C. Vaillant, pp. 272–280. Appleton-Century, New York.

Hornbostel, H. G.

1921–1923   Unpublished notes, drawings, and artifact catalogs on file at Bernice Pauahi Bishop Museum, Honolulu, Hawaii.

Hoskins, J.

1996a   The Heritage of Headhunting: History, Ideology, and Violence on Sumba, 1890–1990. In *Headhunting and the Social Imagination in Southeast Asia*, edited by J. Hoskins, pp. 216–248. Stanford University Press, Stanford, Calif.

1996b   Introduction: Headhunting as Practice and Trope. In *Headhunting and the Social Imagination in Southeast Asia*, edited by J. Hoskins, pp. 1–49. Stanford University Press, Stanford, Calif.

Hossfeld, P. S.

1964   The Aitape Calvarium. *The Australian Journal of Science* 27(6):179.

1965   Radiocarbon Dating and Paleoecology of the Aitape Fossil Human Remains. *Proceedings of the Royal Society of Victoria* 78:161–165.

Houlbrooke, R.

1998   *Death, Religion, and the Family in England, 1480–1750*. Clarendon Press, Oxford, U.K.

Hubert, H., and M. Mauss

1964 [1899]   *Sacrifice: Its Nature and Function*. University of Chicago Press, Chicago.

Hudson, C.

1976   *The Southeastern Indians*. University of Tennessee Press, Knoxville.

Hummel, S.

1961   Die Leichenbestattung in Tibet. *Monumenta Serica* 20:266–281.

Humphreys, S. C., and H. King (editors)

1981   *Mortality and Immortality: The Anthropology and Archaeology of Death*. Academic Press, London.

Hunter-Anderson, R. L., and B. M. Butler

1995   *An Overview of Northern Marianas Prehistory*. Micronesian Archaeological Survey Report No. 31. Division of Historic Preservation, Saipan, Commonwealth of the Northern Mariana Islands.

Huntington, R., and P. Metcalf

1979   *Celebrations of Death: The Anthropology of Mortuary Ritual*. Cambridge University Press, Cambridge.

Hutchinson, D. L., and L. V. Aragon

2002   Collective Burials and Community Memories: Interpreting the Placement of the Dead in the Southeastern and Mid-Atlantic United States with Reference to Ethnographic Cases from Indonesia. In *The Space and Place of Death*, edited by H. Silverman and D. B. Small, pp. 27–54. Archaeological Papers of the American Anthropological Association No. 11. Arlington, Va.

Hutchinson, D. L., C. S. Larsen, M. J. Schoeninger, and L. Norr

1998   Regional Variation in the Pattern of Maize Adoption and Use in Florida and Georgia. *American Antiquity* 63(3):397–416.

Hyndman, D.
1991   The Kam Basin Homeland of the Wopkamin: A Sense of Place. In *Man and a Half: Essays in Pacific Anthropology and Ethnobiology in Honour of Ralph Bulmer*, edited by A. Pawley, pp. 256–265. Polynesian Society Memoirs 48. Polynesian Society, Auckland.

Izumi, S., P. Cuculiza, and C. Kano
1972   *Excavations at Shillacoto, Huanuco, Peru.* University Museum Bulletin No. 3. University of Tokyo, Tokyo.

Jalland, P.
1996   *Death in the Victorian Family.* Oxford University Press, Oxford.

James, D.
1996   Women, Men, and Prestige Speech Forms: A Critical Review. In *Rethinking Language and Gender Research: Theory and Practice*, edited by V. L. Bergvall, J. M. Bing, and A. F. Freed, pp. 98–125. Longman, New York.

Jankowiak, W.
1993   *Sex, Death, and Hierarchy in a Chinese City.* Columbia University Press, New York.

Jankulak, K.
2000   *The Medieval Cult of St Petroc.* Boydell Press, Woodbridge, U.K.

Jessup, D.
1987   *Social and Economic Change in a Post-imperial Society: The Chiribaya Period of Southern Perú.* Dissertation proposal, Department of Anthropology, University of Chicago.

1990a   *Desarrollos Generales en el Intermedio Tardió en el Valle de Ilo, Perú.* Informe Interno del Programa Contisuyu. Submitted to Instituto Nacional de Cultura, Lima.

1990b   Rescate Arqueológico en el Museo de Sitio de San Gerónimo, Ilo. In *Trabajos Arqueológicos en Moquegua, Peru*, edited by L. K. Watanabe, M. E. Moseley, and F. Cabieses, vol. 3, pp. 151–165. 3 vols. Programa Contisuyo del Museo Peruano de Ciencias de la Salud, Southern Peru Copper Corporation, Lima.

1991   General Trends in the Development of the Chiribaya Culture, South-Coastal Perú. Paper presented at the Society for American Archaeology 56th Annual Meeting, New Orleans, La.

Jessup, D., and E. Torres Pino
1990   Sumario de las Excavaciones en el Museo de Sitio, San Gerónimo, Ilo, Peru. Manuscript on file, Department of Anthropology, University of New Mexico, Albuquerque.

Jetsun Pema
1997 [1996]   *Tibet: My Story,* with Gilles Van Grasdorff. Translated by G. Le Roy and J. Mayor. (Originally published as *Tibet, Mon Histoire,* by Éditions Ramsay, Paris.) Element Books, Rockport, Mass.

Jimenez de la Espada, M. (editor)
1965   *Relaciones Geograficas de Indias.* Biblioteca de Autores Españoles, Madrid.

Jochelson, W.
1926   *The Yukagir and the Yukagirized Tungus.* The Jesup North Pacific Expedition, Vol. 9, Memoir of the American Museum of Natural History. G. E. Stechert, New York.

Jolly, M.
1984   The Anatomy of Pig Love. *Canberra Anthropology* 17(1–2):78–108.

Jones, B. A., and M. J. Tomonari-Tuggle
1994   *Archaeological Data Recovery at the Guma Capuchino and South Garapan Sites, Garapan Village, Saipan, Commonwealth of the Northern Mariana Islands.* Report prepared for Historic Preservation Office, Saipan. International Archaeological Research Institute, Honolulu, Hawaii.

Jones, G. D.
1998   *The Conquest of the Last Maya Kingdom.* Stanford University Press, Stanford, Calif.

Joyce, R. A.
1998   Performing the Body in Pre-Hispanic Central America. *Res* 33:147–165.
1999   Social Dimensions of Pre-Classic Burials. In *Social Patterns in Pre-Classic Mesoamerica,* edited by D. C. Grove and R. A. Joyce, pp. 15–47. Dumbarton Oaks, Washington, D.C.

Jungwirth, J.
1971   Die Babenberger-Skelette im Stift Melk und ihre Identifizierung. *Annalen des Naturhistorischen Museums Wien* 75:661–666.

Kaestle, F. A., and K. A. Horsburgh
2002   Ancient DNA in Anthropology: Methods, Applications, and Ethics. *Yearbook of Physical Anthropology* 45:92–130.

Kamp, K. A.
1998   Social Hierarchy and Burial Treatments: A Comparative Assessment. *Cross-Cultural Research* 32(1):79–115.

Kan, S.
1989   *Symbolic Immortality: The Tlingit Potlatch of the Nineteenth Century.* Smithsonian Institution Press, Washington, D.C.

Kantner, J.
1999   Anasazi Mutilation and Cannibalism in the American Southwest. In *The Anthropology of Cannibalism,* edited by L. Goldman, pp. 75–104. Bergin and Garvey, Westport, Conn.

Katzenberg, M. A.
2000   Stable Isotope Analysis: A Tool for Studying Past Diet, Demography, and Life History. In *Biological Anthropology of the Human Skeleton,* edited by M. A. Katzenberg and S. Saunders, pp. 305–327. Wiley-Liss, New York.

Keesing, R. M.
1982   *The Living and the Dead in a Solomon Island Society.* Columbia University Press, New York.

Kehoe, A. B.
1999   A Resort to Subtler Contrivances. In *Manifesting Power: Gender and the Interpretation of Power in Archaeology,* edited by T. L. Sweely, pp. 17–29. Routledge, London.

Kelley, E.
1978   The Temple of the Skulls at Alta Vista, Chalchihuites. In *Across the Chichimec Sea: Papers in Honor of J. Charles Kelley,* edited by E. Kelley and B. C. Hedrick, pp. 102–126. Southern Illinois University Press, Carbondale.

Kendall, D. G.
1971   Seriation from Abundance Matrices. In *Mathematics in the Archaeological and Historical Sciences,* edited by F. R. Hodson, D. G. Kendall, and P. Tautu, pp. 215–252. Edinburgh University Press, Edinburgh.

Kerber, R.
1986   *Political Evolution in the Lower Illinois Valley.* Ph.D. dissertation, Northwestern University, Evanston, Ill.

Kertzer, D. I.
1988   *Ritual, Politics, and Power.* Yale University Press, New Haven, Conn.

Kidder, A. V.
1947   *The Artifacts of Uaxactun, Guatemala.* Carnegie Institution of Washington Publication 576. Washington, D.C.

Kite, B., G. Childs, and P. S. Sherpa
1988   *Myth, Mountains, and Mandalas: Mani Rimdu and Tengboche Monastery through the Eyes of the Dancers.* Tengboche Trust, Kathmandu.

Knapp, A. B. (editor)
1992   *Archaeology, Annales, and Ethnohistory.* Cambridge University Press, Cambridge.

Koch, W.
1976   Zu den Babenbergergräbern in Heiligenkreuz. In *Babenberger Forschungen,* pp. 193–215. Jahrbuch für Landeskunde von Niederösterreich, Neue Folge 42. Vienna.

Kohn, R. J.
2001   *Lord of the Dance: The Mani Rimdu Festival in Tibet and Nepal.* State University of New York Press, Albany.

Kolata, A. L.
1993   *The Tiwanaku: Portrait of an Andean Civilization.* Basil Blackwell, Oxford, U.K. and Cambridge, Mass.

Kolmer, L. (editor)
1997   *Der Tod des Mächtigen: Kult und Kultur des Todes Spätmittelalterlicher Herrscher.* Schöningh, Paderborn, Germany.

Kracke, W.
1978   *Force and Persuasion.* University of Chicago Press, Chicago.
1981   Kagwahiv Mourning I: Dreams of a Bereaved Father. *Ethos* 9:258–275.

Kroeber, A. L.
1925   *Handbook of the Indians of California.* Bureau of American Ethnology Bulletin No. 78. Washington, D.C.
1927   Disposal of the Dead. *American Anthropologist* 29:308–315.
n.d.   *Culture Stratifications in Peru.* Unpublished manuscript on file. Field Museum of Natural History, Chicago.

Kroeber, A. L., and D. Collier
1998   *The Archaeology and Pottery of Nazca, Peru: Alfred L. Kroeber's 1926 Expedition.* Altamira Press, Walnut Creek, Calif.
n.d.   Unpublished fieldnotes and notes to manuscript. Field Museum of Natural History, Chicago.

Kunen, J. L., M. J. Galindo, and E. Chase
2002   Pits and Bones: Identifying Maya Ritual Behavior in the Archaeological Record. *Ancient Mesoamerica* 12(197–211).

Kurashina, H., G. M. Heathcote, and J. Yamauchi
1989   *Hotel Nikko Guam: Data Recovery and Mitigation Procedures in the General Vicinity of Locality Y at Gognga-Gun Beach, Tumon Bay, Guam.* Submitted to Post-Field Summary Report. Unpublished manuscript on file at Guam Historic Preservation Office, Agana Heights, Guam.

Kus, S. M.
1992   Toward an Archaeology of Body and Soul. In *Representations in Archaeology,* edited by J.-C. Gardin and C. S. Peebles, pp. 168–177. Indiana University Press, Bloomington.

Kut, S. T., and J. E. Buikstra
1998   Calibration of C-14 Dates in the Lower Illinois Valley. Paper presented at the 63rd Annual Meeting of the Society for American Archaeology, Seattle, Wash.

Kutcher, N.
1999   *Mourning in Late Imperial China: Filial Piety and the State.* Cambridge University Press, Cambridge.

Kuznar, L. A.
1997   *Reclaiming a Scientific Anthropology.* Altamira Press, Walnut Creek, Calif.

Labarge, M. W.
1968   *Saint Louis: The Life of Louis IX of France.* Macmillan of Canada, Toronto.

Labov, W.
1972   *Sociolinguistic Patterns.* University of Pennsylvania Press, Philadelphia.

Landtman, G.
1927   *The Kiwai Papuans of British New Guinea: A Nature-Born Instance of Rousseau's Ideal Community.* MacMillan, London.

Lanning, E. P.
1967   *Peru before the Incas.* Prentice-Hall, Englewood Cliffs, N.J.

Lapiner, A. C.
1976   *Pre-Columbian Art of South America.* H. N. Abrams, New York.

Larsen, C. S.
1995   Regional Perspectives on Mortuary Analysis. In *Regional Approaches to Mortuary Analysis,* edited by L. A. Beck, pp. 247–264. Plenum Press, New York.

Larson, L. H.
1971   Archaeological Implications of Social Stratification at the Etowah Site, Georgia. In *Approaches to the Social Dimensions of Mortuary Practices,* edited by J. A. Brown, pp. 58–67. Society for American Archaeology, Washington, D.C.

Laufer, B.
1923   *Use of Human Skulls and Bones in Tibet.* Department of Anthropology Publication No. 10. Field Museum of Natural History, Chicago.

Lawrence, C. H.
1984   *Medieval Monasticism: Forms of Religious Life in Western Europe in the Middle Ages.* Longman, New York.

Lebeuf, A. J.
1954   *Histoire de la Ville et de Tous le Diocèse de Paris.* Montlhéry, Paris.

Lechner, K.
1976   *Die Babenberger.* Böhlau, Vienna.

Ledesma, A. de
1975   Mission in the Marianas: An Account of Father Diego Luis de Sanvitores and His Companions, 1669–1670. University of Minnesota Press, Minneapolis.

Lefevre, Y.
1954   L'Elucidarium et les Lucidaires: Mélanges d'Archéologie et d'Histoire des Ecoles Françaises d'Athènes et de Rome. De Boccard, Paris.

Leigh, S. R.
1988   Comparative Analysis of Elizabeth Middle Woodland Artifact Assemblages. In The Archaic and Woodland Cemeteries at the Elizabeth Site in the Lower Illinois River Valley, edited by D. K. Charles, S. R. Leigh, and J. E. Buikstra, pp. 191–217. KAC Research Series 7. Center for American Archeology, Kampsville, Ill.

Leitner, T.
1989   Habsburgs vergessene Kinder. Carl Ueberreuter, Vienna.

Le Nain de Tillemont, L.-S.
1965   Vie de Saint Louis, Roi de France. Renouard, Paris.

Léon-Dufour, X.
1980   Dictionary of the New Testament. 2nd ed. Geoffrey Chapman, London.

Lévesque, R. (editor)
1995   History of Micronesia: A Collection of Source Documents. Vol. 4: Religious Conquest, 1638–1670. Lévesque Publications, Gatineau, Québec.

Levy, J. E.
1995   Heterarchy in Bronze Age Denmark: Settlement Pattern, Gender, and Ritual. In Heterarchy and the Analysis of Complex Societies, edited by R. M. Ehrenreich, C. L. Crumley, and J. E. Levy. Archaeological Publications of the American Anthropological Association No. 6. Washington, D.C.
1999   Gender, Power, and Heterarchy in Middle-Level Societies. In Manifesting Power: Gender and the Interpretation of Power in Archaeology, edited by T. L. Sweely, pp. 62–78. Routledge, London.

Lewis, A. B.
1951   The Melasian People of the South Pacific. Chicago Natural History Museum, Chicago.

Lindenbaum, S.
1979   Kuru Sorcery: Disease and Danger in the New Guinea Highlands. Mayfield, Palo Alto, Calif.

Lipburger, P. M.
1997   De Prodigiis et Ostentis Que Mortem Friderici Imperatoris Precesserunt. Zum Tod Kaiser Friedrichs III. In Der Tod des Mächtigen, edited by L. Kolmer, pp. 125–135. Schöningh, Paderborn, Germany.

Lisowski, F.
1980   The Practice of Cremation in China. Eastern Horizon 19:21–24.

List, C.
1980   Die mittelalterlichen Grablegen der Wittelsbacher in Altbayern. In Die Zeit der frühen Herzöge, edited by H. Glaser, pp. 521–540. Hirmer, R. Piper and Co., Munich.

Lloyd, T. C.
1999   A Comparison of the Two Large Oblong Mounds at the Hopewell Site. Paper

presented at the 64th Annual Meeting of the Society for American Archaeology, Chicago.

2000   Human Remains as Burial Accompaniments at the Hopewell Site. Unpublished article. Department of Anthropology, University of Albany, Albany, New York.

Loeb, E. M.

1924   *Pomo Folkways.* University of California Publications in American Archaeology and Ethnology 14. Berkeley.

Looper, M. G.

1999   New Perspectives on the Late Classic Political History of Quiriguá, Guatemala. *Ancient Mesoamerica* 10:263–280.

López Austin, A.

1988   *The Human Body and Ideology: Concepts of the Ancient Nahuas.* University of Utah Press, Salt Lake City.

Lorrain, C.

2000   Cosmic Reproduction: Economics and Politics among the Kulina of Southwest Amazonia. *Journal of the Royal Anthropological Institute* 6:293–310.

Loseries, A.

1993   Charnel Ground Traditions in Tibet: Some Remarks and Observations. In *Anthropology of Tibet and the Himalaya*, edited by C. Ramble and M. Brauen, pp. 179–197. Volkerkundemuseum der Universitat Zurich, Zurich.

Loving, R.

1976   Use of Bamboo by the Awa. *Journal of the Polynesian Society* 85:521–542.

Lozada Cerna, M. C.

1998   *The Señorío of Chiribaya: A Bio-archaeological Study in the Osmore Drainage of Southern Perú.* Ph.D. dissertation, Department of Anthropology, University of Chicago.

Lozada Cerna, M. C., D. E. Blom, and J. E. Buikstra

1996   Evaluating Verticality through Cranial Deformation Patterns in the South Andes. Paper presented at the Society for American Archaeology 61st Annual Meeting, New Orleans, La.

Lozada Cerna, M. C., and E. Torres Pino

1991   Mortuary Excavations at El Yaral, Southern Perú. Manuscript.

Lucy, S. J.

1997   Housewives, Warriors, and Slaves? Sex and Gender in Anglo-Saxon Burials. In *Invisible People and Processes: Writing Gender and Childhood into European Archaeology*, edited by J. Moore and E. Scott, pp. 150–168. Leicester University Press, London.

1998   *The Early Anglo-Saxon Cemeteries of East Yorkshire: An Analysis and Reinterpretation.* BAR British Series 272. British Archaeological Reports, Oxford.

Lull, V.

1982   Discusión Cronológica de la Cerámica Sepulcral Argárica. *Cypsela* 4:61–67.

1983   *La "Cultura" de El Argar: Un Modelo para el Estudio de las Formaciones Económico-Sociales Prehistóricas.* Akal, Madrid.

2000   Argaric Society: Death at Home. *Antiquity* 74:581–590.

Lull, V., and J. Estévez

1986   Propuesta Metodológica para el Estudio de las Necrópolis Argáricas. In *Homenaje a Luis Siret, 1934–1984*, pp. 441–452. Consejería de Cultura de la Junta de Andalucía, Sevilla.

Lumbholtz, C., and A. Hrdlicka
1898   Marked Human Bones from a Prehistoric Tarasco Indian Burial Place in the State of Michoacan, Mexico. *Bulletin of the American Museum of Natural History* 10:272–280.

Lumbreras, L. G.
1972   *De los Orígenes del Estado en el Perú: Nueva Crónica sobre el Viejo Perú.* 1st edition. Milla Batres, Lima.
1972–1973   Sobre la Problemática Arqueológica de Arica. *Chungará* 1–2:25–27.
1974   *The Peoples and Cultures of Ancient Peru.* Translated by B. J. Meggers. Smithsonian Institution Press, Washington, D.C.

McAnany, P.
1995   *Living with the Ancestors: Kinship and Kingship in Ancient Maya Society.* University of Texas Press, Austin.
1998   Ancestors and the Classic Maya Built Environment. In *Function and Meaning in Classic Maya Architecture*, edited by S. D. Houston, pp. 271–298. Dumbarton Oaks, Washington, D.C.

McAnany, P., R. Storey, and A. K. Lockard
1999   Mortuary Ritual and Family Politics at Formative and Early Classic K'axob, Belize. *Ancient Mesoamerica* 10:129–146.

MacDonald, D. H.
2001   Grief and Burial in the American Southwest: The Role of Evolutionary Theory in the Interpretation of Mortuary Remains. *American Antiquity* 66:704–714.

McGee, R. J.
1990   *Life, Ritual, and Religion among the Lacandon Maya.* Wadsworth Publishers, Belmont, Calif.

McGimsey, C. R.
1995   *Lamellar Flakes and the Illinois Middle Woodland: A Selectionist Perspective.* Ph.D. dissertation, Southern Illinois University at Carbondale.

MacGregor, A.
1985   *Bone, Antler, Ivory, and Horn.* Barnes and Noble Books, Totowa, N.J.

McGregor, J. C.
1958   *The Pool and Irving Villages: A Study of Hopewell Occupation in the Illinois River Valley.* University of Illinois Press, Urbana.

McGuire, R. H.
1988   Dialogues with the Dead: Ideology and the Cemetery. In *The Recovery of Meaning*, edited by M. P. Leone and P. B. Potter, pp. 435–480. Smithsonian Institution Press, Washington, D.C.
1992   *Death, Society, and Ideology in a Hohokam Community.* Westview Press, Boulder, Colo.

McHugh, F.
1999   *Theoretical and Quantitative Approaches to the Study of Mortuary Practice.* BAR International Series 785. British Archaeological Reports, Oxford.

Macintyre, M.
1984   The problem of the Semi-alienable Pig. *Canberra Anthropology* 17(1–2):109–121.

McLaughlin, M.
1994 Consorting with Saints: Prayer for the Dead in Early Medieval France. Cornell University Press, Ithaca, N.Y.

McNeill, J. R.
in prep. Archaeological Investigations in Apotguan, Guam: Agana Beach Condominium Site. Vol. 2: Burial Recovery. Report prepared for Hanil Development Co., Hagatña, Guam. International Archaeological Research Institute, Honolulu, Hawaii.

Mainfort, R. C., Jr.
1989 Adena Chiefdoms? Evidence from the Wright Mound. Midcontinental Journal of Archaeology 14(2):164–178.

Makemson, M.
1951 The Book of the Jaguar Priest. Schuman, New York.

Maraini, F.
2000 [1951] Secret Tibet. Translated by E. Mosbacher and G. Waldman. (Originally published as Segreta Tibet by Leonardo da Vinci, Bari.) Harvill Press, London.

Marshall, L. G.
1989 Bone Modification and the Laws of Burial. In Bone Modification, edited by B. Robson and M. H. Sorg, pp. 7–24. University of Maine Center for the Study of the First Americans, Orono.

Martin, F. M.
1954 Some Subjective Aspects of Social Stratification. In Social Mobility in Britain, edited by D. V. Glass, pp. 51–75. Routledge and Kegan Paul, London.

Massey, V. K.
1989 The Human Skeletal Remains from a Terminal Classic Skull Pit at Colha. Papers of the Colha Project 3. Texas Archaeological Research Laboratory of the University of Texas at Austin and Texas A&M University, Austin.

Massey, V. K., and D. G. Steele
1997 A Maya Skull Pit from Terminal Classic Period, Colha, Belize. In Bones of the Maya: Studies of Ancient Skeletons, edited by S. L. Whittington and D. M. Reed, pp. 62–77. Smithsonian Institution Press, Washington, D.C.

Mays, S.
1998 The Archaeology of Human Bones. Routledge, London.

Menzel, D., J. H. Rowe, and L. Dawson
1964 The Paracas Pottery of Ica: A Study in Style and Time. University of California Publications in American Archaeology and Ethnology 50. University of California Press, Berkeley.

Merbs, C. F.
1967 Cremated Human Remains from Point of Pines, Arizona: A New Approach. American Antiquity 32(4):498–506.

Meskell, L.
1999 Archaeologies of Social Life: Age, Sex, Class, et cetera in Ancient Egypt. Blackwell, Oxford.
2000 Cycles of Life and Death: Narrative Homology and Archaeological Realities. World Archaeology 31:423–441.
2001 The Egyptian Ways of Death. In Social Memory, Identity, and Death: Anthropological Perspectives on Mortuary Rituals, edited by M. S. Chesson, pp. 27–40.

Archaeological Papers of the American Anthropological Association No. 10. Washington, D.C.

Meslin, M., and J.-R. Palanque

1967   *Le Christianisme Antique.* Armand Colin, Paris.

Metcalf, P., and R. Huntington

1991   *Celebrations of Death: The Anthropology of Mortuary Ritual.* 2nd ed. Cambridge University Press, Cambridge.

Meyer, R. J.

2000   *Königs- und Kaiserbegräbnisse im Spätmittelalter.* Beihefte zu J. F. Böhmer, Regesta Imperii 19. Böhlau, Cologne.

Micozzi, M.

1991   *Postmortem Change in Human and Animal Remains: A Systematic Approach.* Charles C. Thomas, Springfield, Ill.

Migot, A.

1955   *Tibetan Marches.* Translated from the French by P. Fleming. Rupert Hart-Davis, London.

Millauer, M.

1830   *Die Grabstätten und Grabmäler der Landesfürsten Böhmens.* Abhandlungen der Königlichen Böhmischen Gesellschaft der Wissenschaften, Neue Folge, Zweiter Band. Gottlieb Haase Söhne, Prague.

Miller, D.

1982   Structures and Strategies: An Aspect of the Relationship between Social Hierarchy and Cultural Change. In *Symbolic and Structural Archaeology,* edited by I. Hodder, pp. 89–98. Cambridge University Press, Cambridge.

Miller, D., and C. Tilley (editors)

1984   *Ideology, Power, and Prehistory.* Cambridge University Press, Cambridge.

Miller, V. E.

1999   The Skull Rack in Mesoamerica. In *Mesoamerican Architecture as a Cultural Symbol,* edited by J. K. Kowalski, pp. 341–360. Oxford University Press, New York.

Mills, W. C.

1916   The Exploration of the Tremper Mound. *Ohio Archaeological and Historical Quarterly* 25:262–398.

1922   Explorations of the Mound City Group. *Ohio Archaeological and Historical Quarterly* 31:453–592.

Milner, G. R., and V. G. Smith

1989   Carnivore Alteration of Human Bone from a Late Prehistoric Site in Illinois. *American Journal of Physical Anthropology* 79:43–49.

Mitchell, D. R.

1994   The Pueblo Grande Burial Artifact Analysis: A Search for Wealth, Ranking, and Prestige. In *The Pueblo Grande Project,* edited by D. R. Mitchell, vol. 7, pp. 129–180. Soil Systems Publications in Archaeology. Soil Systems, Phoenix, Ariz.

Mitchell, D. R., and J. L. Brunson-Hadley (editors)

2001   *Ancient Burial Practices in the American Southwest: Archaeology, Physical Anthropology, and Native American Perspectives.* University of New Mexico Press, Albuquerque.

Mock, S. B.

1998a   Prelude. In *The Sowing and Dawning: Termination, Dedication, and Transforma-*

tion in the Archaeological and Ethnographic Record of Mesoamerica, edited by S. B. Mock, pp. 3–20. University of New Mexico Press, Albuquerque.

1998b The Defaced and the Forgotten: Decapitation and Flaying/Mutilation as a Termination Event at Colha, Belize. In *The Sowing and the Dawning: Termination, Dedication, and Transformation in the Archaeological and Ethnographic Record of Mesoamerica*, edited by S. B. Mock, pp. 113–124. University of New Mexico Press, Albuquerque.

Moholy-Nagy, H., and J. M. Ladd

1992   Objects of Stone, Shell, and Bone. In *Artifacts from the Cenote of Sacrifice, Chichen Itza, Yucatan: Textiles, Basketry, Stone, Bone, Shell, Ceramics, Wood, Copal, Rubber, Other Organic Materials, and Mammalian Remains*, edited by C. C. Coggins, pp. 99–152. Memoirs of the Peabody Museum, Vol. 3, No. 10. Harvard University, Cambridge, Mass.

Moorehead, W. K.

1922   *The Hopewell Mound Group of Ohio*. Field Museum of Natural History Publication 211, Anthropology Series, Vol. 6, No. 5. Chicago.

Morgan, W. N.

1988   *Prehistoric Architecture in Micronesia*. University of Texas Press, Austin.

Morris, E. H., J. Charlot, and A. A. Morris

1931   *Temple of the Warriors at Chichen Itza, Yucatan*. Carnegie Institution, Washington, D.C.

Morris, I.

1991   The Archaeology of Ancestors: The Saxe/Goldstein Hypothesis Revisited. *Cambridge Archaeological Journal* 1(2):147–169.

Morrow, C. A.

1987   Blades and Cobden Chert: A Technological Argument for Their Role as Markers of Regional Identification during the Hopewell Period in Illinois. In *The Organization of Core Technology*, edited by J. K. Johnson and C. A. Morrow, pp. 119–149. Westview Press, Boulder, Colo.

1988   *Chert Exploitation and Social Interaction in the Prehistoric Midwest, 200 B.C.–A.D. 600*. Ph.D. dissertation, Southern Illinois University at Carbondale.

1998   Blade Technology and Nonlocal Cherts: Hopewell(?) Traits at the Twenhafel Site, Southern Illinois. In *Changing Perspectives on the Archaeology of the Central Mississippi Valley*, edited by M. J. O'Brien and R. C. Dunnell, pp. 281–298. University of Alabama Press, Tuscaloosa.

Moseley, M. E.

1992   *The Incas and Their Ancestors: The Archaeology of Peru*. Thames and Hudson, London.

Moser, C. L.

1973   *Human Decapitation in Ancient Mesoamerica*. Studies in Pre-Columbian Art and Archaeology, No. 11. Dumbarton Oaks, Washington, D.C.

Mosteiro da Batalha

1988   *Capela do Fundador/Founder's Chapel*. Museu do Mosteiro de Santa Maria da Vitória, Batalha, Portugal.

Mostny, G.

1957   La Momia del Cerro el Plomo. *Boletin del Museo de Historia Natural* 27(1):1–120.

Mraz, G.
1988   Albrecht VI. In *Die Habsburger*, edited by B. Hamann, pp. 42–43. Ueberreuter, Vienna.

Mumford, S. R.
1989   *Himalayan Dialogue: Tibetan Lamas and Gurung Shamans in Nepal.* University of Wisconsin Press, Madison.

Muñoz, I.
1983   El Poblamiento Aldeano en el Valle de Azapa y sus Vinculaciones con Tiwanaku (Arica-Chile). In *Asentamientos Aldeanos en los Valles Costeros de Arica: Documentos de Trabajo*, vol. 3, pp. 43–93. Instituto de Antropología y Arqueología, Universidad de Tarapacá, Arica, Chile.

Murphy, E. M., and J. P. Mallory
2000   Herodotus and the Cannibals. *Antiquity* 74:388–394.

Naquin, S.
1988   Funerals in North China: Uniformity and Variation. In *Death Ritual in Late Imperial and Modern China*, edited by J. L. Watson and E. S. Rawski, pp. 37–70. University of California Press, Berkeley.

Nash, J.
1985   *In the Eyes of the Ancestors: Belief and Behavior in a Maya Community.* Waveland, Prospect Heights, Ill.

Needham, R.
1976   Skulls and Causality. *Man* 11:71–88.

Neira Avedaño, M., and V. P. Coelho
1972   Enterramientos de Cabezas de la Cultura Nasca. *Revista do Museu Paulista, n.s.* 20:109–142.

Nelson, A. J.
1998   Wandering Bones: Archaeology, Forensic Science, and Moche Burial Practices. *International Journal of Osteoarchaeology* 8(3):192–212.

Ngapo, N. J., K. Chodra, C. T. Phuntso, N. Zhen, C. Xiansheng, J. Chinlei, and D. Luosantselie
1981   *Tibet.* McGraw-Hill, New York.

Nials, F. L., E. E. Deeds, M. E. Moseley, S. G. Pozorski, T. G. Pozorski, and R. Feldman
1979a   El Niño: The Catastrophic Flooding of Coastal Peru, Part I. *Field Museum of Natural History Bulletin* 50(7):4–14.
1979b   El Niño: The Catastrophic Flooding of Coastal Peru, Part II. *Field Museum of Natural History Bulletin* 50(8):4–10.

Niemetz, P.
1974   *Die Grablege der Babenberger in der Abtei Heiligenkreuz.* Heiligenkreuzer Verlag, Heiligenkreuz, Austria.

Norbu, T. J., and C. M. Turnbull
1970   *Tibet.* Simon and Schuster, New York.

Norr, L.
1995   Interpreting Dietary Maize from Bone Stable Isotopes in the American Tropics: The State of the Art. In *Archaeology in the American Tropics: Current Analytical Methods and Applications*, edited by P. W. Stahl, pp. 198–223. Cambridge University Press, Cambridge.

Nuñez Atencio, L.
1972–1973 Carta Repuesta a Luis Guillermo Lumbreras, "Sobre la Problemática Arqueológica de Arica." *Chungará* 1–2:27–32.

Oakdale, S.
2002 Creating a Continuity between Self and Other: First-Person Narration in an Amazonian Ritual Context. *Ethos* 30:158–175.

Odell, G. H.
1985 Micro-wear Analysis of Middle Woodland Lithics. In *Smiling Dan: Structure and Function at a Middle Woodland Settlement in the Illinois Valley*, edited by B. D. Stafford and M. B. Sant, pp. 298–326. Center for American Archeology, Kampsville, Ill.
1994 The Role of Stone Bladelets in Middle Woodland Society. *American Antiquity* 59:102–120.

Ogilvie, M. D., and C. E. Hilton
2000 Ritualized Violence in the Prehistoric American Southwest. *International Journal of Osteoarchaeology* 10:27–48.

Ohler, N.
1990 *Sterben und Tod im Mittelalter.* Artemis, Munich.

Ollier, C. D., and C. F. Pain
1978 Some Megaliths and Cave Burials, Woodlark Island (Murua), Papua New Guinea. *Archaeology and Physical Anthropology in Oceania* 13(1):11–18.

Orbegoso, C.
1998 Excavaciones en la Zona Sureste de la Plaza 3c de la Huaca de la Luna durante 1996. In *Investigaciones en la Huaca de la Luna 1996*, edited by S. Uceda, E. Mujica, and R. Morales, pp. 43–64. Universidad Nacional de Trujillo, Trujillo, Peru.

Orefici, G.
1993 *Nasca: Arte e Societa del Popolo dei Geoglifi.* Jaca Book, Milan.

Orschiedt, J.
1997 Beispiele für Sekundärbestattungen vom Jungpaläolithikum bis zum Neolithicum. *Ethnographisch-Archäologische Zeitschrift* 38:325–345.

Ortner, S. B.
1999 *Life and Death on Mt. Everest: Sherpas and Himalayan Mountaineering.* Princeton University Press, Princeton, N.J.

O'Shea, J. M.
1981 Social Configuration and the Archaeological Study of Mortuary Practices: A Case Study. In *The Archaeology of Death*, edited by R. Chapman, I. Kinnes, and K. Randsborg, pp. 39–52. Cambridge University Press, Cambridge.
1984 *Mortuary Variability: An Archaeological Investigation.* Academic Press, New York.
1995 Mortuary Custom in the Bronze Age of Southeastern Hungary: Diachronic and Synchronic Perspectives. In *Regional Approaches to Mortuary Analysis*, edited by L. A. Beck, pp. 125–145. Plenum Press, New York.
1996 *Villagers of the Maros: A Portrait of an Early Bronze Age Society.* Plenum, New York.

Owen, B. D.
1993 *A Model of Multiethnicity: State Collapse, Competition, and Social Complexity from Tiwanaku to Chiribaya in the Osmore Valley, Peru.* Ph.D. dissertation, Department of Anthropology, University of California–Los Angeles.

Owsley, D. W.
1994 Warfare in Coalescent Traditions Populations of the Northern Plains. In *Skeletal Biology in the Great Plains,* edited by D. W. Owsley and R. L. Jantz, pp. 333–344. Smithsonian Institution Press, Washington, D.C.

Pacheco, P. J.
1989 Ohio Middle Woodland Settlement Variability in the Upper Licking River Drainage. *Journal of the Steward Anthropological Society* 18(1–2):87–117.
1993 *Ohio Hopewell Settlement Patterns: An Application of the Vacant Center Model to Middle Woodland Period Intracommunity Settlement.* Ph.D. dissertation, Ohio State University, Columbus.
1996 Ohio Hopewell Regional Settlement Patterns. In *A View from the Core: A Synthesis of Ohio Hopewell Archaeology,* edited by P. J. Pacheco, pp. 16–35. Ohio Archaeological Council, Columbus, Ohio.
1997 Ohio Middle Woodland Intracommunity Settlement Variability: A Case Study from the Licking Valley. In *Ohio Hopewell Community Organization,* edited by W. S. Dancey and P. J. Pacheco, pp. 41–84. Kent State University Press, Kent, Ohio.

Pader, E. J.
1982 *Symbolism, Social Relations, and the Interpretation of Mortuary Remains.* BAR International Series 130. British Archaeological Reports, Oxford.

Palmqvist, L.
1993 The Great Transition: First Farmers of the Western World. In *People of the Stone Age: Hunter-Gatherers and Early Farmers,* edited by G. Burenhult, pp. 17–38. Harper Collins, New York.

Parker Pearson, M.
1982 Mortuary Practices, Society, and Ideology: An Ethnoarchaeological Study. In *Symbolic and Structural Archaeology,* edited by I. Hodder, pp. 99–113. Cambridge University Press, Cambridge.
1993 The Powerful Dead: Archaeological Relationships between the Living and the Dead. *Cambridge Archaeological Journal* 3:203–229.
1995 Return of the Living Dead: Mortuary Analysis and the New Archaeology Revisited. *Antiquity* 69:1046–1048.
1999 *The Archaeology of Death and Burial.* Texas A&M University Press, College Station.

Parker Pearson, M., and Ramilisonina
1998 Stonehenge for the Ancestors: The Stones Pass on the Message. *Antiquity* 72:308–326.

Paul, A. H.
1990 *Paracas Ritual Attire: Symbols of Authority in Ancient Peru.* University of Oklahoma Press, Norman.

Peebles, C. S.
1971 Moundville and Surrounding Sites: Some Structural Considerations of Mortuary Practices. In *Approaches to the Social Dimensions of Mortuary Practices,* edited by J. A. Brown, pp. 68–91. Society for American Archaeology, Washington, D.C.

Peebles, C. S., and S. M. Kus
1977   Some Archaeological Correlates of Ranked Societies. *American Antiquity* 42:421–448.

Perino, G.
1968   The Pete Klunk Mound Group, Calhoun County, Illinois: The Archaic and Hopewell Occupations, with an Appendix on the Gibson Mound Group. In *Hopewell and Woodland Site Archaeology in Illinois*, edited by J. A. Brown, pp. 9–124. Illinois Archaeological Survey Bulletin 6. University of Illinois, Urbana.

1973   The Late Woodland Component at the Pete Klunk site, Calhoun County, Illinois. In *Late Woodland Site Archaeology in Illinois*, pp. 58–89. Bulletin 9. Illinois Archaeological Survey, Springfield.

n.d.a   The Gibson Mounds Hopewell Project, Calhoun County, Illinois. Unpublished manuscript.

n.d.b   The Bedford Mound Group, Pike County, Illinois. Unpublished manuscript.

Peter-Röcher, H.
1997   Menschliche Skelettreste in Siedlungen und Höhlen. Kritische Anmerkungen zu herkömmlichen Deutungen. *Ethnographisch-Archäologische Zeitschrift* 38:315–324.

Peters, A. H.
1991   Ecology and Society in Embroidered Images from the Paracas Necrópolis. In *Paracas Art and Architechture: Object and Context in South Coastal Peru*, edited by A. Paul, pp. 240–313. University of Iowa Press, Iowa City.

Pezzia Assereto, A.
1968   *Ica y el Perú Precolombino*. Vol. 1: *Arqueología de la Provincia de Ica*. Editora Ojeda, Ica, Peru.

Pickering, R. B.
1985   Human Osteological Remains from Alta Vista, Zacatecas: An Analysis of the Isolated Bone. In *The Archaeology of West and Northwest Mexico*, edited by M. S. Foster and P. C. Weigand, pp. 289–326. Westview Press, Boulder, Colo.

Pietrusewsky, M.
1973   A Multivariate Analysis of Craniometric Data from the Territory of Papua and New Guinea. *Archaeology and Physical Anthropology in Oceania* 8(1):12–23.

Pietrusewsky, M., M. T. Douglas, and R. M. Ikehara-Quebral
1997   An Assessment of Health and Disease in the Prehistoric Inhabitants of the Mariana Islands. *American Journal of Physical Anthropology* 104:315–342.

2003   *Archaeological Investigations in Apotguan, Guam: Agana Beach Condominium Site*. Vol. 3: *An Osteological Investigation and Comparison with Other Micronesian Series*. Draft report prepared for Hanil Development Co., Hagåtña, Guam. International Archaeological Research Institute, Honolulu, Hawaii.

Pijoan Aguadé, C. M., and J. Mansilla Lory
1997   Evidence for Human Sacrifice, Bone Modification, and Cannibalism in Ancient México. In *Troubled Times: Violence and Warfare in the Past*, edited by D. L. Martin and D. W. Frayer, pp. 217–238. Gordon and Breach, Amsterdam.

Piña Chan, R.
1970   *Informe Preliminar de la Reciente Exploracíon del Cenote Sagrado de Chichén Itzá*. Instituto Nacional de Antropología e Historía, Mexico City.

Pollock, D.
1993   Death and the Afterdeath among the Kulina. *Latin American Anthropology Review* 5:61–64.

Polo de Ondegardo, J.
1916 [1585]   *Instruccion Contra las Ceremonias y Ritos que Usan los Indios Conforme al Tiempo de su Gentilidad*. Coleccion de Libros y Documentos Referentes a la Historia del Peru, Lima.

Ponce Sangines, C., and E. Linares Iturralde
1966   *Comentario Antropologico Acerca de la Determinacion Paleo-serologica de Grupos Sanguineos en Momias Prehispanicas del Altiplano Boliviano*. Academia Nacional de Ciencias de Bolivia, La Paz.

Poole, F. J. P.
1982   The Ritual Forging of Identity: Aspects of Person and Self in Bimin-Kuskusmin Male Initiation. In *Rituals of Manhood*, edited by G. H. Herdt, pp. 99–154. University of California, Los Angeles.

Potts, D. T.
2002   The Domestication of Death. *Review of Archaeology* 23(1):17–22.

Proskouriakoff, T.
1962   Civic and Religious Structures of Mayapán. In *Mayapán, Yucatan, Mexico*, edited by H. E. D. Pollock, R. L. Roys, T. Proskouriakoff, and A. L. Smith, pp. 87–164. Carnegie Institution, Washington, D.C.
1970   On Two Inscriptions at Chichen Itza. In *Monographs and Papers in Maya Archaeology*, edited by W. R. Bullard, pp. 450–467. Papers of the Peabody Museum of Archaeology and Ethnology, Vol. 61. Harvard University, Cambridge, Mass.

Proulx, D. A.
1968   *Local Differences and Time Differences in Nasca Pottery*. University of California Publications in Anthropology 5. University of California Press, Berkeley.
1971   Headhunting in Ancient Peru. *Archaeology* 24(1):16–21.
1989   Nasca Trophy Heads: Victims of Warfare or Ritual Sacrifice? In *Cultures in Conflict: Current Archaeological Perspectives*, edited by D. C. Tkaczuk and B. C. Vivian, pp. 73–85. Proceedings of the 20th Annual Chacmool Conference. Archaeological Association, University of Calgary, Calgary.
2001   Ritual Uses of Trophy Heads in Ancient Nasca Society. In *Ritual Sacrifice in Ancient Peru*, edited by E. P. Benson and A. G. Cook, pp. 119–136. University of Texas Press, Austin.

Prufer, O. H.
1964   The Hopewell Complex of Ohio. In *Hopewellian Studies*, edited by J. R. Caldwell and R. L. Hall, pp. 35–83. Scientific Papers 12. Illinois State Museum, Springfield.
1965   *The McGraw Site: A Study in Hopewellian Dynamics*. Scientific Publications of the Cleveland Museum of Natural History, Cleveland, Ohio.
1997   How to Construct a Model. In *Ohio Hopewell Community Organization*, edited by W. S. Dancey and P. J. Pacheco, pp. 105–128. Kent State University Press, Kent, Ohio.

Prutz, H.
1879   *Kaiser Friedrich I, Grabstätte: Eine kritische Studie*. Ernst Gruihn, Danzig, Poland.

Pugh, T.
2001   Architecture, Ritual, and Social Identity at Late Postclassic Zacpetén, Petén, Guatemala: Identification of the Kowoj. Ph.D. dissertation, Southern Illinois University at Carbondale.

Quirke, S., and J. Spencer
1992   The British Museum Book of Ancient Eygpt. British Museum Press, London.

Rainville, L.
1999   Hanover Deathscapes: Mortuary Variability in New Hampshire, 1770–1920. Ethnohistory 46(3):541–597.

Rakita, G. F. M.
2001   Social Complexity, Religious Organization, and Mortuary Ritual in the Casas Grandes Region of Chihuahua, Mexico. Ph.D. dissertation, University of New Mexico, Albuquerque.

Randsborg, K.
1973   Wealth and Social Structure as Reflected in Bronze Age Burials—A Quantitative Approach. In The Explanation of Culture Change: Models in Prehistory, edited by C. Renfrew, pp. 565–570. Duckworth, London.
1975   Population and Social Variation in Early Bronze Age Denmark: A Systemic Approach. In Population, Ecology, and Social Evolution, edited by S. Polgar, pp. 139–166. Mouton, The Hague.
1984   Women in Prehistory: The Danish Example. Acta Archaeologica 55:143–154.

Rappaport, R. A.
1968   Pigs for the Ancestors. Yale University Press, New Haven, Conn.

Ravesloot, J. C.
1988   Mortuary Practices and Social Differentiation at Casas Grandes, Chihuahua, Mexico. Anthropological Papers of the University of Arizona 49. University of Arizona Press, Tucson.

Rawski, E. S.
1988   A Historian's Approach to Chinese Death Ritual. In Death Ritual in Late Imperial and Modern China, edited by J. L. Watson and E. S. Rawski, pp. 228–253. University of California Press, Berkeley.

Read, K. A.
1998   Time and Sacrifice in the Aztec Cosmos. Indiana University Press, Bloomington.

Redfield, R.
1941   The Folk Culture of Yucatan. Chicago University Press, Chicago.

Redfield, R., and A. Villa Rojas
1934   Chan Kom: A Maya Village. Carnegie Institution of Washington Publication 448. Carnegie Institution, Washington, D.C.

Reeder, G.
2000   Same-Sex Desire, Conjugal Constructs, and the Tomb of Niankhknum and Khnumhotep. World Archaeology 32:193–208.

Rega, E.
1997   Age, Gender, and Biological Reality in the Early Bronze Age Cemetery at Mokrin. In Invisible People and Processes: Writing Gender and Childhood into European Archaeology, edited by J. Moore and E. Scott, pp. 229–247. Leicester University Press, London.

Reinhard, J.
1992   Sacred Peaks of the Andes. *National Geographic* 181(3):83–111.
1997   Sharp Eyes of Science Probe the Mummies of Peru. *National Geographic* 191(1):36–43.
1999   Frozen in Time. *National Geographic* 196(5):36–55.

Reinman, F. M.
1977   *An Archaeological Survey and Preliminary Test Excavations on the Island of Guam, Mariana Islands, 1965–1966.* Miscellaneous Publications No. 1. Micronesian Area Research Center, University of Guam, Mangilao.

Reiss, J. W., and M. A. Stubel
1880–1887   *The Necropolis of Ancon in Peru: A Contribution to Our Knowledge of the Cultures and Industries of the Empire of the Incas, Being the Results of Excavation Made on the Spot.* Ascher, Berlin.

Ribeiro, B.
1979   *Diário do Xingu.* Paz e Terra, São Paulo.

Rice, D. S.
1986   The Petén Postclassic: A Settlement Perspective. In *Late Lowland Maya Civilization*, edited by J. A. Sabloff and E. W. Andrews IV, pp. 301–344. University of New Mexico Press, Albuquerque.
1989   Osmore Drainage, Peru: The Ecological Setting. In *Ecology, Settlement, and History in the Osmore Drainage, Peru*, edited by D. S. Rice, C. Stanish, and P. R. Scarr, pp. 17–33. International Series 545. British Archaeological Reports, Oxford.
1993   Late Intermediate Period Domestic Architecture and Residential Organization at La Yaral. In *Domestic Architecture, Ethnicity, and Complementarity in the South-Central Andes*, edited by M. S. Aldenderfer, pp. 66–82. University of Iowa Press, Iowa City.

Rice, D. S., and P. M. Rice
1981   Muralla de León: A Lowland Maya Fortification. *Journal of Field Archaeology* 8:271–288.

Rice, D. S., P. M. Rice, and T. Pugh
1997   Settlement Continuity and Change in the Central Petén Lakes Region: The Case of Zacpetén. In *Anatomía de Una Civilización: Aproximaciones Interdisciplinarias a la Cultura Maya*, edited by A. Ciudad. Sociedad Española de Estudios Mayas, Madrid.

Rice, P. M.
1986   The Petén Postclassic: Perspectives from the Central Petén Lakes. In *Late Lowland Maya Civilization*, edited by J. A. Sabloff and E. W. Andrews IV, pp. 251–299. University of New Mexico Press, Albuquerque.
1999   Rethinking Classic Lowland Maya Pottery Censers. *Ancient Mesoamerica* 10:25–50.

Riché, P.
1973   *La Vie Quotidienne dans l'Empire Carolingien.* Hachette, Paris.

Ricketson, O. G., and E. H. B. Ricketson
1937   *Uaxactun, Guatemala: Group E—1926–1931.* Carnegie Institution of Washington Publication 477. Carnegie Institution, Washington, D.C.

Riddell, F. A.
1986   *Report of Archaeological Fieldwork, Acarí Valley and Yauca Valley, Arequipa,*

Peru, April–May and July–August, 1985. California Institute for Peruvian Studies, Turlock, Calif.

Rieth, T.

1998   Taphonomic Observations on Historic Crania from Papua New Guinea. Ms. on file, New Guinea Research Program, Department of Anthropology, Field Museum, Chicago.

Riley, E. B.

1925   *Among Papuan Headhunters.* Seeley, Service and Co., London.

Rivero de la Calle, M.

1975   *Estudio Antropológico de Dos Momias de la Cultura Paracas.* Universidad de la Habana, Centro de Información Científica y Técnica, La Habana, Cuba.

Rivers, W. H. R.

1914   *The History of Melanesian Society,* vol. 2. Cambridge University Press, Cambridge.

Riviere, P.

2000   "The More We Are Together . . ." In *The Anthropology of Love and Anger,* edited by J. Overing and A. Passes, pp. 252–267. Routledge, New York.

Roark, R. P.

1965   From Monumental to Proliferous in Nasca Pottery. *Ñawpa Pacha* 3:1–92.

Robicsek, F., and D. M. Hales

1984   Maya Heart Sacrifice: Cultural Perspective and Surgical Technique. In *Ritual Human Sacrifice in Mesoamerica: A Conference at Dumbarton Oaks, October 13th and 14th, 1979,* edited by E. P. Benson and E. H. Boone, pp. 49–89. Dumbarton Oaks, Washington, D.C.

Robin, C.

1989   *Preclassic Maya Burials at Cuello, Belize.* BAR International Series 480. British Archaeological Reports, Oxford.

Robinson, W. J., and R. Sprague

1965   Disposal of the Dead at Point of Pines, Arizona. *American Antiquity* 30(4):442–453.

Rockmore, M. R.

1998   *The Social Development of the Itzá Maya: A Reassessment of the Multiple Lines of Evidence.* Master's thesis, Southern Illinois University at Carbondale.

Romain, W. F.

1994   Hopewell Geometric Enclosures: Symbols of an Ancient World View. *Ohio Archaeologist* 44(2):37–43.

1996   Hopewellian Geometry: Forms at the Interface of Time and Eternity. In *A View from the Core: A Synthesis of Ohio Hopewell Archaeology,* edited by P. J. Pacheco, pp. 194–209. Ohio Archaeological Council, Columbus.

2000   *Mysteries of the Hopewell: Astronomers, Geometers, and Magicians of the Eastern Woodlands.* University of Akron Press, Akron, Ohio.

Rostworowski de Diez Canseco, M.

1977   *Etnía y Sociedad: Costa Peruana Prehispánica.* Instituto de Estudios Peruanos, Lima.

1981   *Señoríos Indígenas de Lima y Canta.* Instituto de Estudios Peruanos, Lima.

1989   *Costa Peruana Prehispánica.* Instituto de Estudios Peruanos, Lima.

1991   *Las Macroetnías en el Ambito Andino.* Allpanchis 35/36 Vol. 1. Instituto Pastoral Andina, Lima.

Rothenberg, P. S.
1998   Race, Class, and Gender in the United States: An Integrated Study. 4th ed. St. Martin's Press, New York.

Rowe, J. H.
1963   Urban Settlements in Ancient Peru. Ñawpa Pacha 1:1–27.

Roys, R. L.
1962   Literary Sources for the History of Mayapán. In Mayapán, Yucatan, Mexico, edited by H. E. D. Pollock, R. L. Roys, T. Proskouriakoff, A. L. Smith, pp. 25–87. Carnegie Institution of Washington Publication 619. Carnegie Institution, Washington, D.C.

Rush, A. C.
1941   Death and Burial in Christian Antiquity. Catholic University of America Press, Washington, D.C.

Russell, M. D.
1987   Mortuary Practices at the Krapina Neanderthal Site. American Journal of Physical Anthropology 72:381–397.

Russell, S.
1998   Tiempon i Manmofo'na: Ancient Chamorro Culture and History of the Northern Mariana Islands. Micronesian Archaeological Survey Report No. 32. Division of Historic Preservation, Saipan, Commonwealth of the Northern Mariana Islands.

Sahlins, M.
1981   Historical Metaphors and Mythical Realities. Association for the Study of Anthropology in Oceania, Special Publication No. 1. University of Michigan Press, Ann Arbor.
1985   Islands of History. University of Chicago Press, Chicago.

Salin, E.
1949   La Civilisation Mérovingienne Vol. 2. Picard, Paris.

Salomon, F.
1995   "The Beautiful Grandparents": Andean Ancestor Shrines and Mortuary Ritual as Seen through Colonial Records. In Tombs for the Living: Andean Mortuary Practices, edited by T. D. Dillehay, pp. 315–353. Dumbarton Oaks, Washington, D.C.

Sancho de la Hoz, P.
1917 [c.1525]   An Account of the Conquest of Peru. Cortes Society, New York.

Sandness, K. L.
1992   Temporal and Spatial Dietary Variability in the Prehistoric Lower and Middle Osmore Drainage: The Carbon and Nitrogen Isotope Evidence. Master's thesis, University of Nebraska, Lincoln.

Sanger, D.
1973   Who Were the Red Paints? In Maine Prehistory: A Selection of Short Papers, edited by D. Sanger and R. G. MacKay. University of Maine, Orono.

Sangren, P. S.
1987   History and Magical Power in a Chinese Community. Stanford University Press, Stanford, Calif.

Santos Ramirez, R.
1983   Rescate e Investigación Arqueológica en Ilo, Moquegua. Praxis 2:8–13.

Saul, F.
1975   The Maya and Their Neighbors as Recorded in Their Skeletons. In The Maya and

Their Neighbors, pp. 35–40. Peabody Museum of Ethnology and Archaeology, Harvard University, Cambridge, Mass.

Saunders, S. R., and A. Herring (editors)

1995   *Grave Reflections: Portraying the Past through Cemetery Studies*. Canadian Scholar's Press, Toronto.

Savage, S. H.

2001   Some Recent Trends in the Archaeology of Predynastic Egypt. *Journal of Archaeological Research* 9:101–155.

Saville, W. J. V.

1926   *In Unknown New Guinea*. Seeley, Service and Co., London.

Sawyer, A. R.

1966   *Ancient Peruvian Ceramics: The Nathan Cummings Collection*. The Metropolitan Museum of Art, New York.

1972   The Feline in Paracas Art. In *The Cult of the Feline: A Conference in Pre-Columbian Iconography*, edited by E. P. Benson, pp. 91–116. Dumbarton Oaks, Washington, D.C.

Saxe, A. A.

1970   *Social Dimensions of Mortuary Practices*. Ph.D. dissertation, University of Michigan, Ann Arbor.

Saxe, A. A., and P. L. Gall

1977   Ecological Determinants of Mortuary Practices: The Temuan of Malaysia. In *Cultural-Ecological Perspectives on Southeast Asia: A Symposium*, edited by W. Wood, pp. 74–82. Center for International Studies, Ohio University, Athens.

Schaafsma, P.

1994   The Prehistoric Kachina Cult and Its Origins as Suggested by Southwestern Rock Art. In *Kachinas in the Pueblo World*, edited by P. Schaafsma, pp. 63–79. University of New Mexico Press, Albuquerque.

Schäfer, D.

1920   Mittelalterlicher Brauch bei der Überführung von Leichen. *Sitzungsberichte der Preussischen Akademie der Wissenschaften*, S:478–498.

Schaff, P.

1956   *A Select Library of the Nicene and Post-Nicene Fathers of the Christian Church*. First Series 1. 10 vols. Eerdmans, Grand Rapids, Mich.

Schaller, H. M.

1993   Der Kaiser stirbt. In *Tod im Mittelalter*, edited by A. Borst, G. v. Graevenitz, A. Patschovsky, and K. Stierle, pp. 59–75. Universitätsverlag, Konstanz, Germany.

Schele, L., and D. A. Freidel

1990   *A Forest of Kings: The Untold Story of the Ancient Maya*. Morrow, New York.

Schele, L., and P. Mathews

1998   *The Code of Kings: The Language of Seven Sacred Maya Temples and Tombs*. Scribner, New York.

Schele, L., and M. E. Miller

1986   *The Blood of Kings: Dynasty and Ritual in Maya Art*. Kimball Art Museum, Ft. Worth, Tex.

Schiffer, M. B.
1987   *Formation Processes of the Archaeological Record.* University of New Mexico Press, Albuquerque.

Schobinger, J.
1966   *La "Momia" del Cerro el Toro.* Taller Grafico, Mendoza, Argentina.
1991   Sacrifices of the High Andes. *Natural History* 4(April):63–66.

Schoeninger, M. J., M. J. DeNiro, and H. Tauber
1983   Stable Nitrogen Isotope Ratios of Bone Collagen Reflect Marine and Terrestrial Components of Prehistoric Human Diet. *Science* 220:1381–1383.

Schramm, P. E., and F. Mütherich
1962   *Denkmale der Deutschen Könige und Kaiser: Ein Beitrag zur Herrschergeschichte von Karl dem Grossen bis Friedrich II.* Prestel Verlag, Munich.

Schreiber, K. J.
1998   Afterword: Nasca Research since 1926. In *The Archaeology and Pottery of Nazca, Peru: Alfred L. Kroeber's 1926 Expedition,* by Alfred L. Kroeber and Donald Collier, edited by P. H. Carmichael, pp. 261–270. Altamira Press, Walnut Creek, Calif.

Schubart, H., V. Pingel, and O. Arteaga
2000   *Fuente Alamo. Las Excavaciones Arqueológicas 1977–1991 en el Poblado de la Edad del Bronce.* Junta de Andalucía, Consejería de Cultura, Seville.

Schukraft, H.
1989   *Die Grablegen des Hauses Württemberg.* Theiss, Stuttgart.

Searle, J. R.
1995   *The Construction of Social Reality.* The Free Press, New York.

Seligmann, C. G.
1910   *The Melanesians of British New Guinea.* University Press, Cambridge.

Sempowski, M. L.
1986   Differential Mortuary Treatment of Seneca Women: Some Social Inferences. *Archaeology of Eastern North America* 14:35–44.

Shanks, M., and C. Tilley
1982   Ideology, Symbolic Power and Ritual Communication: A Reinterpretation of Neolithic Mortuary Practices. In *Symbolic and Structural Archaeology,* edited by I. Hodder. Cambridge University Press, Cambridge.
1987   *Re-Constructing Archaeology: Theory and Practice.* Cambridge University Press, Cambridge.

Sharer, R. J.
1978   Archaeology and History at Quiriguá, Guatemala. *Journal of Field Archaeology* 5:51–70.

Sharer, R. J., W. L. Fash, D. W. Sedat, L. P. Traxler, and R. Williamson
1999   Continuities and Contrasts in Early Classic Architecture of Central Copán. In *Mesoamerican Architecture as a Cultural Symbol,* edited by J. K. Kowalski, pp. 220–249. Oxford University Press, New York.

Shay, T.
1985   Differentiated Treatment of Deviancy at Death as Revealed in Anthropological and Archaeological Material. *Journal of Anthropological Archaeology* 4:221–241.

Sheets, P. D., J. M. Ladd, and D. Bathgate
1992   Chipped-Stone Artifacts. In *Artifacts from the Cenote of Sacrifice, Chichen Itza,*

Yucatan: Textiles, Basketry, Stone, Bone, Shell, Ceramics, Wood, Copal, Rubber, Other Organic Materials, and Mammalian Remains, edited by C. C. Coggins, pp. 153–178. Memoirs of the Peabody Museum of Archaeology and Ethnology. vol. 3, no. 10. Harvard University, Cambridge, Mass.

Shen, Tsung Lien, and Shen Chi Liu
1953   *Tibet and the Tibetans*. Stanford University Press, Stanford, Calif.

Shennan, S.
1975   The Social Organization at Branc. *Antiquity* 49:279–288.
1982   From Minimal to Moderate Ranking. In *Ranking Resource and Exchange: Aspects of the Archaeology of Early European Society*, edited by C. Renfrew and S. Shennan, pp. 27–32. Cambridge University Press, Cambridge.

Shetrone, H. C.
1926   Explorations of the Hopewell Group of Prehistoric Earthworks. *Ohio Archaeological and Historical Quarterly* 35:1–227.

Shimada, I.
1994   *Pampa Grande and the Mochica Culture*. University of Texas Press, Austin.

Shipman, P., G. Foster, and M. Schoeninger
1984   Burnt Bones and Teeth: An Experimental Study of Color, Morphology, Crystal Structure, and Shrinkage. *Journal of Archaeological Science* 11:307–325.

Shryock, A. J.
1987   The Wright Mound Re-examined: Generative Structures and the Political Economy of a Simple Chiefdom. *Midcontinental Journal of Archaeology* 12(2):243–268.

Sievert, A. K.
1992   *Maya Ceremonial Specialization: Lithic Tools from the Sacred Cenote at Chichen Itza, Yucatan*. Prehistory Press, Madison, Wis.

Silverman, H.
1993   *Cahuachi in the Ancient Nasca World*. University of Iowa Press, Iowa City.

Silverman, H., and D. A. Proulx
2002   *The Nasca*. Blackwell Publishers, Malden, Mass., and Oxford, U.K.

Silverman, H., and D. B. Small (editors)
2002   *The Space and Place of Death*. Archeological Papers of the American Anthropological Association 11. Arlington, Va.

Siret, H., and L. Siret
1887   *Les Premiers Ages du Métal dans le Sud-Est de l'Espagne*. Anvers, Belgium.

Siret, L.
1913   *Questions de Chronologie et D'Ethnographie Ibériques*. Paul Geuthner, Paris.

Smith, A. L.
1950   *Uaxactun, Guatemala: Excavations of 1931–1937*. Carnegie Institution of Washington Publication 588. Carnegie Institution, Washington, D.C.

Smith, G. E., and W. R. Dawson
1924   *Egyptian Mummies*. Kegan Paul International, London.

Smith, M. E.
1992   Braudel's Temporal Rhythms and Chronology Theory in Archaeology. In *Archaeology, Annales, and Ethnohistory*, edited by A. B. Knapp, pp. 23–34. Cambridge University Press, Cambridge.

Smith, W., R. B. Woodbury, and N. F. S. Woodbury
1966   *The Excavation of Hawikuh by Frederick Webb Hodge: Report of the Hendricks-Hodge Expedition, 1917–1923.* Museum of the American Indian, Heye Foundation, New York.

Sofaer Derevenski, J.
1997   Age and Gender at the Site of Tiszapolgár-Basatanya, Hungary. *Antiquity* 71:875–889.
2000   Rings of Life: The Role of Early Metalwork in Mediating the Gendered Life Course. *World Archaeology* 31:389–406.

Soustelle, J.
1984   Ritual Human Sacrifice in Mesoamerica: An Introduction. In *Ritual Human Sacrifice in Mesoamerica,* edited by E. H. Boone, pp. 1–5. Dumbarton Oaks, Washington, D.C.

Spencer, C. S.
1982   *The Cuicatlán Cañada and Monte Albán: A Study of Primary State Formation.* Academic Press, New York.

Spenneman, D. H. R.
1987   Cannibalism in Fiji: The Analysis of Butchering Marks on Human Bones and the Historical Record. *Domodomo* 1–2:29–46.
1990   Don't Forget the Bamboo: On Recognizing and Interpreting Butchery Marks in Tropical Faunal Assemblages. *Tempus:*(2)108–134.
1994   On the Diet of Pigs Foraging on the Mudflats of Tongatapu: An Investigation in Taphonomy. *Archaeology in New Zealand* 37:104–110.

Spier, L.
1928   *Havasupai Ethnography.* Anthropological Papers of the American Museum of Natural History No. 29, Part 3. New York.
1933   *Yuman Tribes of the Gila River.* University of Chicago Press, Chicago.

Spoehr, A.
1957   *Marianas Prehistory: Archaeological Survey and Excavations on Saipan, Tinian, and Rota.* Fieldiana: Anthropology, Vol. 48. Field Museum of Natural History, Chicago.

Sproles, G. B.
1985   Behavioral Science Theories of Fashion. In *The Psychology of Fashion,* edited by M. R. Solomon, pp. 55–70. Lexington Books, Lexington, Mass.

Squier, E. G., and E. H. Davis
1848   *Ancient Monuments of the Mississippi Valley.* Smithsonian Contributions to Knowledge Vol. 1. Smithsonian Institute, Washington, D.C.

Stanish, C.
1989   An Archaeological Evaluation of an Ethnohistorical Model in Moquegua. In *Ecology, Settlement, and History in the Osmore Drainage, Peru,* edited by D. S. Rice, C. Stanish, and P. R. Scarr, pp. 303–320. International Series 545. British Archaeological Reports, Oxford.
1992   *Ancient Andean Political Economy.* University of Texas Press, Austin.

Stanish, C., and D. S. Rice
1989   The Osmore Drainage, Peru: An Introduction to the Work of Programa Contisuyu. In *Ecology, Settlement, and History in the Osmore Drainage, Peru,* edited by D. S.

Rice, C. Stanish and P. R. Scarr, pp. 1–14. International Series 545. British Archaeological Reports, Oxford.

Steensberg, A.
1980   *New Guinea Gardens.* Academic Press, New York.

Steuer, H.
1968   Zur Bewaffnung und Sozialstruktur der Merowingerzeit. *Nachrichten aus Niedersachsens Urgeschichte* 37:18–87.

Stodder, A. L. W., and T. Rieth
2003   The Middens of Aitape: Contextualizing Human Remains from the North Coast of Papua New Guinea. Paper presented at the 68th Annual Meeting of the Society for American Archaeology, Milwaukee, Wis.

Stone, A. C.
2000   Ancient DNA from Skeletal Remains. In *Biological Anthropology of the Human Skeleton,* edited by M. A. Katzenberg and S. R. Saunders, pp. 351–371. Wiley-Liss, New York.

Stoodley, N.
1999   *The Spindle and the Spear: A Critical Enquiry into the Construction and Meaning of Gender in the Early Anglo-Saxon Burial Rite.* BAR British Series 288. British Archaeological Reports, Oxford.

Strong, W. D.
1929   *Aboriginal Society in Southern California.* University of California Press, Berkeley.
1957   *Paracas, Nazca, and Tiahuanacoid Cultural Relationships in South Coastal Peru.* Memoirs of the Society for American Archaeology 13. Salt Lake City, Utah.

Stross, B.
1998   Seven Ingredients in Mesoamerican Ensoulment. In *The Sowing and the Dawning: Termination, Dedication, and Transformation in the Archaeological and Ethnographic Record of Mesoamerica,* edited by S. Mock, pp. 31–39. University of New Mexico Press, Albuquerque.

Strouhal, E.
1992   *Life of the Ancient Egyptians.* American University in Cairo Press, Cairo.

Struever, S.
1968   *A Re-examination of Hopewell in Eastern North America,* University of Chicago Press, Chicago.

Stuart, D.
1995   *A Study of Maya Inscriptions.* Ph.D. dissertation, Vanderbilt University, Nashville, Tenn.

Stuart, D., L. Schele, and N. Grube
1989   *A Mention of 18 Rabbit on the Temple 11 Reviewing Stand.* Copan Notes 62. Instituto de Antropología e Historia and Copán Mosaics Project, Austin, Tex.

Sullivan, M. B., and K. Schram
1989   Investigation of Exudate Formation of Prehistoric Human Mummified Remains from the American Southwest. In *Recent Advances in the Conservation and Analysis of Artifacts,* edited by J. Black, pp. 267–272. Summer School Press, University of London, London.

Sullivan, T. D.
1974   The Rhetorical Orations, or Huehuetlatolli. In *Sixteenth-Century Mexico: The*

Work of Sahagún, edited by M. S. Edmonson, pp. 79–110. University of New Mexico Press, Albuquerque.

Sutter, R. C.
1997   *Dental Variation and Biocultural Affinities among Prehistoric Populations from the Coastal Valleys of Moquegua, Peru, and Azapa, Chile.* Ph.D. dissertation, University of Missouri–Columbia.

Swadling, P., N. Araho, and B. Ivuyo
1991   Settlements Associated with the Inland Sepik-Ramu Sea. *Bulletin of the Indo-Pacific Prehistory Association* 11:92–112.

Swadling, P., J. Chappell, G. Francis, N. Araho, and B. Ivuyo
1989   A Late Quaternary Inland Sea and Early Pottery in Papua New Guinea. *Archaeology in Oceania* 24:106–109.

Tainter, J. A.
1975a   *The Archaeological Study of Social Change: Woodland Systems in West-Central Illinois.* Ph.D. dissertation, Northwestern University, Evanston, Ill.
1975b   Social Inference and Mortuary Practices: An Experiment in Numerical Classification. *World Archaeology* 7:1–15.
1977a   Modeling Change in Prehistoric Social Systems. In *For Theory Building in Archaeology*, edited by L. R. Binford, pp. 327–351. Academic Press, New York.
1977b   Woodland Social Change in West-Central Illinois. *Mid-Continental Journal of Archaeology* 2:67–98.
1978   Mortuary Practices and the Study of Prehistoric Social Systems. In *Advances in Archaeological Method and Theory*, vol. 1, edited by M. B. Schiffer, pp. 105–141. Academic Press, New York.

Tarlow, S.
1997   An Archaeology of Remembering: Death, Bereavement, and the First World War. *Cambridge Archaeological Journal* 7:105–121.
1999   *Bereavement and Commemoration: An Archaeology of Mortality.* Blackwell, Oxford.

Tartaglia, L. J.
1980   A Revised C14 Chronology for Northern Chile. In *Prehistoric Trails of Atacama: Archaeology of Northern Chile*, edited by C. W. Meighan and D. L. True, pp. 5–22. Institute of Archaeology, University of California, Los Angeles.

Taussig, M.
1999   *Defacement: Public Secrecy and the Labor of the Negative.* Stanford University Press, Stanford, Calif.

Tayles, N., and K. Roy
1989   The Human Population. In *Aftena: The Prehistory of Southwest Saipan*, edited by R. McGovern-Wilson, pp. 115–158. Report prepared for InterPacific Resorts, Inc., and Historic Preservation Office, Saipan, CMNI. Anthropology Department, University of Otago, Dunedin, New Zealand.

Taylor, A. C.
1993   Remembering to Forget: Identity, Mourning, and Memory among the Jivaro. *Man* 28:653–678.

Tedlock, D.
1979   Zuni Religion and World View. In *Handbook of North American Indians.* Vol. 9:

Southwest, edited by A. Ortiz, pp. 499–508. Smithsonian Institution, Washington, D.C.

1996   *Popul Vuh: The Definitive Edition of the Maya Book of the Dawn of Life and the Glories of Gods and Kings*. Simon and Schuster, New York.

Tello, J. C.

1918   *El Uso de las Cabezas Humanas Artificialmente Momificadas y Su Representación en el Antiguo Arte Peruano*. Casa Editora de Ernesto R. Villarán, Lima.

1926   Los Descubrimientos del Museo de Arqueologia Peruana en la Peninsula de Paracas. *Atti del XXII Congresso Internazionale degli Americanisti* 1:679–690.

Terrell, J. E., and R. L. Welsch

1997   Lapita and the Temporal Geography of Prehistory. *Antiquity* 71:548–572.

Thomas, C.

1894   *Report on the Mound Explorations of the Bureau of Ethnology*. Government Printing Office, Washington, D.C.

Thompson, E. H.

1992   The Sacred Well of the Itzas. In *Artifacts from the Cenote of Sacrifice, Chichen Itza, Yucatan: Textiles, Basketry, Stone, Bone, Shell, Ceramics, Wood, Copal, Rubber, Other Organic Materials, and Mammalian Remains*, edited by C. C. Coggins, pp. 1–8. Memoirs of the Peabody Museum of Archaeology and Ethnology, Vol. 3, No. 10. Harvard University, Cambridge, Mass.

Thompson, J. E. S.

1970   *Maya History and Religion*. 1st ed. University of Oklahoma Press, Norman.

Thompson, J. E. S., and N. Hammond

1977   *Social Process in Maya Prehistory: Studies in Honour of Sir Eric Thompson*. Academic Press, New York.

Thompson, L. M.

1932   *Archaeology of the Mariana Islands*. Bernice Pauahi Bishop Museum Bulletin No. 100. Bernice Pauahi Bishop Museum, Honolulu, Hawaii.

1945   *The Native Culture of the Marianas Islands*. Bernice Pauahi Bishop Museum Bulletin No. 185. Bernice Pauahi Bishop Museum, Honolulu, Hawaii.

Thurston, A.

1987   *Enemies of the People: The Ordeal of the Intellectuals in China's Great Cultural Revolution*. Harvard University Press, Cambridge, Mass.

Thwaites, R. G. (editor)

1896–1901   *The Jesuit Relations and Allied Documents*. Burrow, Cleveland, Ohio.

Tieszen, L. L., and T. Fagre

1993   Carbon Isotopic Variability in Modern and Archaeological Maize. *Journal of Archaeological Science* 20(1):25–40.

Tilley, C.

1984   Ideology and the Legitimation of Power in the Middle Neolithic of Southern Sweden. In *Ideology, Power, and Prehistory*, edited by D. Miller and C. Tilley, pp. 111–146. Cambridge University Press, Cambridge.

1994   *A Phenomenology of Landscape: Places, Paths, and Monuments*. Berg, Oxford.

Tomczak, P. D.

1995   *Paleodietary Analysis of Chiribaya Alta: The Stable Isotope and Trace Element Evidence*. Master's thesis, Department of Anthropology, University of Chicago, Chicago.

2001   *Prehistoric Socio-economic Relations and Population Organization in the Lower Osmore Valley of Southern Perú.* Ph.D. dissertation, University of New Mexico, Albuquerque.

Topic, J. R., and T. L. Topic
1997   La Guerra Mochica. *Revista Arqueológica "SIAN"* (Universidad Nacional de Trujillo) 4:10–12.

Toth, N., and M. Woods
1989   Molluscan Shell Knives and Experimental Cut-Marks on Bones. *Journal of Field Archaeology* 16(2):250–255.

Toulouse, J. H.
1944   Cremation among the Indians of New Mexico. *American Antiquity* 10:65–74.

Toulouse, J. H., and R. L. Stephenson
1960   *Excavations at Pueblo Pardo, Central New Mexico.* Museum of New Mexico, Santa Fe.

Toussaint-Devine, M. J.
1984   *The Representation of Human Decapitation and Trophy Heads in Colima Ceramics.* Master's thesis, Arizona State University, Tempe.

Townsend, R. F.
1985   Deciphering the Nazca World: Ceramic Images from Ancient Peru. *Museum Studies* (Art Institute of Chicago) 11:117–139.

Tozzer, A. M.
1907   *A Comparative Study of the Mayas and Lancandones: Archaeological Institute of America, Report of the Fellow in Archaeology 1902–1907.* Macmillan, New York.
1941   *Landa's Relación de las Cosas de Yucatán: A Translation.* Papers of the Peabody Museum of American Archaeology and Ethnology 18. Harvard University, Cambridge, Mass.
1957   *Chichen Itza and Its Cenote of Sacrifice.* Memoirs of the Peabody Museum 11–12. Harvard University, Cambridge, Mass.

Travassos, E.
1993   A Tradiçaõ Guerreira nas Narrativas e nos Cantos Caiabis. In *Karl Von den Steinen: Um Século de Antropologia no Xingu,* edited by V. P. Coelho, pp. 447–484. Editora da Universidade de São Paulo, São Paulo, Brazil.

Treffort, C.
1996   *L'Église Carolingienne et la Mort.* Collection d'Histoire et d'Archéologie Médiévales. Presses Universitaires de Lyon, Lyon, France.

Trompf, G.
1991   *Melanesian Religion.* Cambridge University Press, Cambridge.

Trudgill, P.
1983   *On Dialect: Social and Geographical Perspectives.* Blackwell, Oxford.

Tse-Tung, M.
1971   Serve the People. In *Selected Reading from the Works of Mao Tse-Tung,* pp. 369–373. Foreign Language Press, Peking.

Tucci, G.
1973   *Transhimalaya.* Translated from the French by J. Hogarth. Barrie and Jenkins, London.
1980 [1970]   *The Religions of Tibet.* Translated by G. Samuel. (Originally published as "Die Religionen Tibets" in *Die Religionen Tibets und der Mongolie* by Guiseppe

Tucci and Walter Heissig, W. Kohlhammer, Stuttgart.) Routledge and Kegan Paul, London.

1987 [1956]   *To Lhasa and Beyond.* Translated by M. Carelli. (First published as *A Lhasa e Oltre.*) Snow Lion Publication, by arrangement with Oxford and IBH Publishing, Ithaca, N.Y.

Tufinio, M.

2001   Excavaciones en la Plaza 3C. In *Investigaciones en la Huaca de la Luna 1999*, edited by S. Uceda, E. Mujica, and R. Morales, pp. 65–83. Universidad Nacional de Trujillo, Trujillo, Peru.

Tung, T.

2003   *A Bioarchaeological Perspective on Wari Imperialism: A View from Heartland and Hinterland Skeletal Populations.* Ph.D. dissertation, University of North Carolina–Chapel Hill.

Turner, C. G.

1993   Human Dentition from the Akari Site, Madang, Papua New Guinea, with Observations on the Oldest Known Interproximal Tooth Groove in Australmelanesia. *Bulletin of the Indo-Pacific Prehistory Association* 13(4):15–19.

Turner, C. G., and J. A. Turner

1995   Cannibalism in the Prehistoric American Southwest: Occurrence, Taphonomy, Explanation, and Suggestions for Standardized World Definition. *Anthropological Sciences* 103(1):1–22.

1999   *Man Corn: Cannibalism and Violence in the Prehistoric American Southwest.* University of Utah Press, Salt Lake City.

Turner, V.

1995 [1969]   *The Ritual Process: Structure and Anti-structure.* Aldine De Gruyter, New York.

Ubbelohde-Doering, H.

1966   *On the Royal Highway of the Inca.* Praeger, New York.

Uceda, S., and J. Canziani

1993   Evidencias de Grandes Precipitaciones en Diversas Etapas Constructivas de la Huaca de la Luna, Costa Norte del Perú. *Bulletin de l'Institut Français d'Études Andines* 22(1):313–343.

Ucko, P. J.

1969   Ethnography and Archaeological Interpretation of Funerary Remains. *World Archaeology* 1:262–280.

Uhle, M.

1914   The Nazca Pottery of Ancient Peru. *Proceedings of the Davenport Academy of Sciences* 13:1–46.

1919   Arqueologia de Arica y Tacna. *Boletin de la Sociedad Ecuatoriana de Estudios Historicos Americanos* 3(7–8):1–48.

1922   *Fundamentos Etnicos y Arqueologia de Arica y Tacna.* Sociedad Ecuatoriana de Estudios Historicos Americanos, Quito, Ecuador.

1974   Los Aborigenes de Arica y el Hombre Americano. *Chungará* 3:13–22.

Underhill, R. M.

1939   *Social Organization of the Papago Indians.* Columbia University Press, New York.

Up de Graff, F. W.
1923   *Head Hunters of the Amazon.* Duffield, New York.

Uriarte, M. T.
2001   Unity in Duality: The Practice and Symbols of the Mesoamerican Ballgame. In *The Sport of Life and Death: The Mesoamerican Ballgame,* edited by E. M. Whittington, pp. 40–49. Mint Museum of Art, Charlotte, N.C.

Valera, B.
1945 [c.1590]   *Las Costumbres Antiguas del Peru y la Historia de los Incas.* Los Pequenos Libros de Historia Americana. Miranda, Lima.

Valli, E., and D. Summers
1994   *Caravans of the Himalaya.* National Geographic Society, Washington, D.C.

van Gennep, A.
1960 [1908]   *The Rites of Passage.* University of Chicago Press, Chicago.

Van Nest, J., D. K. Charles, J. E. Buikstra, and D. L. Asch
2001   Sod Blocks in Illinois Hopewell Mounds. *American Antiquity* 66(4):633–650.

Verano, J. W.
1986   A Mass Burial of Mutilated Individuals at Pacatnamu. In *The Pacatnamu Papers,* edited by C. B. Donnan and G. A. Cock, vol. 1, pp. 117–138. Museum of Cultural History, Los Angeles.

1995   Where Do They Rest? The Treatment of Human Offerings and Trophies in Ancient Peru. In *Tombs for the Living: Andean Mortuary Practices,* edited by T. D. Dillehay, pp. 189–227. Dumbarton Oaks, Washington, D.C.

1997   Human Skeletal Remains from Tomb I, Sipán (Lambayeque River Valley, Peru), and their Social Implications. *Antiquity* 71(273):670–682.

1998a   Sacrificios Humanos, Desmembramientos, y Modificaciones Culturales en Restos Osteológicos: Evidencias de las Temporadas de Investigación 1995–96 en la Huaca de la Luna. In *Investigaciones en la Huaca de la Luna 1996,* edited by S. Uceda, E. Mujica, and R. Morales, pp. 159–171. Universidad Nacional de Trujillo, Trujillo, Peru.

1998b   Anexo 3: Análisis del Material Óseo de la Plaza 3B. In *Investigaciones en la Huaca de la Luna 1996,* edited by S. Uceda, E. Mujica, and R. Morales, pp. 81. Universidad Nacional de Trujillo, Trujillo, Peru.

2000   Human Sacrifice at the Pyramid of the Moon, Northern Peru. Report submitted to the National Geographic Committee for Research and Exploration, October 10, 2000, Washington, D.C.

2001a   The Physical Evidence of Human Sacrifice in Ancient Peru. In *Ritual Sacrifice in Ancient Peru,* edited by E. Benson and A. Cook, pp. 165–184. University of Texas Press, Austin.

2001b   War and Death in the Moche World: Osteological Evidence and Visual Discourse. In *Moche Art and Archaeology in Ancient Peru,* edited by J. Pillsbury, pp. 111–125. National Gallery of Art, Washington, D.C.

Verano, J. W., and M. Tufinio
2005   Plaza 3C. In *Investigaciones en la Huaca de la Luna 2000,* edited by S. Uceda, E. Mujica, and R. Morales. Universidad Nacional de Trujillo, Trujillo, Peru.

Verano, J. W., S. Uceda, C. Chapdelaine, R. Tello, M. I. Paredes, and V. Pimentel
1999   Modified Human Skulls from the Urban Sector of the Pyramids of Moche, Northern Peru. *Latin American Antiquity* 10(1):59–70.

Verdery, K.
1999   *The Political Lives of Dead Bodies: Reburial and Post-socialist Change.* Columbia University Press, New York.

Villa, P.
1992   Cannibalism in Prehistoric Europe. *Evolutionary Anthropology* 1(3):93–104.

Villa, P., C. Bouville, J. Courtin, D. Helmer, E. Mahieu, P. Shipman, G. Belluomini, and M. Branca
1986   Cannibalism in the Neolithic. *Science* 233:431–437.

Viveiros de Castro, E.
1992   *From the Enemy's Point of View.* University of Chicago Press, Chicago.
1998   Cosmological Deixis and Amerindian Perspectivism. *Journal of the Royal Anthropological Institute* 4:469–488.

Vogt, E. Z.
1976   *Tortillas for the Gods: A Symbolic Analysis of Zinacanteco Rituals.* Harvard University Press, Cambridge, Mass.
1993   *Tortillas for the Gods: A Symbolic Analysis of Zinacanteco Rituals.* Reprint ed., University of Oklahoma Press, Norman.
1998   Zinacanteco Dedication and Termination Rituals. In *The Sowing and the Dawning: Termination, Dedication, and Transformation in the Archaeological and Ethnographic Record of Mesoamerica,* edited by S. B. Mock, pp. 21–30. University of New Mexico Press, Albuquerque.

Vones, L.
1996   Ludwig IX (1226–1270). In *Die französischen Könige des Mittelalters,* edited by J. Ehlers, H. Müller, and B. Schneidmüller, pp. 176–193. C. H. Beck, Munich.

Vreeland, J. M., and A. Cockburn
1980   Mummies of Peru. In *Mummies, Disease, and Ancient Cultures,* edited by A. Cockburn and E. Cockburn, pp. 135–176. Abridged ed. Cambridge University Press, Cambridge.

Waddell, L. A.
1972 [1895] *Tibetan Buddhism with Its Mystic Cults, Symbolism, and Mythology.* (Originally published as *The Buddhism of Tibet, or Lamaism,* by W. H. Allen, London.) Dover Publications, New York.

Wakeman, F.
1988   Mao's Remains. In *Death Ritual in Late Imperial and Modern China,* edited by J. L. Watson and E. S. Rawski, pp. 254–288. University of California Press, Berkeley.

Walker, P. L., and M. J. DeNiro
1986   Stable Nitrogen and Carbon Isotope Ratios in Bone Collagen as Indices of Prehistoric Dietary Dependence on Marine and Terrestrial Resources in Southern California. *American Journal of Physical Anthropology* 71(1):51–61.

Walker, W. H.
1998   Where Are the Witches in Prehistory? *Journal of Archaeological Method and Theory* 5(3):245–308.

Wallace, A. F. C.
1970   *The Death and Rebirth of the Seneca.* Knopf, New York.

Wallace, S. E.
1985   *Medieval Burial Practice and Skeletal Remains in Soissons, France.* Unpublished Master's thesis, Wesleyan University, Middletown, Conn.

Watson, J. L.
1985   Standardizing the Gods: The Promotion of T'ien Hou (Empress of Heaven) along the South China Coast, 960–1960. In *Popular Culture in Late Imperial China,* edited by D. Johnson, A. J. Nathan, and E. Rawski, pp. 292–324. University of California Press, Berkeley.
1988a   The Structure of Chinese Funerary Rites: Elementary Forms, Ritual Sequence, and the Primacy of Performance. In *Death Ritual in Late Imperial and Modern China,* edited by J. L. Watson and E. S. Rawski, pp. 3–19. University of California Press, Berkeley.
1988b   Funerary Specialists in Cantonese Society: Pollution, Performance, and Social Hierarchy. In *Death Ritual in Late Imperial and Modern China,* edited by J. L. Watson and E. S. Rawski, pp. 109–134. University of California Press, Berkeley.
Watson, R. S.
1988   Remembering the Dead: Graves and Politics in Southeastern China. In *Death Ritual in Late Imperial and Modern China,* edited by J. L. Watson and E. S. Rawski, pp. 203–227. University of California Press, Berkeley.
1994   Making Secret Histories: Memory and Mourning in Post-Mao China. In *Memory, History, and Opposition under State Socialism,* edited by R. S. Watson, pp. 65–85. SAR Advanced Seminar Series. School of American Research, Santa Fe, N.Mex.
Weglian, E.
2001   Grave Goods Do Not a Gender Make: A Case Study from Singen am Hohentwiel, Germany. In *Gender and the Archaeology of Death,* edited by B. Arnold and N. L. Walker, pp. 137–155. Altamira Press, Walnut Creek, Calif.
Weiss, P.
1932   Restos Humanos de Cerro Colorado. *Revista del Museo Nacional* 1(2):90–102.
1961   *Osteología Cultural: Practicas Cefalicas.* Part 2: *Tipología de las Deformaciones Cefálicas.* Estudio Cultural de los Tipos Cefálicos y de Algunas Enfermedades Oseas. Universidad Nacional Mayor de San Marcos, Lima.
Weiss-Krejci, E.
2001   Restless Corpses: "Secondary Burial" in the Babenberg and Habsburg Dynasties. *Antiquity* 75:769–780.
Welsch, R.
1998   *An American Anthropologist in Melanesia: The Diaries of Albert B. Lewis.* University of Hawaii Press, Honolulu.
Welsh, W. B. M.
1988   *An Analysis of Classic Lowland Maya Burials.* BAR International Series 409. British Archaeological Reports, Oxford.
White, J. P. (editor)
1972   *Ol Tumbuna: Archaeological Excavations in the Eastern Central Highlands, Papua New Guinea.* Terra Australis 2. Department of Prehistory, Research School of Pacific Studies, Australian National University, Canberra.
White, T. D.
1992   *Prehistoric Cannibalism at Mancos 5MTUMR-2346.* Princeton University Press, Princeton, N.J.
Whitley, J.
2002   Too Many Ancestors. *Antiquity* 76:119–126.

Whittle, A.
2001   Different Kinds of History: On the Nature of Lives and Change in Central Europe, c. 6000 to the Second Millennium B.C. In *The Origin of Human Social Institutions*, edited by W. G. Runciman, pp. 39–68. Oxford University Press, Oxford.

Whittlesey, S. M.
1978   *Status and Death at Grasshopper Pueblo: Experiments towards an Archaeological Theory of Correlates.* Ph.D. dissertation, University of Arizona, Tucson.

Whittlesey, S. M., and J. J. Reid
2001   Mortuary Ritual and Organizational Inferences at Grasshopper Pueblo, Arizona. In *Ancient Burial Practices in the American Southwest: Archaeology, Physical Anthropology, and Native American Perspectives*, edited by D. R. Mitchell and J. L. Brunson-Hadley, pp. 68–96. University of New Mexico Press, Albuquerque.

Whyte, M. K.
1988   Death in the People's Republic of China. In *Death Ritual in Late Imperial and Modern China*, edited by J. L. Watson and E. S. Rawski, pp. 289–316. University of California Press, Berkeley.

Wiant, M. D., and C. R. McGimsey (editors)
1986   *Woodland Period Occupations of the Napoleon Hollow Site in the Lower Illinois Valley.* Center for American Archeology, Kampsville, Ill.

Wilcox, D. R.
1991   Hohokam Social Complexity. In *Chaco and Hohokam: Prehistoric Regional Systems in the American Southwest*, edited by P. L. Crown and W. J. Judge, pp. 253–275. School of American Research, Santa Fe, N.Mex.

Wilkerson, S. J. K.
1991   And Then They Were Sacrificed: The Ritual Ballgame of Northeastern Mesoamerica through Time and Space. In *The Mesoamerican Ballgame*, edited by S. J. K. Wilkerson. University of Arizona Press, Tucson.

Willard, T. A.
1926   *City of the Sacred Well.* Century Co., New York.

Williams, F. E.
1941   Natives of Lake Kutubu, Papua. *Oceania* 12:49–74.

Williams, S., and L. A. Beck
2001   Introduction. Cultural Interactions with Human Remains. Paper presented at the 66th Annual Meeting of the Society for American Archaeology, New Orleans, La.

Williams, S. R., K. Forgey, and E. Klarich
2001   An Osteological Study of Nasca Trophy Heads Collected by A. L. Kroeber during the Marshall Field Expeditions to Peru. *Fieldiana* (Field Museum of Natural History, Chicago) Vol. 33, publication 1516.

Willoughby, C. C.
1922   *The Turner Group of Earthworks, Hamilton County, Ohio.* Papers of the Peabody Museum of American Archaeology and Ethnology, Vol. 8, No. 3. Harvard University, Cambridge, Mass.

Wilson, G.
1939   Nyakyusa Conventions of Burial. *Bantu* 13:1–31.

Wolfram, W., and N. Schilling-Estes
1998   *American English Dialects and Variation.* Blackwell, Malden, Mass.

Wren, L.
1991   The Great Ball Court Stone from Chichen Itza. In *Sixth Palenque Round Table,* edited by V. M. Fields, pp. 51–55. University of Oklahoma Press, Norman.

Wright, G. A.
1990   On the Interior Attached Ditch Enclosures of the Middle and Upper Ohio Valley. *Ethnos* (1–2):92–107.

Wrong, G. M. (editor)
1939   *The Long Journey to the Country of the Hurons, by Father Gabriel Sagard.* Publications of the Champlain Society No. 25. Toronto.

Young, B.
1977   Paganisme, Christianisme, et Rites Funéraires Mérovingiens. *Archéologie Médiévale* 7:5–81.

Zegwaard, G. A.
1959   Headhunting Practices of the Asmat of Netherlands New Guinea. *American Anthropologist* 61:1020–1041.

Zotz, T.
1996   Phillip III (1270–1285). In *Die französischen Könige des Mittelalters,* edited by J. Ehlers, H. Müller, and B. Schneidmüller, pp. 195–201. C. H. Beck, Munich.

Zuidema, R. T.
1972   *Meaning in Nazca Art: Iconographic Relationships between Inca, Huari, and Nazca Cultures in Southern Peru.* Goteborg Etnografiska Museum, Goteborg, Sweden.

Index

Gordon F. M. Rakita is assistant professor of anthropology at the University of North Florida. He is a co-editor of *Style and Function: Conceptual Issues in Evolutionary Archaeology* (2001).

Jane E. Buikstra is professor of bioarchaeology and director of the Center for Bioarchaeological Research at the School of Human Evolution and Social Change, Arizona State University. She is the author or editor of several books, including *The Bioarchaeology of Tuberculosis* (University Press of Florida, 2003).

Lane A. Beck is associate curator at the Arizona State Museum and associate professor of anthropology at the University of Arizona. She is the editor of *Regional Approaches to Mortuary Analysis* (1995).

Sloan R. Williams is associate professor of anthropology at the University of Illinois–Chicago and has written extensively on the human genetics of ancient populations.

Printed in the USA
CPSIA information can be obtained
at www.ICGtesting.com
LVHW052306290823
756688LV00020BA/197